Fifth Edition

Mental Health Concepts

D0060995

This book is dedicated to my children:
Mick, Anne, Malik, and Jané.

Fifth Edition

Mental Health Concepts

Claire G. Waughfield, MSN, RN, CS, APN

Contributor:

Teresa S. Burckhalter, MSN, RN, C
Nursing Instructor
Technical College of the Lowcountry
Beaufort, South Carolina

DELMAR

THOMSON LEARNING — Australia Canada Mexico Singapore Spain United Kingdom United States

DELMAR

THOMSON LEARNING ™

Mental Health Concepts, Fifth Edition

by Claire G. Waughfield

Health Care Publishing Director:
William Brottmiller

Executive Editor:
Cathy L. Esperti

Acquisitions Editor:
Matthew Kane

Developmental Editor:
Marjorie A. Bruce

Editorial Assistant:
Shelley Esposito

Executive Marketing Manager:
Dawn F. Gerrain

Channel Manager:
Jennifer McAvey

Marketing Coordinator:
Kip Summerlin

Production Coordinator:
Anne Sherman

Art/Design Coordinator:
Connie Lundberg-Watkins

Project Editor:
Mary Ellen Cox

For more information contact Delmar,
5 Maxwell Rd., P.O. Box 8007
Clifton Park, NY 12065

Or you can visit our Internet site at
http://www.delmar.com

For permission to use material from this text or product, contact us by
Tel   (800) 730-2214
Fax   (800) 730-2215
www.thomsonrights.com

Library of Congress Cataloging-in-Publication Data
Waughfield, Claire, G.
    Mental health concepts / Claire G. Waughfield ; contributor, Teresa S. Burckhalter — 5th ed.
        p. cm.
    ISBN 0-7668-3830-7 (alk. paper)
    1. Psychiatric nursing. 2. Mental health.
    I. Burckhalter, Teresa S. II. Title
    [DNLM: 1. Mental Disorders—therapy—nurses' instruction. 2. Mental Disorders—prevention & control—nurses' instruction. 3. Stress, Psychological —prevention & control—nurses' instruction. 4. Mental Health—nurses' instruction.]
RC440.W37 2001
616.89—dc21   2001047700

NOTICE TO THE READER

Contents

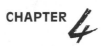

CHAPTER ## Effective Communication 83

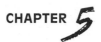

CHAPTER ## Relieving Anxiety 112

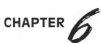

CHAPTER ## Psychotherapies 137

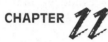

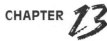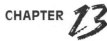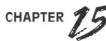

List of Tables

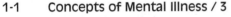

Preface

Mental Health Concepts, fifth edition, is a comprehensive and unique text written specifically for practical/vocational nursing students, but can also be used by any beginning health care providers. The simplicity and conciseness of the text mean that it is easily applicable in various health care settings. The engaging and straight-forward writing style lends itself to ease in reading. Difficult to comprehend material is presented so it can be easily understood, but still remains comprehensive in scope. Throughout, the text emphasizes the responsibilities of the licensed practical/vocational nurse in providing care to clients with specific mental disorders.

The goal of the text is to help learners achieve accurate knowledge and a clear understanding of the concepts of mental health to enable them to provide safe, competent, and effective client care. The fifth edition continues to present the stress and coping model as an approach to holistic care covering life span and developmental issues. The content is theoretically sound and has a basis in scientific research.

Mental Health Concepts encourages health care providers to assess their own mental health and develop a personal plan for improved mental health. They are also encouraged to continue to expand their learning about, and understanding of, the mental health discipline.

CHANGES FOR THE FIFTH EDITION

■ Content was updated/added in the following areas:

- legal issues
- confidentiality of client information
- community health services
- therapeutic communication
- meaning and development of self-concept over the lifespan
- Cognitive-Behavioral Therapy (CBT)
- group therapy
- maladaptive behaviors, including social phobia/anxiety disorder, depression in the elderly, bipolar disorder, dissociative identity disorder, impulse control disorder, and attention deficit/hyperactive disorder
- alcoholism
- drug use/abuse
- human sexuality: gender identity disorder (GID)
- violence: self-directed, other-directed (domestic violence)
- pain as the 5th vital sign; alternative (complementary) approaches to pain management
- medications and side effects

■ reorganized chapters to improve sequencing of topics

■ added chapter outlines as an overview to content and for quick review

■ Key Terms added at beginning of chapters

■ nursing diagnoses updated to "Nursing Diagnoses: Definitions & Classification, 2001-2002", NANDA, 2001

■ DSM references updated to DSM-IV-TR, American Psychiatric Association, 2000

■ persons receiving care are referred to consistently as clients, except in historical references where the term patient is used

■ review questions were revised/added to reflect changes in content and to increase effectiveness of testing comprehension/understanding; new questions in "Apply Your Learning" are at a higher level to help users develop problem-solving skills

■ updated nursing care plans that provide specific interventions for nursing clients with major psychiatric disorders

It is the author's hope that *Mental Health Concepts* will promote safe, therapeutic, and effective care of people across the life span in a time of rapidly increasing scientific knowledge of the brain and an increased understanding of persons with acute and chronic mental illness.

ABOUT THE AUTHOR

Claire G. Waughfield has many years of experience in teaching mental health concepts to nursing students, as well as practicing psychiatric nursing in both clinical and management roles. Currently, she is a clinical nurse specialist in the psychiatric ambulatory care clinic at the Roudebush Veterans Affairs Medical Center, Indianapolis. Ms. Waughfield is also an assistant clinical professor at the Indiana University graduate program for psychiatric/mental health nursing. Before this, she was the unit director of the inpatient psychiatric unit at Indiana University Hospital, Indianapolis, former coordinator of the nursing program and homemakers–home health aide program at Danville Area Community College, Danville, Illinois, and former director of the Illinois Migrant Council, Hoopston, Illinois. Ms. Waughfield earned a bachelor of arts degree from Eastern Illinois University, a bachelor of science in nursing degree from Governor's State University, Park Forest South, Illinois, and a master of science degree with a major in psychiatric/mental health nursing from Indiana University, Indianapolis. She has certification as a clinical specialist in adult psychiatric and mental health nursing and is an advanced practice nurse.

ACKNOWLEDGMENTS

No book is ever written by the author alone. It takes a great many people to put it all together and applaud the small victories. My sincere thanks goes to:

Randy E. Morton who nurtured me with his friendship, wisdom, and insight, Jaéla Lashéa for her happy, whimsical ways, and Dave Gullans who provided valuable assistance in preparing the manuscript.

A special thank you is extended to my colleagues at Indiana University and the advanced practice nurses at Roudebush VA for their support and encouragement. Participation with the psychiatric/mental health team has expanded my knowledge and assisted me to develop more effective client intervention strategies. And finally, I express appreciation to the clients who have shared their unique and painful experiences and their journeys to self-awareness.

Special mention goes to Gena Duncan, RN, MSEd, MS of Lutheran College, Fort Wayne, Indiana, who authored the nursing care plans in selected chapters.

I also want to thank Teresa S. Burckhalter, MSN, RN, C of the Technical College of the Lowcountry in Beaufort, South Carolina, for revising the review questions and adding new questions to help readers develop critical thinking skills and integrate their learning.

Finally, sincere appreciation is expressed to the reviewers for their contributions to this edition:

Teresa S. Burckhalter, MSN, RN, C
Nursing Instructor, Technical College of the Lowcountry
Beaufort, SC

Iva Burgan, MSN, RN, FNP-C (Deceased)
Former Director of Vocational Nursing, Coastal Bend College
Alice, TX

Janet Dicke, RN
Instructor of Nursing, Rochester Community and
   Technical College
Rochester, MN

Sandra Foltz, MSN, RN
Professor of Nursing, Sinclair Community College
Lebanon, OH

Sheila Guidry, BSN, MSN, DSN
Nursing Department, Wallace Community College
Selma, AL

Patricia Richter Sipe, RN, Med
Associate Professor, Nursing, Howard Community College
Columbia, MD

History, Trends, and Standards

OUTLINE

KEY TERMS

bedlam

mesmerized

stigma

standards of care

commitment

gravely disabled

competency

guardian

conservator

right to refuse treatment

involuntary admission

confidentiality

OBJECTIVES

After studying this chapter, the student should be able to:

- State the changes in attitude and treatment concerning persons with mental illness that have occurred from primitive times to the present.
- Match pioneers in mental health care with their contributions and beliefs.
- Identify legislation enacted to improve mental health care.
- List ten services offered by comprehensive community mental health centers.
- Explain how changes in mental health care affect the role of the nurse.
- Explain the purpose of standards for nursing care.
- Identify legal rights of persons with mental illness.

CONCEPTS OF MENTAL ILLNESS FROM PRIMITIVE TIMES THROUGH THE MILLENNIUM

Primitive Times

It is impossible to estimate the extent to which mental illness affected primitive people. However, there is evidence that it did exist and that attempts were made to treat it. Mental illness was thought to be caused by evil spirits entering and taking over the body. Medicine men attempted to drive these evil spirits from the body through the use of incantations and magic (Table 1-1).

TABLE 1-1 Concepts of Mental Illness

TIME PERIOD	CONCEPTS OF MENTAL ILLNESS
PRIMITIVE TIMES	Evil spirits possess the body and must be driven from the body
ANCIENT CIVILIZATION	Thought to be natural phenomenon; humanistic approach Hippocrates attempted to classify behavior
MIDDLE AGES	Superstition, witchcraft, and torture
RENAISSANCE	Decline in belief of possession by evil spirits Mental problems irreversible Scientific inquiry; humanism
EIGHTEENTH CENTURY	Reform movement; chains removed Need for medical care recognized First patients with mental illness treated in hospitals
NINETEENTH CENTURY	Research began Legislation concerning mental health enacted Hospitals for persons with mental illness established with long-term custodial care First psychiatric training school in United States established in Massachusetts Rush—the Father of American psychiatry
TWENTIETH CENTURY	Start of mental health movement Large state hospitals built Psychoanalysis More legislation concerning mental health enacted Community health care centers established Holistic concept of care and short-term care introduced Goal to return client to society Human services programs established Focus on prevention Individuals, families, communities viewed as *consumers* of mental health services Explosion of scientific knowledge Collaborative Care for neurobiological disorders

Some primitive tribes rejected their persons with mental illness and drove them from the community. Other tribes allowed persons with mental illness to stay as long as they were not completely incapacitated or their behavior did not create fear. Some tribes encouraged disturbed individuals to act out their difficulties and to confide in the witch doctor.

Ancient Civilization

The ancient Greeks, Romans, and Arabs viewed mental deviations as natural phenomena and treated persons with mental illness humanely. Although emotional problems were thought to be related to disturbances in the brain, some distinction was made between functional and organic disorders. Care consisted of sedation with opium, music, good physical hygiene, nutrition, and activity. The Greek philosopher Plato (429–348 B.C.) and the Greek physician Hippocrates (460–377 B.C.), known as the Father of Medicine, were concerned about the treatment of persons with mental illness. Hippocrates described a variety of personalities and attempted to classify people according to their behavior. Aristotle (354–322 B.C.), a Greek philosopher, studied anatomy and concluded that the mind was associated with the heart. Galen, a Greek physician and writer during the second century A.D., disagreed with Aristotle. In his writings, Galen declared the mind to be associated solely with the brain.

Middle Ages (A.D. 500–1450)

When the Roman Empire fell in A.D. 476, the humanitarian ideas concerning persons with mental illness were forgotten. The work reverted to superstition, mysticism, witchcraft, and magic. Little was done to treat mental illness. Sometimes, patients were humanely cared for by members of religious orders. However, persons with mental illness were usually locked in asylums where flogging, starvation, torture, and bloodletting were common. Within families, persons with mental illness were hidden or banished to roam the streets.

The Renaissance (Fourteenth to Seventeenth Century)

The belief that mental illness was caused by evil spirits possessing the body continued for much of the Renaissance period. If persons with mental illness were considered a menace to society, they were put in prison. Otherwise, society protected itself by locking persons with mental illness in asylums where nonprofessional people were paid to care for them. Mental illness was considered irreversible. Persons with mental illness were beaten for disobedience and confined to cages or closets. They were often subjected to cruel forms of torture.

Generally, patients with a mental illness were viewed as incompetent, defective, and potentially dangerous. They had no rights and were left in social isolation to communicate primarily with other patients with mental illness. Their caretakers were untrained and often punitive. As a result, the persons with mental illness tended to become more ill and less able to function in society.

The Bethlehem Royal Hospital, the first mental hospital in England, was opened during the seventeenth century. It was the second such hospital in Europe. Patients were treated as animals and were kept chained in cages. For a small fee, the public was allowed to wander through the hospital and view the patients. "Bedlam," as it was called, is the Cockney pronunciation for Bethlehem. The meaning of the word **bedlam** is tumult or frenzy.

A Swiss physician named Paracelsus (1493–1541) rejected the belief that evil spirits caused mental illness. Like the ancient Greeks and Romans, he believed that mental illness was a natural phenomenon. The idea that evil spirits possessed the body began to decline. Scientific inquiry, along with objective study of behavior, began to grow. A rational explanation for irrational behavior was sought. Authorities were divided into two groups—the psychics and the organics. The psychics believed that mental illness was a result of personal guilt; it was a possible atonement for sin. The organics felt that mental illness was caused by internal organs and that bloodletting would release enough blood and pressure to change behavior. It was not until the middle of the eighteenth century that any real advancement was made in the treatment and care of persons with mental illness.

The Eighteenth Century

Franz Mesmer (1733–1815), an Austrian physician, was a pioneer in the therapeutic approach to maladaptive behavior. He believed that the universe was filled with magnetic forces. Mesmer professed that persons with mental illness could be cured by having them hold rods filled with iron filings in water. This supposedly brought people into balance with the universe. Although Mesmer's techniques were later revealed as false, his idea of suggestive power has carried over to some modern psychotechniques. The term **mesmerized** is from Mesmer. To be mesmerized is to be placed in a hypnotic trance.

A French physician, Philippe Pinel (1745–1826), began the movement toward more humane treatment of persons with mental illness when he removed the chains from twelve male patients at Bicêtré Hospital near Paris in 1792. Pinel disavowed punitive treatment of patients with mental illness. He recognized the need for medical care and advocated freedom, useful work, and kindness for these individuals. He attempted to classify persons with mental illness according to their observable behaviors and sought to devise specific treatment for each classified type.

During colonial times in America, persons with mental illness were punished at the stocks or whipping posts. Often considered witches, they were burned at the stake, hung, or tortured.

During the Revolutionary War period, the persons with mental illness in America were treated for the first time as patients in a hospital setting. The first hospital in America to admit patients with mental illness was the Pennsylvania Hospital located in Philadelphia. The first American textbook on psychiatry was written during this period by Benjamin Rush. Rush (1745–1813) was a physician who used a humanistic approach in the treatment of mental illness. Rush, who was also a signer of the Declaration of Independence, is considered by many to be the Father of American Psychiatry.

The Nineteenth Century

Jean Martin Charcot (1825–1893), a French neurologist, was a major influence during the nineteenth century in the treatment of persons with mental illness. Charcot used suggestive power in the form of hypnotism to treat hysteria (Figure 1-1). He also diagnosed and located neurological disturbances in patients.

The establishment of American hospitals for the care of persons with mental illness was due largely to the work of Dorothea Lynde Dix. Dorothea Dix (1802–1887) was a Boston schoolteacher who spent much of her life working for better conditions for persons with mental illness. She traveled throughout the country in an effort to have legislation enacted for improved care for persons with mental illness. As a result of her efforts, many hospitals were built in the United States, Canada, and other countries.

Humane treatment of persons with mental illness became more widespread in the late nineteenth century. Nurses showed interest in improving the care of persons with mental illness. Research on how syphilis affected the mind was begun. It was also discovered that some bizarre behavior was due to vitamin deficiencies. With advances in medicine, the concept of mental illness and those afflicted with it became more accepted and tolerated.

The first psychiatric training school in the United States was established in 1882 at McLean Hospital, Waverly, Massachusetts. However, in 1939, only half of all nursing schools provided psychiatric nursing courses. Participation in a psychiatric nursing course did not become a requirement for a nursing license until 1955.

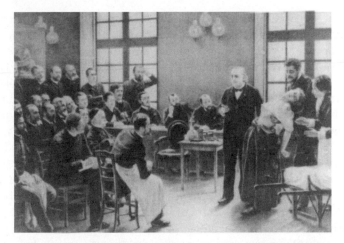

FIGURE 1-1 Charcot demonstrating hypnotism in treatment of hysteria about 1887 at Salpêtrière. (Photo painting by A. Brouillet, National Library of Medicine, Bethesda, MD.)

The Twentieth Century

Twentieth-century reforms in psychiatric care began in 1908 with the publication of a book entitled *A Mind That Found Itself,* by Clifford Beers. In the book, Beers describes his experiences and observations during his three years in mental institutions. The suffering of persons with mental illness as portrayed in the book promoted the mental health movement. It made the public aware of the need for better care of persons with mental illness. Beers came from a wealthy and influential family. In 1909, he used this influence to organize the National Society for Mental Hygiene (now known as the National Association for Mental Health).

Large state hospitals were built as a result of the public's increased awareness of the problems of persons with mental illness. These state hospitals usually were established away from large cities, where clients could receive fresh air and sunshine. Few people were released from the hospitals once they were admitted. However, the public's conscience was eased.

In 1920, an Austrian neurologist, Sigmund Freud (1856–1939), made a significant contribution to the understanding and treatment of mental illness. Freud conducted a series of studies and determined a need for deeper probing into the psychological side of the individual. His belief in the power of unconscious memories and repressed emotions led him to develop the theory and practice of psychoanalysis. Because of his work, he is called the Founder of Psychoanalysis. Freud believed that each life event was determined by prior mental events. He studied the dreams, memories, and fantasies of his clients in a search for unconscious impulses and conflicts. Freud identified three major divisions of the self or mind: the id, superego, and ego. Freud also presented a theory of psychosexual personality development (Chapter 5).

In 1937, an International Committee for Mental Hygiene met in Paris, France, marking the beginning of international concern for mental health. The World Federation for Mental Health was formed in 1948. By 1961, The World Psychiatric Association was organized.

World War II brought the immensity of the mental health problem into view. The public was shocked when vast numbers of young men were rejected for service and many more were discharged because of mental problems. Also, many veterans returning from the war required treatment for mental problems. State hospitals were grossly inadequate. Obviously, new and better treatment was needed.

Mental Health Legislation

Following World War II, the Hill-Burton Act, which allotted funds for building psychiatric units, was passed by Congress. In 1946, the National Mental Health Act provided federal funds to begin training programs for mental health professions. This act established the National Institute for Mental Health (1948) and provided grants for education and research (Table 1-2).

TABLE 1-2 Mental Health Organizations, Legislation, 1909–1992

1909	National Society for Mental Hygiene	Studied nursing care of insane Provided reforms in psychiatric care Set up programs to treat afflicted servicemen
1940		Railroading patients into hospitals with wrongful commitment
1946	National Mental Health Act	Provided funds for professional training programs
1947	International Committee or Mental Hygiene Hill-Burton Act	Sparked international concern for mental health Provided funds for building psychiatric units
1948	World Federation for Mental Health	Provided grants for education and research
1948	National Institute of Mental Health	Provided grants for education and research

(Continues)

TABLE 1-2 (Continued)

1952	Draft Act Governing Hospitalization of the Mentally Ill	Terminology changed from insane to mentally ill; certification to commitment
1955	Joint Commission on Mental Illness and Health	Studied and evaluated needs and resources available
1961	World Psychiatric Association	Looked at social consequence of mental disorders
1963	The Mental Retardation Facilities and Community Mental Health Centers Construction Act	Federal funds provided to match local and state monies; purpose was to decentralize mental health care
1964	Economic Opportunity Act	Designed to help the poor and disadvantaged reach their full social potential Emphasized improved social environment to prevent mental health problems
1967	Mental Health Amendment	Provided grants for construction and staffing of mental health centers
1968	Community Mental Health Centers Act Amendment	Provided community services and facilities for treatment of drug addicts and alcoholics
1968	Alcoholic and Narcotic Addiction Rehabilitation Amendment	Provided funds to develop treatment and rehabilitation for alcoholics and drug abusers Provided grants for special training
1970	Community Health Centers Amendment	Provided for extended programs, construction grants, and increased construction through acquisition of land
1975	Community Health Centers Amendment	Community mental health programs to include special programs for children and the elderly Continuation of funding for existing mental health centers
1980	Mental Health Systems Act	Addresses mental health rights and advocacy for the mentally ill
1990	The Americans with Disabilities Act (PL 101-336)	Prohibits discrimination based on disabilities, including mental disabilities

In response to the public's new interest and concern about mental illness, Congress created the Joint Commission on Mental Illness and Health in 1955. This commission studied and evaluated the needs of persons with mental illness and resources available for coping with the problem. The report, submitted by the commission to Congress in 1961, revealed three distinct areas of concern: manpower, facilities, and cost. The commission also made recommendations for solving these problems. However, even with increased allocation of resources, the long history of negative social perceptions about persons with mental illness has led to the stigma in today's society.

COMPREHENSIVE COMMUNITY MENTAL HEALTH

In 1963, Congress enacted the Mental Retardation Facilities and Community Mental Health Centers Construction Act. This act authorized federal funds to match local and state monies to build community health centers. It was believed that community agencies could more easily locate and treat people with mental problems by decentralizing mental health care and bringing services closer to the people. Community health centers were designed to offer such services as inpatient and outpatient treatment, partial hospitalization, emergency services, and consultation and educational services (Table 1-3). Centers were considered comprehensive if they also offered additional services such as diagnosis and rehabilitation care before and after hospitalization, training of professional and paraprofessionals, and research and evaluation. Because of limited monies, however, few of the agencies existing today are actually comprehensive.

Later legislation added funds to help staff the centers. In 1968, amendments were added to the Community Mental Health Centers Act to provide funds to develop community services and facilities for treating and rehabilitating drug addicts and alcoholics. There are also a number of court cases that have helped to identify rights of persons with mental illness (Table 1-4).

The Economic Opportunity Act of 1964 was designed to help the poor and disadvantaged reach their full social potential. This was a step toward placing full emphasis on the prevention of mental disorders through improvement of the social environment. The development of social psychiatry added the public health point of view to psychiatry. Social psychiatry closely examines the social environment of people who are mentally ill or have a high potential for mental illness. The goal is prevention.

In the early 1970s, care of persons with mental illness shifted from the hospital to the community. These services included:

Group home	Home for persons with mental illness who require supervision yet are in transition toward independent living in the community.
Foster home	Person with mental illness lives in a family that is supervised by a case manager. Room and board is provided for their length of stay.
Day care center	Independent living with therapeutic support during daytime hours (client resides in own home).
Halfway house	Transitional living from hospital to community. Each resident has responsibilities in the house, and counseling is available. Staffing is on site 24 hours.
Crisis center	Person with mental illness who is decompensating can reside at the center for one to two weeks and participate in the program. Medication and counseling are provided. Closer supervision occurs.
Hot line	Crisis intervention service with a specific listing: a hot line. Specially trained crisis clinicians are available 24 hours per day and 7 days per week. If it is a suicidal crisis, the crisis clinician will obtain as much identifying information as possible (name, address, telephone number), call 911, and keep the caller on the line until rescue personnel arrive.

TABLE 1-3 Services Offered by Comprehensive Community Mental Health Centers

PRIMARY

Inpatient services (short-term hospitalization)

Partial hospitalization/day treatment programs

Outpatient services

    Residential programs

    Rehabilitation programs

    Supportive guidance

Emergency services (24-hour interventions)

Education/consultation (community)

ADDITIONAL SERVICES

Research and evaluation

Vocational rehabilitation programs

Diagnostic services

Education of professionals/paraprofessionals

TABLE 1-4 Specific Court Cases Dealing with the Rights of the Persons with Mental Illness

Rouse vs. Cameron 373 F.2d 451 (D.C. Cir. 1966)	Right to treatment issues; if involuntarily committed and not treated, it is deprivation of civil rights
Nason vs. Bridgewater 233 N.E.2d 908 (Mass. 1968)	Right to treatment; not custodial care
Wyatt vs. Stickney 344 F.Supp 373 (M.D. Ala.1972)	Established constitutional rights of involuntary client to individualized treatment, qualified staff, a humane place
Donaldson vs. O'Connor 493 F.2d 507 (5th Cir. 1974)	Constitutional right to treatment; client awarded compensatory and punitive damages
Tarasoff vs. The Regents of the University of California 17 Cal3d 425 (1976)	Duty to warn of threats to harm others
Foucha vs. Louisiana 60 USLN 4359 (1992)	A person who is no longer mentally ill and dangerous no longer requires hospitalization

Private psychiatric hospitals were established, and units for psychiatric services were developed in general hospitals. Some private insurance companies established coverage for psychiatric care.

Much has been learned since 1970, especially in the area of chronic mental illness. Several very effective drugs have been developed. Although there are serious side effects, drugs along with counseling and supervision offer the best hope for persons with serious and persistent mental illness. New theories about the cause of mental illness have been presented.

CURRENT TRENDS

Releasing persons with mental illness from state hospitals was based on humanitarian ideals. It was to provide more personalized and humane care to persons whose civil rights had long been denied. However noble the move was meant to be, it has not proved totally successful. Some people adjusted very well to the community after being discharged from state institutions, but for some others the quality of life did not improve. Some former clients went home until their families burned out and they were turned into the streets. Some went into their own apartments but were later evicted because of failure to pay rent or because of bizarre behavior that bothered other residents. Many of those who got jobs soon lost them because of their behavior or because of excessive time off.

Unfortunately, persons with mental illness do not always recognize their problems and tend not to seek help. Because of current legislation, there are limited ways to force treatment and there is no control over those who periodically do come to a mental health center. If medication is given to them, there is no way to be certain how it is taken or even if it is taken. As a result, many of today's homeless population are actually persons with chronic mental illness. Only a small percentage of the 2.5 million persons with chronic mental illness are being treated on a regular basis. The Kassebaum-Kennedy-Haslert Bill (1996) is a health insurance congressional reform bill that deals with mental health parity. Currently, annual and lifetime caps are imposed on mental illness. Private health insurance contracts have imposed a low ceiling ($50,000 or less) for mental health, whereas a limit of $1 million is set for physical health care. This reform bill states that insurance payments for mental health/illness can be no more restrictive than those imposed on other services. Benefits would be felt most by adults with severe mental illness, children with serious emotional disturbances, and people with major mental health problems.

Deinstitutionalization has fallen far short of its goal, and currently mental health care is very fragmented. The fault, however, is not totally with the idea of deinstitutionalization. Many communities were ill prepared to cope with the former clients. They offered few actual services and insufficient housing for low-income people.

In 1980, Congress passed the Mental Health Systems Act, which called for more money for the community centers and for specialized services for persons with mental illness. The next year it passed the Omnibus Budget Reconciliation Act, which lumped all mental health services together with alcohol and drug problems. Later, all mental health funding was cut by 30 percent. This meant that there were no funds to carry out the Mental Health Systems Act of the previous year. Even though a small percentage of clients are still hospitalized, many states continue to send the major portion of all funding for mental health to the state institutions.

Since persons with mental illness do not readily seek help, the problem will remain even if funding becomes adequate. Mental health services will have to be provided in a more imaginative and progressive manner.

Persons with mental illness need a satisfactory and useful life within their own social environment. Therefore, emphasis is being placed on community living for these clients, where they are helped to participate in a variety of activities. Activities of daily living and social skills training become a part of the hospitalized client's life. Clients are taught reality living activities such as dressing, grooming, and manners. This new approach improves clients' morale and increases cooperation. Individual counseling is initiated, and supportive contact is made with clients.

The approach to mental health has been redesigned to emphasize human services programs. Training procedures and use of personnel were reassessed. To provide services to all levels of the population, it was necessary to recruit and train workers. This led to the *paraprofessional* (a trained aide who helps a professional person). It has even been suggested by some authorities that mental health workers will have to go into the community to find and treat clients if deinstitutionalization is to work.

With changes in mental health care, the role of the nurse has also changed. Nurses are now more involved members of the health care team. Nurses in mental health are involved in an *eclectic approach*; that is, they draw from various sources for the best care for the client. Nurses develop open communication with a variety of people: the professional nurse, psychiatrist, clinical psychologist, social worker, physical therapist and occupational therapist. They utilize available therapeutic services. Nurses express their feelings and findings at interdisciplinary staffing meetings and draw from their own experience to help develop client care plans.

Today, mental health nursing is concerned with the whole person. Custodial care is no longer the only nursing concern. Mental health nursing permeates all settings and recognizes the diverse needs of the clients (Table 1-5).

TABLE 1-5 Comprehensive Care of Persons with Mental Illness

CONTINUITY	CONSTANCY	CONSISTENCY
ASSESSMENT	Physical, psychological, social	
INTERVENTIONS	Provide coping strategies Explore problem-solving techniques Symptom recognition Environmental limit-setting Foster positive experiences	
EDUCATION	For client and family/significant other Understanding of diagnosis Recognition of the symptoms of relapse Knowledge of medication and side effects Provide support group information	

The primary sources of knowledge of mental illness today are newspapers, television, films, and books. Occasionally, the mass media have contributed to the **stigma** of mental illness through negative and inaccurate information and name-calling (psycho, lunatic, fruitcake, maniac, wacko), which sets up potentially harmful consequences. Frequently, people with mental illness have been portrayed as violent and dangerous, and thus, there are unfavorable expectations about mental illness. The National Alliance of the Mentally Ill (NAMI) is a strong consumer group that educates and advocates for persons with mental illness. The group is composed of family members that are supportive to each other's plight, and members volunteer their time to lobby for pertinent issues.

STANDARDS OF CARE

The nurse's responsibilities are determined by legislation, agency policy, and standards set by the profession. Legislation is enacted to provide safe practitioners. **Standards of care** focus on practice and fulfill the professions obligation to provide service and to continually improve that service. Standards provide a means of determining the quality of nursing that the client receives, whether such services are provided by the professional nurse, the practical nurse, or the nursing assistant. The nurse, working in a mental health care setting, is responsible for providing high-quality care as identified by the standards of psychiatric nursing within the nurse's legal role. The American Nurses' Associations booklet *Standards of Psychiatric–Mental Health Nursing Practices* (Kansas City, MO: American Nurses' Association, 1994) lists the standards of psychiatric–mental health nursing practice. (See Appendix.)

LEGAL RIGHTS OF CLIENTS

All states have revised laws to protect the rights of persons with mental illness (Figure 1-2). For example, in 1977, the state of New Mexico enacted the Mental Health and Developmental Disability Code. This code revised existing state laws for hospitalization and treatment of mentally disabled persons. The code specifically states client rights; what is to be included in treatment plans; steps to be followed in an **involuntary admission**; the rights of persons who voluntarily admit themselves; consent of treatment; treatment of minors; the meaning of confidentiality; and the right to obtain care, regardless of ability to pay. Many laws are state-mandated especially with regard to seclusion/ restraints (see Chapter 13). Most admissions to mental health facilities are now voluntary. A voluntary admission occurs when

1. The right to appropriate treatment in settings and under conditions most supportive and least restrictive to personal liberty

2. The right to an individualized written treatment plan, periodic review of treatment, and revision of plan

3. The right to ongoing participation in the planning of services and the right to a reasonable explanation of general mental condition, treatment objective, adverse effects of treatment, reasons for treatment, and available alternatives

4. The right to refuse treatment except in an emergency or as permitted by law

5. The right not to participate in experimentation

6. The right to freedom from restraint or seclusion

7. The right to a humane treatment environment

8. The right to confidentiality of records

9. The right to access to records except data provided by third parties or unless access would be detrimental to health

10. The right of access to telephone use, mail, and visitors

11. The right to know these rights

12. The right to initiate grievances when rights are infringed

13. The right to referral when discharged

FIGURE 1-2 Bill of Rights for Clients (From Mental Health System Act, 1980, 96th Congress, Public Law 96-398, Section 9501, Amendment to Senate Bill 1177, September 23, 1980.)

the client agrees to an admission to the hospital inpatient unit for assessment and treatment. The admission paperwork is willingly signed. Clients can still be committed by the courts. **Commitment** is sought when a client is assessed as being harmful to self or others, or gravely disabled. Recent violent acts or threats of violence to self (suicide) or others (homicide) are reported. If a person presents as a danger, anyone can initiate the commitment process. This will place a hold on the person for a number of hours (24) until a hearing on the commitment is held. This is called an *involuntary commitment*. However, just because someone is known to be mentally ill, he or she cannot be picked up and placed on an inpatient psychiatric unit. Regulations are now more stringent. The individual committed by the court has a right to treatment—not just custodial care. The health care facility can be held liable if treatment is not provided. Court cases showing that treatment was not provided have resulted in the release of the client. The courts can look at competency versus incompetency of the individual. **Competency** is defined as the capability to make reasonable, rational decisions and manage daily life circumstances. At times, the court may appoint a **guardian** or conservator. A guardian is legally responsible for the physical needs of another, in this case the client. A **conservator** is a person who has the legal responsibility for another's finances. The conservator disperses money to the client and keeps accurate records of expenditures (Figure 1-3).

Clients have a **right to refuse treatment**. All health care facilities must obtain informed consent from clients before beginning treatment. They must be provided with information that will enable them to make valid decisions concerning any proposed treatment. A client has the right to refuse treatment or later, withdraw from treatment. To make an informed decision about treatment, the risks, benefits, and options of the proposed treatment plan must be presented to the client so that he or she can weigh the advantages and disadvantages and consent to follow the treatment plan. Commitment to an institution does not automatically mean loss of the right to make a valid decision. Clients can also be held involuntarily if they are deemed to be suicidal, homicidal, or gravely disabled. This is to keep the client and others safe.

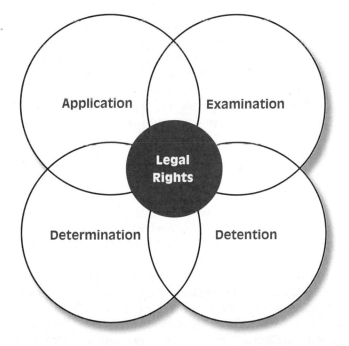

FIGURE 1-3 Legal rights: A four-step commitment process.

Clients have a right to humane treatment. This means they have the right to receive quality care in an environment that promotes their recovery. They also must be treated with respect and dignity. Personnel are legally liable for acts that do not conform with these rights. A nurse who observes cruelty to a client or other degrading acts and does not report them is as legally liable as the person committing the act. Currently, there are clear, well-defined client abuse guidelines that are closely adhered to in hospitals and mental health facilities.

Clients have the right to be treated as individuals. Some states have proclaimed that clients legally have the right to their own clothes and belongings while hospitalized. Clothes and belongings help the client to maintain identity. Maintaining identity is important when everything around the client is changing. It is an accepted fact that change itself causes stress. When dealing with a person who is already overwhelmed, it is imperative that care be taken by health care workers to avoid creating more stress. Therapeutic relationships are based on trust; therefore, confidentiality is an important concept. Confidentiality safeguards information from being disclosed to others. It applies in all practice settings. Frequently, the client's medical records are requested by employers, legal systems, or insurance companies. Family members call and request information. A release of information (ROI) specifying the particular person/group (i.e., wife, probation officer) to whom information can be given, must be signed by the client and be on file before any information can be released. The client's right to confidentiality is protected by law.

An issue in the twenty-first century is computer security. Computer records are confidential and safe but available. Sensitive information can be shared only with those who are authorized. To ensure confidentiality, always log off the computer when you walk away from it and never share your password.

SUMMARY

Mental illness has existed from primitive times. It was once thought to be caused by evil spirits entering and taking over the body. Medicine men, through incantations and magic, sought to drive the evil spirits from the body. Ancient Greeks, Romans, and Arabs believed that mental illness was a natural phenomenon and treated persons with mental illness humanely. After the fall of the Roman Empire, humanitarian ideas gave way to mysticism, witchcraft, and magic. Little was done to treat mental illness. Patients were locked in institutions where flogging, starvation, torture, and bloodletting were common. Toward the end of the Renaissance, the belief that evil spirits possessed the body began to decline and scientific inquiry increased. Objective study of behavior grew.

Philippe Pinel began the movement toward more humane treatment of persons with mental illness when he removed the chains from patients and advocated freedom, useful work, and kindness for the patient. Dorothea Lynde Dix was instrumental in having legislation enacted to improve conditions for patients with mental illness in America.

During the Revolutionary period, Benjamin Rush wrote the first American textbook on psychiatry. He is often referred to as the Father of American Psychiatry. The first psychiatric training school in the United States was established at McLean Hospital in Massachusetts in 1882. Early in the twentieth century, large state hospitals were built to house persons with mental illness. These hospitals provided fresh air and sunshine but little cure. In 1920, Sigmund Freud made a significant contribution to the understanding and treatment of mental illness with his work in psychoanalysis.

World War II brought the immensity of the mental health problem to the public's attention. Legislation was enacted to meet the need for better mental health care for returning veterans. The early 1960s saw an increased focus on the establishment of better care for persons with mental illness. Human services programs were introduced. Community health centers were provided to take the place of the obsolete state hospitals. Care of persons with mental illness shifted from the hospital to the community. Recent trends provide for the prevention and treatment of mental illness. These recent changes have brought about a change in nursing. The nurse has become more involved as a member of the health care team. Mental health is now concerned with the whole person. The goal is to restore persons with mental illness to an adequate level of functioning so that they may have satisfying and productive lives.

Nursing responsibilities are determined by legislation, agency policy, and standards of care set by the profession. Standards are set to continually improve practice. The nurse caring for individuals with mental illness has an obligation to give high-quality care as identified by the standards of psychiatric nursing within his or her legal role. The American Nurses' Association gives eleven standards for psychiatric–mental health nursing practice.

Persons with mental illness are demanding their rights. All states have enacted legislation protecting their rights. Clients have the right to therapeutic treatment, informed consent, humane care, and to be treated as individuals. As expanding knowledge of the brain continues, two pertinent areas of serious challenge remain: the provision of quality health care for persons with mental illness and the accessibility of that quality care to all people.

SUGGESTED ACTIVITIES

■ Assess your own attitudes concerning persons with mental illness. Include personal feelings and stereotypes.

■ Evaluate your local hospital's care of persons with mental illness. Write your impressions in one or two paragraphs.

■ Read about the life of Pinel, Dix, or Beers and plan a panel discussion in class.

■ Write a report on legislation passed in your state that has affected the care of persons with mental illness.

REVIEW

KNOW AND COMPREHEND
A. Multiple choice. Select the one best answer.

1. History first indicates evidence of mental illness during which of the following time periods?
   ❑ A. World War I
   ❑ B. the fall of the Roman Empire
   ❑ C. primitive times
   ❑ D. medieval times

2. The Father of American Psychiatry is
   ❑ A. Hippocrates.
   ❑ B. Sigmund Freud.
   ❑ C. Benjamin Rush.
   ❑ D. Philippe Pinel.

3. The ancient Greeks, Romans, and Arabs thought that mental illness was
   ❑ A. caused by evil spirits entering the body.
   ❑ B. a punishment for sins.
   ❑ C. a natural phenomenon.
   ❑ D. the result of witchcraft.

4. Post–World War II legislation that allocated funds for building psychiatric units was the
   ❑ A. National Mental Health Act.
   ❑ B. Economic Opportunity Act.
   ❑ C. Mental Retardation Facilities Act.
   ❑ D. Hill-Burton Act.

5. Community mental health centers were established to provide all of the following services except to
   ❏ A. offer consultation and educational services.
   ❏ B. offer outpatient care.
   ❏ C. bring mental health care closer to the people.
   ❏ D. provide local options for inpatient care.

6. Legislation that authorized federal funds to match local and state monies to build community health centers is the
   ❏ A. Mental Retardation Facilities and Community Mental Health Centers Construction Act.
   ❏ B. National Mental Health Act.
   ❏ C. Joint Commission on Mental Illness and Health.
   ❏ D. Hill-Burton Act.

7. Legislation designed to help the poor and disadvantaged reach their full potential is the
   ❏ A. National Mental Health Act.
   ❏ B. Economic Opportunity Act.
   ❏ C. Mental Retardation Facilities Act.
   ❏ D. Mental Health Amendment.

8. Recent trends in mental health care delivery focus on all of the following except
   ❏ A. prevention of mental illness.
   ❏ B. returning the client to an adequate level of functioning.
   ❏ C. community care.
   ❏ D. confining clients to state institutions.

9. A nurse who observes cruelty to a client and does not report it is
   ❏ A. legally guilty of cruelty.
   ❏ B. morally guilty of cruelty.
   ❏ C. just minding her own business.
   ❏ D. morally responsible to stop the cruelty herself.

10. A client who is legally committed to an institution
   ❏ A. has the right to treatment.
   ❏ B. automatically loses his or her right to make decisions.
   ❏ C. must accept prescribed treatment.
   ❏ D. may receive only custodial care.

APPLY YOUR LEARNING
B. Multiple Choice. Select the one best answer.

1. The practical nurse prepares a presentation for high school teachers regarding services offered by the local community mental health center. Which of the following services would be important to include in the presentation?
   - ❏ A. family planning services
   - ❏ B. crisis intervention and hot lines
   - ❏ C. treatment of sexually transmitted diseases
   - ❏ D. career development services

2. The nurse's neighbor asks, "Why aren't people with mental illness kept in hospitals anymore?" Which response by the nurse is most accurate?
   - ❏ A. "Clients have a right to treatment in the least restrictive setting. Hospitals are very restrictive."
   - ❏ B. "Because of the nursing shortage, there aren't enough nurses to take care of hospitalized clients anymore."
   - ❏ C. "Our nation has fewer persons with mental illness; therefore, fewer hospital beds are needed."
   - ❏ D. "Psychiatric hospitals are no longer popular as the result of negative stories in the press."

3. The clients described below all have serious and persistent mental illness, receive services from the local community mental health center, and live in the community. Which client may need involuntary hospitalization?
   The client who:
   - ❏ A. mumbles responses to auditory hallucinations.
   - ❏ B. begins drinking alcohol after one year of sobriety.
   - ❏ C. decides to stop taking medication prescribed by the MD.
   - ❏ D. shouts at drivers while standing in the middle of a busy city street.

4. A nurse's assistant in a psychiatric hospital suggests to the nurse, "We don't have time to help clients fill out their menu choices everyday. Let's just ask the dietary department to send the same tray to each client." Which response by the nurse would be *most* appropriate?
   - ❏ A. "Thanks for the idea, but it's important to treat clients as individuals. Giving menu choices is one way we can respect clients' individuality."
   - ❏ B. "Thanks for the suggestion, but the National Institute for Mental Health requires us to offer menu choices to clients."

❏ C. 'Thanks, that's a really good idea. We can announce the new policy at the community meeting today."

❏ D. 'Thanks for the suggestion, but that idea will not work for our clients who also have diabetes mellitus.'

5. The practical nurse subscribes to a nursing journal and reads it each month. What is the nurse's rationale for this activity?

❏ A. The cost of the journal is a tax-deductible professional expense for the nurse.

❏ B. Journals are the only source of new information for practicing nurses.

❏ C. Reading a journal promotes the nurse's continued professional growth and development.

❏ D. Reading journals is required for maintaining the nurse's licensure in most states.

6. The nurse's next door neighbor is admitted to the psychiatric unit. Which action by the nurse would recognize the client's rights? ·

❏ A. Say to the client "I'm sorry you've developed a mental illness."

❏ B. Ask the supervisor to be assigned to the client's care daily.

❏ C. Tell the client "I'm required to keep all information confidential."

❏ D. Avoid talking to the client at all times.

7. In the hospital elevator, the nurse overhears a group of health care professionals discussing a client with mental illness. The nurse should first:

❏ A. keep the overheard information confidential.

❏ B. immediately notify the nursing supervisor.

❏ C. inform the group they are violating the client's rights.

❏ D. notify the state board of nursing regarding the misconduct.

B. Match the contribution in column I with the name in column II.

Column I	Column II
	a. Clifford Beers

1. published the first American textbook on psychiatry
2. believed all illness was controlled by the stars and planets
3. used hypnotism to treat hysteria
4. worked for passage of legislation to improve care of persons with mental illness in America
5. authored a book that made the public aware of the need for better care for persons with mental illness
6. developed a technique called psychoanalysis
7. believed that the universe was filled with magnetic forces and that persons with mental illness could be cured by bringing them into balance with the universe
8. began the movement toward humane treatment of persons with mental illness by removing chains from patients

a. Clifford Beers
b. Jean Martin Charcot
c. Dorothea Lynde Dix
d. Sigmund Freud
e. Franz Mesmer
f. Paracelsus
g. Philippe Pinel
h. Benjamin Rush

C. Briefly answer the following:

1. Explain changes in mental health care with the creation of community mental health centers.

2. Explain the purposes of standards for nursing care.

3. Explore the quality and accessibility of care for persons with mental illness in your particular community. Prepare a brief report and include proactive plans.

Stress and Mental Health

OUTLINE

KEY TERMS

mental health

mental illness

Diagnostic and Statistical Manual of Mental Disorders, Fourth
   Edition, Text Revision 2000 (DSM-IV-TR)

stress

adaptation

nursing process

   assessment

   nursing diagnosis

   planning

   implementation

   intervention

   evaluation

burnout

OBJECTIVES

After studying this chapter, the student should be able to:

- State the characteristics of a healthy personality.
- Name the three stages of the general adaptation syndrome.
- List four factors that affect a person's ability to cope with stress.
- Name four rules of good health that help to maintain coping ability.
- Identify classifications of mental illness.

There are two major contributions of nursing to the health care system: the concept of holistic beings and a dedication to the promotion
of a high degree of wellness. Nurses who are committed to these ideals,
whether primarily engaged in mental or physical care, accept responsibility for fostering mental health and preventing mental illness. This
is not an easy task, and it is made even more difficult by the lack of a
single definition for mental health. The factors that promote mental
health are disputed even more. Many authorities even deny the existence of mental illness unless there is a definite change in the brain
cells. Some authorities define mental health as a responsibility. They
consider a person who accepts responsibility for his or her own behavior to be mentally healthy. Other people relate mental health to
self-awareness. Still others consider **mental health** to be learned

behavior. There is also disagreement on what may be termed healthy behavior. Acts that are unacceptable at one time may be considered acceptable or normal at another time. What is punished by one group may be approved by another group.

Even though mental health cannot be universally defined, most agree that it is a positive state. This means that it is more than the absence of disease. The person with mental health usually is considered to be self-directive. Generally, the person has a feeling of well-being, is productive, and enjoys life. He or she sets goals and realistic limits for activities.

Healthy people have the stability to accept and express love freely. There is a reaching out to help others. These people can stand alone when necessary or accept help from others without losing independence. Flexible and willing to try new things, they are eager to learn about themselves and the world around them. Qualities of mental health include:

- Has success experience

- Is flexible

- Forms close relationships

- Makes appropriate judgments

- Solves problems

- Copes with daily stressors

- Has positive sense of self

- Modulates and regulates mood and affect

Two factors influencing the way an individual functions are inherited characteristics or potential and the psychosocial environment, which includes nurturing received in childhood and circumstances encountered in life. Almost everyone displays some characteristics that would be considered unhealthy under certain circumstances. Occasionally, everyone feels depressed, dependent, or unenthusiastic. To be considered ill, however, the individual must exhibit more of the abnormal behaviors, display them more consistently than most people, and be unable to carry out activities of daily living (ADL).

Other mental health difficulties that pose major social, health, and economic problems in the United States include alcoholism, alienation, rebellion, drug abuse, racism, violence, and suicide. Many people need help in coping with the added stresses of disease or disaster. Million of others, though not considered to have a mental illness, consistently function under anxiety.

CLASSIFICATION OF MENTAL ILLNESS

For ease in studying, mental disorders are usually classified. For many years, all mental disorders were covered in the following general categories: Mental retardation (encompassed all developmental disabilities); organic brain syndrome (included conditions resulting in behavioral changes that could be traced to organic causes); psychoses (included diseases that resulted in severe abnormal behavior accompanied by a withdrawal from reality); psychoneuroses (included forms of abnormal behavior milder than psychosis; the person with a neurosis was more in contact with the real world than was the psychotic individual); personality disorders, or dysfunctional behaviors (behaviors that interfered with the individual's ability to function effectively in society); psychophysiological disorders (included conditions in which physical symptoms developed because of emotional problems).

These categories caused some difficulties because the boundaries were not clear and symptoms overlapped. In 1954, the *Diagnostic and Statistical Manual of Mental Disorders (DSM)* was published by the American Psychiatric Association in an attempt to assist in the formation of reliable, accurate and objective diagnoses. The current manual, *DSM-IV-TR (2000)* assigns a specific number to each diagnostic category (i.e., 300.02 Generalized Anxiety Disorder) and specifies the severity of the symptoms (mild, moderate, severe) and the course of the disease (partial or full remission). It guides the clinician through a multiaxial system. (See Appendix C.) An example follows:

Axis I: Major psychiatric disorder (i.e., Major Depressive Disorder–recurrent moderate)

Axis II: Personality disorders (i.e., Borderline Personality Disorder) and development disorders

Axis III: General medical conditions (GMC) (i.e., hypertension, diabetes)

Axis IV: Psychosocial and environmental stressors (i.e., recent divorce)

Axis V: Global assessment of functioning (GAF) rated at 0–100 utilizing specific criteria and assessment at current time of the evaluation (i.e., GAF 55)

Some psychiatric clients may not have an Axis II or III. It will be documented as "none, deferred, or ø."

STRESS THEORY

According to Hans Selye, **stress** is a nonspecific response to any demand made on the body. Demands may range from a disappointment to a severe illness. Some stress is necessary, but too much stress may send the body into a state of exhaustion. Coping with stress requires a great deal of energy; the supply of this energy is limited.

A person's response to stress is only one theory used to explain mental illness. However, it provides a useful framework for the study and practice of mental health nursing. The theory of stress developed by Selye provides the framework for this book. The stress framework is based on these assumptions:

- People are unique. Although people have the same physiological reactions to stress, they differ in their use of coping energy, the amount of energy available, their coping mechanisms, and available support.

- People become conditioned to coping with stress. Therefore, more effective methods can be learned.

- People are holistic. They are unified biological, spiritual, social, and emotional beings. Psychological and physical stress cannot be separated. What affects one aspect of an individual affects all other aspects.

- The person's internal and external environments are constantly changing. To remain in physiological and psychological balance, one must constantly adapt to these changes.

- Illness is a result of disruption in the stress adaptation mechanism (the person's ability to adjust to change).

- It is the nurse's responsibility to teach effective coping skills, provide physical and emotional support, and minimize stress in the client's environment.

Physiological Effects of Stress

The term *adaptive energy* was coined by Seyle to indicate a force that the individual uses to adapt to stress. Adaptive energy is different from caloric energy, which is replenished by food. Seyle found that demands, which he called *stressors*, cause chemical and structural changes that are manifestations of the body's attempt to maintain homeostasis (Figure 2-1). According to Seyle, these variations represent the general adaptation syndrome (GAS), which responds to any stimulus. He divides the general adaptation syndrome into three stages: the crisis stage, the adaptation stage, and the exhaustion stage.

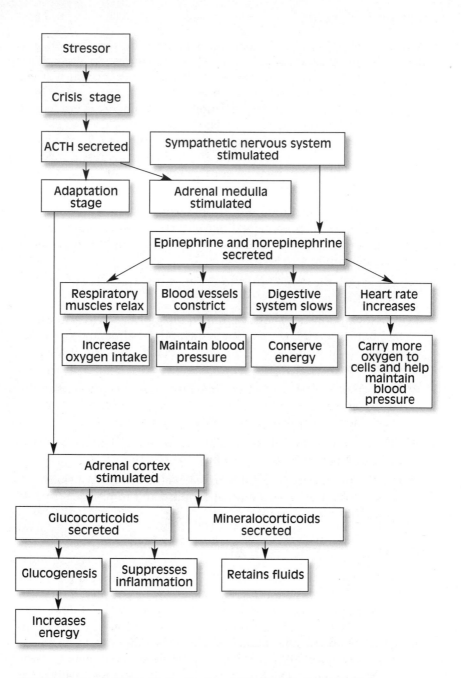

FIGURE 2-1 Physiological effects of the general adaptation syndrome.

In the crisis or alarm stage, the body mobilizes its forces to handle the stressors. The sympathetic nervous system is stimulated. Almost immediately, large amounts of the neurohormones epinephrine and norepinephrine are secreted into the bloodstream. The adrenal medulla is also stimulated, increasing and prolonging the epinephrine in the bloodstream. The heart rate increases and the blood vessels constrict to maintain adequate pressure. The respiratory muscles relax to increase the oxygen supply, and the digestive system, temporarily unneeded, decreases activity. These actions are presumably to save energy, but they may result in some annoying symptoms such as pale, cool skin; shivering; and sweating of the palms and soles. The person under severe stress may experience a pounding heart, dilated pupils, insomnia, dry mouth, nausea, and diarrhea.

In the **adaptation** or resistance stage, the adrenal cortex secretes increased amounts of glucocorticoids and mineralocorticoids. The mineralocorticoids help save fluids and sodium. The glucocorticoids suppress inflammation, mobilize fatty acids, and increase glucose levels, providing fuel or energy. Protein is broken down and changed to amino acids, and the lysosome membrane is stabilized to prevent cell destruction. If stress is prolonged or overwhelming and the adaptive energy is insufficient, the body enters into the third stage, exhaustion. This stage cannot tolerated for extended periods of time. If relief is not obtained, mental illness occurs. The symptoms in this stage are similar to those in the alarm period. The body's ability to adjust is gone. The adaptive mechanism breaks down and the body is no longer able to cope with stress.

Coping Mechanisms

Stress is an automatic response and cannot be avoided. However, people can learn to conserve their adaptive energy. This is important because the energy supply is limited. How much is used for coping depends on conditioning. *Conditioning* occurs when one is continuously taught a behavior until it becomes automatic. Because of conditioning, some people handle a great deal of stress while others find a minimum of stress intolerable. Other factors affecting a person's ability to cope with stress include:

- How the danger is viewed
- The individual's immediate needs
- The amount of support received from others
- The individual's belief about his or her ability to handle the stressful event

■ Previous success or failure in coping

■ Amount of stressors adding up over time or occurring at the same time that the individual must handle

Coping measures that use a minimal amount of energy are called *adaptive measures*. Coping measures that require a great amount of energy are called *maladaptive measures*. Generally, measures that deal directly with the stressful event or its symptoms are adaptive. Measures used to avoid conflict are considered less effective and may be maladaptive (Table 2-1). Adaptive measures that may be used when stressful events are confronted include:

■ Utilizing support people

■ Relaxing to alleviate tense muscles

■ Problem solving

■ Changing behavior

■ Developing more realistic goals

Measures used to avoid stress may include utilizing some defense mechanisms, extreme sleepiness, or depression. People who try to avoid stress may rely on rituals such as constant handwashing, or they may simply deny the stressful experience. Some people tend to transfer stress to an organ, and this stress response can contribute to and complicate physiological disorders such as asthma, heart failure, rheumatoid arthritis, ulcers, and perhaps even cancer. Still others may withdraw from their stressors through the excessive use of alcohol, drugs, or promiscuous sexual behavior.

TABLE 2-1 Levels of Adaptation to the Stress Response

ADAPTIVE COPING MEASURES	LESS ADAPTIVE MEASURES	MALADAPTIVE MEASURES
Relaxation	Some defense mechanisms	Neurosis
Problem solving	Avoidance	Somatic disorders
Behavioral change	Denial	Excessive use of
Developing more	Sleepiness	alcohol or drugs
realistic goals	Pointless activity	Some mental
	Physical withdrawal	mechanisms
		Excessive eating
		Fantasy
		Ritualistic behavior

The psychotic person has a lack of sufficient adaptive energy. According to stress theory, this person finds stress so overwhelming that he or she withdraws from reality into a private world where there is comfort and little stress.

STRESS AND THE NURSING PROCESS

The **nursing process** is a method of achieving client care through deliberate systematic and individualized procedures. It serves as a guide in determining and organizing needs, setting priorities, and implementing and evaluating intervention. It provides a systematic approach to the utilization of the stress theory. The nursing process consists of the following steps: assessment, nursing diagnosis, outcome identification/planning, implementation, and evaluation.

Assessment

Assessment is the first step of the nursing process. The LPN/LVN gathers important data that is subjective (client's reporting) and objective (nurse's findings/observations). Assessment is an ongoing process that begins with the initial contact, usually when the client is admitted to the hospital. Determining the client's stress level and coping mechanisms is part of the nurse's assessment of the client. In order to assess effectively, the nurse observes and communicates with the client and the client's family. He or she then shares this information with the professional nurse and other health care team members. Through observation, the nurse may be able to determine the following about the client:

- Self-image
- Level of anxiety: the client's individual signs and symptoms and causes of anxiety
- Level of coping: the client's perception of adaptive versus maladaptive coping mechanisms
- Degree of contact with and orientation to the outside world
- Reaction to unfamiliar sights and sounds in the environment

Through communication, the nurse may learn the client's

- Knowledge of agency or hospital routines
- Interpretation of his or her health status
- Prior health habits
- Distressful symptoms

- Duration of the presenting problem
- Interpersonal relationships, especially with family members
- Degree of contact with reality
- Usual coping mechanisms

The information obtained through observation and communication is then used to determine possible causes of stress. Note the following examples.

Example 1:

> Mr. Jones is admitted to the hospital for a cholecystectomy. He appears very distressed. His wife tells the nurse that they have no insurance. They have been saving to buy a house, but now the money will be needed to pay the hospital bill.

Cause of Stress. Surgery is itself a stressor. Also, studies have shown that financial worries rank high as stressors for people being admitted to the hospital. People are able to cope with a certain amount of stress. However, when stressors accumulate, physical and psychological symptoms may appear.

Example 2:

> Judy Ann, aged two, is admitted to the hospital with diarrhea and vomiting. Her mother states that Judy Ann has not used a bottle for about a year. Judy Ann sucks her thumb and cries for a bottle when her mother is gone.

Cause of Stress. In addition to stress caused by internal or external trauma, loss of usual coping resources can cause stress. Judy Ann may insist on her bottle because of the stress created by being separated from her mother, whom Judy Ann feels protects her from distressful events.

Example 3:

> Mrs. Thomas tells the nurse that she is frightened about impending labor. She asks if it is really as painful as everyone says. She states that she does not know how she will cope if it is painful because she cannot stand pain.

Cause of Stress. Mrs. Thomas is conditioned to maladaption. Conditioning can turn an otherwise tolerable stress into a pathogenic (disease-causing) stress.

Determining the underlying cause of stress is an important part of assessment. When the problem and possible causes of stress have been determined, the next step is to plan care to meet the needs of the client.

Nursing Diagnosis

A **nursing diagnosis** is a basis of choosing a nursing intervention that will achieve client outcomes. Formulating a nursing diagnosis is the RN's primary responsibility; however, the LPN/LVN gives pertinent information from the assessment findings to the RN. The North American Nursing Diagnosis Association (NANDA) has compiled standardized nursing diagnosis (see Appendix A).

Outcome Identification/Planning

Planning involves determining goals, priorities, and nursing actions to help the client. Nursing goals are desired changes that meet the needs of the client. After goals are set, their order of priority is considered. The action that would best achieve the desired results is then determined.

Helping Mr. Jones obtain his home or pay his hospital bill would be beyond the scope of nursing and should not appear in the nursing care plan as a goal. In some instances, however, a referral to the social services department might be appropriate. An example of a nursing goal for Mr. Jones would be to enhance his usual adapting/coping mechanisms to enable him to handle the added stress of surgery. Providing support is one way of enhancing coping mechanisms. Considering the resources available, the nurse could provide the needed support or encourage Mrs. Jones to provide it. Since Mrs. Jones is also having difficulty coping, the action most likely to succeed is the nurse providing the care and support directly.

Implementation

Implementation puts into action interventions prescribed in the planning phase. An **intervention** is the actual nursing measure used to help the client. All interventions have a rationale based on sound nursing knowledge and theory. Interventions help the client meet basic needs and include all actions taken to relieve stress and restore the client's homeostasis. Supervision of activities of daily living is one way the nurse intervenes to help relieve the client's stress. Other ways are encouraging client participation in diversional activities, administration of medications, and manipulation of the client's environment. Clients sometimes require controls on their activities. Other times, tasks are specifically assigned to them. Encouraging clients to socialize is an important intervention. People who are able to socialize usually adapt better than those who are not able to socialize.

The nurse may also be involved in supportive counseling, either individually or as a cotherapist in a group. Teaching new coping mechanisms, following the prescribed course of treatment, and helping clients achieve homeostasis are other responsibilities that may be assigned to the nurse.

For Mr. Jones, appropriate nursing interventions might be to spend time with him, to encourage him to talk about his anxieties, and to demonstrate an understanding and empathetic attitude toward him.

Evaluation

Evaluation involves determining whether the nursing intervention has been successful. The evaluation examines the goals and outcomes to determine whether they were achieved. It also includes the client's response to the intervention and the accuracy of the risk factors. Mr. Jones appeared depressed when he was admitted. The success of the nursing intervention would be evaluated by observing Mr. Jones's subsequent behavior. For example, if he talked more, smiled, exhibited increased energy, or appeared more hopeful of the future, the nurse could assume that the intervention was successful.

Evaluation of client progress is the responsibility of all members of the health team. In the nursing process, the licensed practical nurse (LPN) functions under the direction of the registered nurse (RN). The responsibilities of the LPN involve direct client care, so they vary according to the situation and the client's needs. Being in direct contact with clients puts the LPN in a position to see the day-to-day changes that determine the effectiveness of the plan, but the registered nurse is responsible for the overall assessment and plan of care. In the hospital you will hear this process referred to as total quality improvement (TQI) which is a part of quality assurance (QA).

The nurse can profoundly affect client progress because of his or her involvement and interaction. It is through contact with professionals and paraprofessionals that the client gains support and learns to see himself or herself as important. Knowledge that others genuinely care and expect improvement encourages the client's recovery.

STRESS AND THE NURSE

Constant contact with highly stressed clients is a stressor for the nurse. It may eventually overwhelm the nurse. This phenomenon is termed **burnout**. At best, it results in ineffective relationships. The nurse may become angry, display an attitude that the clients deserve their problems, or emotionally withdraw from the clients. To avoid burnout, the nurse may need to physically withdraw from the stressful situation and engage in other diversional activities, such as walking, relaxation breathing, and meditation (Figure 2-2).

Even a well-adjusted person may have trouble thinking clearly or making constructive decisions during a crisis. Depending on the degree of stress perceived, there may be a heightened awareness of self, tension, and a feeling of ineffectiveness. There may also be depression and a lack of energy. Well-adjusted people use internal and external resources to conserve energy by making a realistic assessment of the problem. They also recognize and accept situations that cannot be changed and find alternate actions for those that can be changed.

Nurses owe it to themselves and their clients to follow rules of good health in order to prevent physical illness. A physically ill person has less ability to cope. A nurse who is unable to handle his or her own stressors adequately is unable to help others. The nurse should get adequate rest, proper nutrition, and plenty of exercise and engage in wholesome, enjoyable activities. He or she should work on strengthening personal adaptive methods.

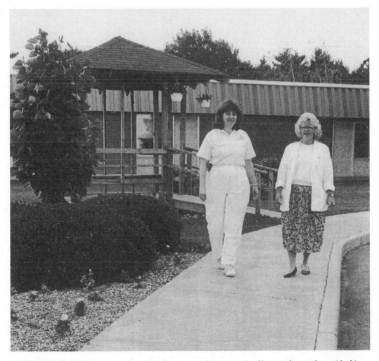

FIGURE 2-2 Nurses enjoying a pleasant diversional activity.

SUMMARY

There is little agreement on a definition for mental health. There is also little agreement on what may be termed a healthy personality. Most authorities believe that mental health is a positive quality— more than the absence of disease. The two factors influencing the way an individual functions are heredity and the psychosocial environment.

Mental health problems are a major social difficulty. Mental illness is classified in diagnostic categories for ease of study.

According to Hans Seyle, stress is a nonspecific response to any stimulus. Symptoms that occur are the result of the body's attempt to adapt to stress. The body's attempt to adapt to stress is called the general adaptation syndrome (GAS). Stress response is automatic, but people can learn to conserve energy. Factors that affect a person's ability to cope include conditioning, degree of perceived danger, immediate needs, support received from others, beliefs about one's ability to handle the stressful situation, previous successes and failures, and the degree of accumulated or concurrent stress. Coping measures that the person uses to confront the stressful event are generally adaptive. Coping measures that avoid stress are less adaptive, or maladaptive.

The nursing process is a method of achieving client care through deliberate, systematic, and individualized procedures. It serves as a guide in determining and organizing care to lessen stress and enhance the client's ability to cope with stress. However, the nurse's mandate, "Know thyself" can contribute to important self-care to avoid burnout.

SUGGESTED ACTIVITIES

- Visit a local mental health center or acute care facility and talk to a nurse about his or her duties.
- Discuss the meaning of mental health with a group of students.
- Have a class discussion about current attitudes toward persons with mental illness.
- Recall the last time you experienced stress. Make a list of the coping mechanisms you used to deal with the situation and their effectiveness.
- Read one or more of the following books:

Szasz, T. S. (1974). *The myth of mental illness: Foundations of a theory of personal conduct.* New York: Harper & Row.

Glasser, W. (1975). *Reality therapy: A new approach to psychiatry.* New York: Harper & Row.

Seyle, H. (1978). *The stress of life.* New York: McGraw-Hill.

REVIEW

KNOW AND COMPREHEND
A. Multiple choice. Select the one best answer.

1. Findings associated with the stress response, which indicate the body is trying to effectively cope, include attempts to
   - ❑ A. run from the impending threat.
   - ❑ B. conserve energy.
   - ❑ C. identify the impending danger.
   - ❑ D. shield the person from unpleasant experiences.

2. The purpose of the first stage of the General Adaptation Syndrome is to
   - ❑ A. alert the individual to danger.
   - ❑ B. determine the extent of the danger.
   - ❑ C. mobilize energy needed for adaptation.
   - ❑ D. shield the individual from unpleasant experiences.

3. The physiological changes during the second General Adaptation Syndrome stage are caused by hormones from the
   - ❑ A. thyroid.
   - ❑ B. thymus.
   - ❑ C. pituitary.
   - ❑ D. adrenals.

4. Coping mechanisms used to deal directly with stress are classified as
   - ❑ A. adaptive.
   - ❑ B. dysfunctional.
   - ❑ C. stressors.
   - ❑ D. maladaptive.

5. For which of the following reasons does the nurse encourage use of coping mechanisms that require minimal amounts of energy?
   - ❑ A. excessive energy slows the heart rate
   - ❑ B. adaptive energy is limited
   - ❑ C. sleep is impossible during stress
   - ❑ D. the appetite is decreased during stress

6. *Burnout* may be associated with all of the following except
   ❏ A. physical exhaustion because of overwork.
   ❏ B. making decisions during a crisis.
   ❏ C. the nurse who acts in a forgetful, hostile manner.
   ❏ D. being overwhelmed by stress.

APPLY YOUR LEARNING
B. Multiple choice. Select the one best answer.

1. The nurse gathers data regarding a newly admitted hospital client. Which of the findings below should alert the nurse that the client may be coping poorly with stress?

   The client:
   ❏ A. reports sleeping 14 to 16 hours per day for the past 3 months.
   ❏ B. states, "I realize I'm not able to play 18 holes of golf anymore. Now I play 9."
   ❏ C. comments, "I've asked my brother for help until I'm feeling stronger."
   ❏ D. says, "I've asked my supervisor to reduce my work schedule to 20 hours a week."

2. In which part of the nursing care plan would the nurse expect to find the following?

   Seat client in dining room at a table with other clients, tid.
   ❏ A. data collection
   ❏ B. planning
   ❏ C. intervention
   ❏ D. evaluation

3. In which part of the nursing care plan would the nurse expect to find the following?

   Client will begin a conversation with one staff member per day.
   ❏ A. data collection
   ❏ B. planning
   ❏ C. intervention
   ❏ D. evaluation

4. A nurse has worked on an acute, inpatient psychiatric unit for the past three years. Which of the following would suggest that the nurse may have experienced burnout?

The nurse:
❏ A. argues daily with co-workers about assignments.
❏ B. plans a long weekend trip to the beach.
❏ C. trades weekend assignments with a co-worker.
❏ D. registers for a course on meditation.

5. A nurse wants to find a description of the characteristics of schizophrenic disorders. Which resource would have the most complete information?
❏ A. a medical-surgical nursing textbook
❏ B. the journal *Psychology Today*
❏ C. *Taber's Cyclopedic Medical Dictionary*
❏ D. *Diagnostic and Statistical Manual of Mental Disorders*

C. Briefly answer the following:

1. List four characteristics of the healthy personality.

2. Name the three stages of the general adaptation syndrome.

3. List four factors that affect a person's ability to cope with stress.

4. Name four rules of good health the nurse needs to follow to maintain coping ability.

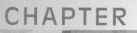

Understanding Self and Others

OUTLINE

KEY TERMS

heredity base	enuresis
psychosocial environment	senior citizen
self-concept	motivation
failure to thrive	self-actualization
separation anxiety	defense mechanisms
autonomy	self-awareness
conscience	self-fulfilling prophecy

OBJECTIVES

After studying this chapter, the student should be able to:

- Define self-concept.
- Name the two important factors in personality development.
- State the significant contributions made to the study of growth and development by Erikson, Maslow, and Sullivan.
- Identify development tasks for each stage of the life cycle as proposed by Erikson.
- List the needs of people as denoted by Maslow.
- Identify the common mental mechanisms.
- List three advantages of increased self-awareness.

The nurse-client relationship is the basis of nursing. It is through this relationship that the nurse assesses the client's needs, assists in determining the care to be given, and evaluates this care. For the client, this relationship depends, in part, on the nurse's knowledge of human needs and behaviors. An understanding of how personality develops and the ability to recognize behavior and motives as they actually exist are essential to developing a helping relationship.

PERSONALITY DEVELOPMENT

An individual's personality develops throughout the life cycle. It is dependent on two interacting factors, the **heredity base** or *potential* and the **psychosocial environment**. Each individual has a unique makeup that is contained within the genes from conception. This makeup sets the direction and ultimate potential, or ceiling, for the individual's achievements. Whether an individual fulfills his or her potential is dependent on the nurturing, support, and opportunities available in the environment and the type and number of stressors encountered throughout the life cycle.

SELF-CONCEPT

Self-concept refers to the way in which a person feels, views, or thinks of himself or herself. The self-concept is strong but not static. It

TABLE 3-1 Statements Made by Significant Others May Affect the Child's Developing Self-Concept

STATEMENTS THAT MAY HAVE A POSITIVE EFFECT ON THE CHILD'S SELF-CONCEPT	STATEMENTS THAT MAY HAVE A NEGATIVE EFFECT ON THE CHILD'S SELF-CONCEPT
"Something is troubling you. Would you like to talk about it?" "Right now I really need to finish this job, but I will be glad to listen to you in a few minutes."	"Do not bother me. Can't you see I am busy?"
"You may find it works better if you do it this way." "You seem to be having a problem with that. How can I help?"	"That is not the way to do it. Can't you do anything right?"
"What would you think about adding this scarf to that dress?" "What do you think about wearing your blue dress tonight? It looks so pretty on you."	"You are not going out dressed like that are you? You never did have any fashion sense."
"What you did was very wrong." "I am really upset with your behavior."	"You are a bad boy."
"I'd like to show you one way I have found that seems to be more efficient." "I found if I do it this way I get the job done thoroughly. It helps me remember all the details so I do not have to do it again."	"Every time you do something, I have to do it over again."
"Thank you for helping me." "I love you." "You are very special."	"Did you get that done yet?" "Sometimes you make me so angry."

continues to develop as the child interacts with others. What significant others tell the child, as well as all of the child's experiences, successes, and failures, helps to mold and change the self-concept. Children are extremely sensitive to the attitudes of those around them. They feel good when they sense satisfaction but have bad feelings about themselves when they experience anxiety. Mild anxiety is a motivator for action. Babies learn that crying will bring relief for stress. Frequent feelings of anxiety, however, lead children to see themselves as bad. If children are told they are good, they believe it; but if they are constantly criticized or ignored, their self-concepts are poor (Table 3-1).

There are many theories of personality development, and none has the answer to all aspects of the personality. Each stage of development prepares the personality for the principal development of the next stage. If the tasks of a particular developmental stage are not completed, it will hinder or limit successful life experiences.

This chapter is based on the combined work of Erikson, Maslow, and Sullivan (Table 3-2). These men were selected because their theories better fit the framework for this book. Freud's theories and psychoanalysis are discussed in Chapter 5.

TABLE 3-2 Selected Theories of Personality Development

THEORISTS	IDEAS ON PERSONALITY DEVELOPMENT
Erik Erikson	1. Develops over the life span 2. Affected by the environment 3. Divided into stages 4. Each stage has a specific task to be accomplished 5. Goal is task accomplishment
Abraham Maslow	1. Develops over the life span 2. Affected by the environment 3. Divided into needs, which are used as motivators 4. Goal is self-actualization
Harry Stack Sullivan	1. Develops over the life span 2. Maternal relationships very significant 3. Satisfying interpersonal relationships important to growth 4. Anxiety stimulates growth 5. Overwhelming stress retards growth 6. The goal is security

Erik Erikson's work was done in early 1900. Until that time, Freud had been the leading theorist. Unlike Freud, Erikson looked at growth potential rather than pathology. Where Freud thought personality developed by the age of five, Erikson carried his theory throughout the life cycle. He recognized stages and named certain developmental tasks that must be accomplished during each of the stages. The stages are infancy, toddler, preschool, school age, adolescence, adult, and old age (Table 3-3).

TABLE 3-3 Developmental Tasks in the Life Cycle

AGE	ERIKSON'S DEVELOPMENTAL TASKS	SPECIFIC DEVELOPMENTAL TASKS
Infancy (Birth to 18 months)	**Trust** versus **mistrust**	Differentiate self from the environment Begin to develop a self-concept Develop trust Develop a relationship with a caring person or persons Learn to sit, stand, and walk Learn to feed self
Toddler (18 months to 3 years)	**Autonomy** versus **shame** and **doubt**	Develop autonomy (self-determination, independence) Begin to develop an identity Develop motor skills Learn to control bowel movements Learn to talk
Preschool (3 to 6 years)	**Initiative** versus **guilt**	Develop a conscience Develop initiative Begin to relate to others socially Learn sexual role identity Begin to fantasize about the future Adjust to prolonged absence from parent (if the child goes to nursery school)
School Age (6 to 12 years)	**Industry** versus **inferiority**	Develop pleasure in work completed Learn and validate social role Learn to relate to age-mates Develop musculature for sports and school activities Adjust to prolonged absence from home Adjust to a structured schedule Achieve independence in personal care Increase learning skills

(Continues)

TABLE 3-3 (Continued)

AGE	ERIKSON'S DEVELOPMENTAL TASKS	SPECIFIC DEVELOPMENTAL TASKS
Adolescence (12 to 18 years)	Identity versus **role diffusion**	Acquire a sense of identity Establish a new role Achieve more mature relationships with friends Accept changed body image Accept new sexual feelings Achieve emotional independence Develop intellectual skills Clarify values
Young Adult (18 to 35 years)	Intimacy versus isolation	Adjust to college or employment Select a lifestyle Accept adult responsibility Achieve economic independence Establish an intimate relationship Select a mate Establish a home Accept a new social role as parent or mate
Middle Adult (35 to 65 years)	Generativity versus **stagnation**	Achieve economic security Help children to become responsible citizens Assess accomplishment Adjust to children leaving the home Adjust to new lifestyle Accept the physical changes of middle age Develop leisure-time activities
Senescence (65 years to death)	Integrity versus **despair**	Adjust to decreased health Accept a new identity Get life in order Accept dependence as needed Accept reality of own death Adjust to death of spouse and friends Adjust to retirement Review life Establish relationships with peers Adjust to new lifestyle, if necessary

Abraham Maslow is recognized as the founder of humanistic psychology. He stressed the need to provide nurturance, acceptance, love, a feeling of belonging, and a sense of self-worth. He developed a hierarchy of needs to serve in motivating behavior. Like Erikson, he viewed personality development as a lifelong process and believed that it was affected by the environmental conditions under which the person lived.

Harry Stack Sullivan was a neo-Freudian. Like Freud, he believed in the significance of the maternal relationship in personality development. He felt security was the major goal in life and that it was achieved through satisfying interpersonal relationships. He felt anxiety stimulated growth, but overwhelming stress was to be avoided.

ERIKSON'S DEVELOPMENTAL TASKS

Infancy (Birth to Eighteen Months)

Newborns are well aware of their environments, can see within 7 to 10 inches, and can hear and discriminate among sounds. Newborns also have a preference for particular visual and auditory stimuli. They like complex patterns, curved lines, and the human face. They follow brightly colored objects with their eyes and pay more attention to the high-pitched female voice. Music seems to have a soothing effect on them. Infants require stimuli for their continued growth. As they grow older, the stimuli must become more varied and complex (Figure 3-1).

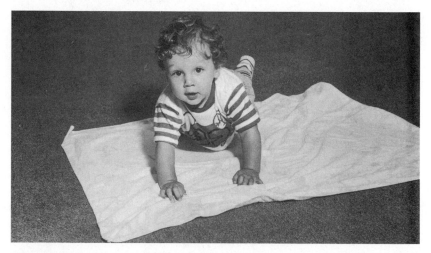

FIGURE 3-1 Stimuli must become more varied and complex as the baby grows.

Newborn infants are particularly sensitive to tactile stimuli and cannot be spoiled by attention. Cuddling, stroking, rocking, and talking to them are essential to optimal growth. Neglecting infants who are wet, hungry, or otherwise unhappy, causes added stress and inhibits development.

Newborns are almost totally dependent on their environment and do not see themselves as separate and distinct from it. They respond to the environment in a general manner rather than a specific way. When newborns are hungry, hot, hurt, or otherwise uncomfortable, they experience stress. They react by crying and vigorously moving their arms or legs. Their reaction to all uncomfortable stimuli is the same.

Infants' crying and moving behavior cue the caring person, usually the parent, to act. If the action relieves stress, infants begin to associate that person with relief and to see that person as good. Because infants cannot separate themselves from their environments, they also see themselves as good. This is the beginning of the self-concept.

At one time it was thought that infants were totally dependent. They were simply receivers of stimuli. Now it is known that children are born with certain temperaments. These temperaments influence the infants' environments. Research has shown that infants can and do affect child-parent relationships. Dr. Berry Brazelton was the pioneer in recognizing the individuality of infants and their ability to influence their environment. Infants' reactions to parental attention may actually help to generate inadequate or inconsistent parenting patterns. A temperament leading to poor parenting can quickly initiate a cycle of maladaptive behaviors on the part of the parent and child. This may lead to poor self-concept and a mistrust of the environment.

The developmental task identified for the infant by Erikson is the learning of trust. As mentioned previously, experience with the caring person is the basis for developing trust. As children grow and learn to differentiate themselves from the environment and meet new challenges, trust becomes very important. Children must trust enough to feel comfortable in new situations, and they must still trust others to meet their needs.

Failure to Thrive. Anxiety is manifested in the infant by sleep and feeding problems and excessive crying. Extreme stress may develop into a condition called **failure to thrive** in which the infant fails to gain weight. There are some physical reasons that infants do not gain weight, and these should be ruled out first by the physician. The term *failure to thrive*, however, is frequently used to identify infants who fail to grow and develop when there is no physical cause. If not reversed, this condition can lead to death. It is estimated that 50 percent of infants who fail to thrive do so because of poor family relationships.

Parents may feel inadequate. They may not react to the infant because the infant's responses do not meet with parent expectations, or they may simply lack knowledge of the child's psychosocial needs. Nurses may find it necessary to make the parents aware of the need to hold and talk to their infants. It is important to promptly and consistently meet infants' needs.

Separation Anxiety. Separation anxiety is the feeling the child has when separated from a familiar face. It usually occurs around the sixth month and extends into the toddler years. The child experiences feelings of distress and responds by screaming. He or she may withdraw or refuse to eat. There may be sleep disturbances. If the separation is short, no permanent damage results, but if separation continues, the child may become depressed. He or she may regress to an earlier stage of development or may even fail to thrive.

When parent and child are reunited, the child may act as if the parent were a stranger. The child seems not to trust any longer. It is for this reason that parents are encouraged to remain with their hospitalized infants. Separation anxiety seems to occur less in infants who have had several care-givers.

Toddler (Eighteen Months to Three Years)

Young toddlers have long trunks and short legs. Because their brains are three-quarters the size of the adult brain, they are top heavy, and their weak abdominal muscles give them a potbellied look. As each year passes, children's legs grow longer. Their muscles grow stronger, and they begin to take on the trimmer, childlike appearance.

Toddlers are self-centered and possessive. They cannot share toys with which they are playing, but older toddlers may, primarily to please a parent, pick out another toy and offer it. Children in this group have short attention spans, and they want everything immediately. They are easily frustrated if they do not get their way.

Erikson calls this period the *stage of autonomy versus shame and doubt.* **Autonomy** is characterized by independence in some activities of daily living such as moving, feeding self, and partially dressing and undressing. The establishment of bowel control is also a measure of autonomy. Children's frequent use of the word *no* is another measure of autonomy. As they learn that they have some control over the environment, their negativism is their way of challenging authority and determining their own limits. Toddlers also engage in rituals that must be strictly adhered to. This ritualistic behavior provides some predictability and security to their changing lives.

A sense of identity is gradually emerging during this time. Toddlers see themselves as independent individuals. As motor skills develop, they begin to realize they can function with some autonomy. Though toddlers enjoy their independence, they couple the enjoyment with a fear of giving up dependence. They are constantly struggling with when to let go and when to hold on. Toddlers often dawdle because they want to please their parents, but at the same time they want to assert themselves. Sometimes this dependence is transferred to objects like pillows, blankets, or dolls. Because these objects are movable and can be carried around by children, they fit better into their growing world (Figure 3-2).

As mobility and curiosity increase, children need new stimuli to prevent boredom. For this reason, toddlers often get into dangerous situations. It is important that parents give toddlers some freedom, but it is also critical that consistent and realistic restrictions be placed on the children. It is through these restrictions that children learn the boundaries of safety and acceptable behavior. Self-doubt is more apt to occur when children do not have these parental controls. Frequent criticism and constant disapproval, however, often lead to shame. Consistency is important. Toddlers engage in rituals and routines to provide their own consistent environment.

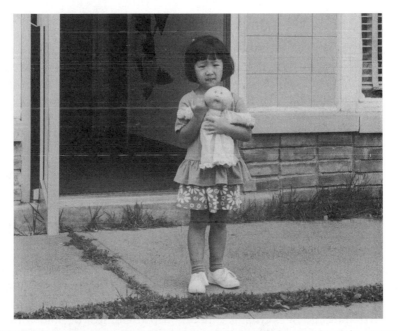

FIGURE 3-2 This toddler clings to a doll as she learns to gain some independence in her widening world.

Fears. As children grow, they are confronted with increasing challenges, and new challenges lead to fears. Each age group has its particular fears. For toddlers, darkness can be frightening. Parental support and understanding, along with a security blanket, are needed. Nightlights can also help alleviate this fear.

Stranger anxiety is a continuation of separation anxiety seen in younger children. Toddlers usually react in more subtle ways by clinging to the parent and refusing to cooperate. When parents are going away, they need to provide a consistent substitute or nurse who will use supportive behaviors with children. The parent substitute or nurse who is a stranger needs to recognize this fear and approach the child slowly, smiling and speaking softly. The use of toys also helps to alleviate some of the anxiety. In fact, play therapy is the best way of communicating with the child. It is advantageous to have the parent remain as long as possible.

Sibling rivalry also creates anxiety in toddlers. Children are not accustomed to sharing their parents with anyone else; therefore, they may feel they have lost their parents' love or that the new child is taking their place. They may regress to the infant's level of behavior in an attempt to regain their parents' love. They may also react with anger and aggression toward the "intruder." Toddlers are capable of real harm if the situation is not recognized and dealt with.

A new infant can easily take all of the parents' time, and the toddler just seems to get in the way. The stress the toddler feels at being pushed aside can be diminished if the parents find some special time just for him or her. There are things the young child can do to help with the infant's care, and he or she should be encouraged to participate according to ability. Frequent references to "our baby" may also help in making the toddler feel that he or she is still a part of the family.

Preschool (Three to Six Years)

Erikson terms the preschool period *initiative versus guilt*. Since preschoolers have achieved some autonomy and mastered the ability to ambulate, they are ready to meet the new challenges in their ever-widening sphere. Initiative is needed for further exploration of the environment. Preschoolers have a consuming curiosity and question everything incessantly. They run, jump, and climb, always exploring the limits of their world. The restrictions that the parent or caring person places on the child, however, continue to be important. Without restrictions, the child is unable to develop a sense of right and wrong. At first, the child does what is expected because of fear of punishment. The rules are eventually internalized and become values. The values then develop into what is commonly called a **conscience**. Too much restriction, though, may result in the child's fear of further exploration and of trying new experiences. This child is unable to successfully accomplish the developmental task of initiative and experiences guilt in normal activities and interpersonal relationships. For this reason, it is important that the child be allowed to explore within limits of safety. It is also important that initiative be encouraged and questions answered simply and truthfully so that growth will continue.

At the age of three, the child begins to socialize. At the first the child plays next to other children and later with them. Play is important to the preschooler. It relieves anxiety, stimulates cognition and imagination, and increases motor skills.

Aggressive behavior is common. Children enjoy roughhouse play with parents or friends, and they may be destructive to their own toys. With consistent and firm limits, along with parental support and understanding, children will learn to control their behavior.

Sometime during this stage, children begin to fantasize about the future (Figure 3-3). These daydreams may eventually lead to the choice of adult roles. Preschoolers may also have frightening nightmares

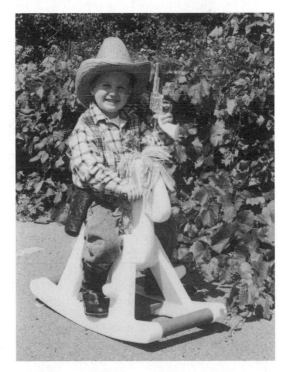

FIGURE 3-3 This preschool child enjoys dressing up as a cowboy and pretending he is riding his horse.

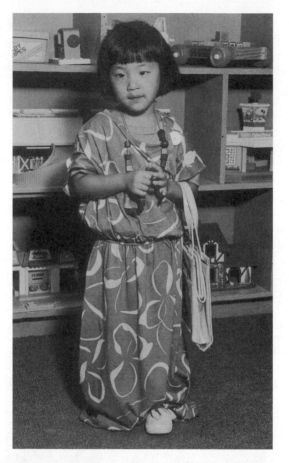

FIGURE 3-4 This preschooler enjoys dressing up as her mother.

because their imaginations are so vivid. During periods of semisleep, before they wake completely, children may see monsters in their dreams. They then need reassurance and comforting from their parents. A night-light may also help. Preschoolers enjoy participating in adult activities and should be given simple responsibilities. They also enjoy mimicking adults and may be seen dressing up or talking like their parents (Figure 3-4). Some significant relationships with other adults may develop.

Enuresis. **Enuresis** is the involuntary wetting of the bed or clothes after the child has been toilet trained. It is a condition seen in the preschooler and young school-age child. There are physical reasons, but sometimes bed-wetting can be attributed solely to stress. The exact cause needs to be determined. The preferred treatment is behavior modification and sometimes medication on a short-term basis.

School Age (Six to Twelve Years)

School is important for the cognitive processes of thought, reasoning, comprehension, and memory development. Because of the length of time children spend in school, it has a great impact on their personalities as well. It is in school that children continue growth toward independence and rely more on teachers and peers than on parents. Through their teachers and primarily their friends, children have an opportunity to test and modify their ideas, feelings, and behaviors. Relating to friends helps children learn to cooperate, compromise, and compete.

At first, friendship associations are informal and loosely structured; eventually, they become more organized. Same-sex clubs and secret societies evolve, and some very good and lasting friendships develop (Figure 3-5). Same-sex friends discuss parental relationships and problems with siblings, thus providing support for each other. They also validate each other's goals and desires.

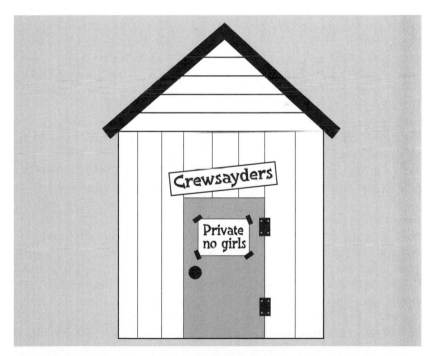

FIGURE 3-5 School-age children enjoy secret clubs involving the same sex.

According to Erikson, this is the stage of *industry versus inferiority*. If children receive recognition for work well done and are accepted by their peers, the children's self-concepts are enhanced. If they fail, children begin to feel inferior.

Normally young school-age children enjoy learning. They apply themselves to the accomplishment of intellectual and motor skills and receive satisfaction from their successes. If they fail to achieve a sense of industry, resulting in feelings of inferiority, children may then continue to be reluctant to try new tasks as they grow to adulthood.

Parents need to encourage their children's intellectual pursuits and praise their accomplishments. Because school-age children will try to meet them, parental expectations need to be realistic. Assigning children to do simple chores around the house not only teaches skill but also helps children develop a sense of responsibility as a family member. By giving their children allowances, parents help them learn judgment and money management.

Children continue to need limits set by parents, as well as punishment for infractions of the rules. Discipline needs to be consistent and appropriate to the situation and age of the children. There also needs to be follow-through. For example, children are given five-minute time-outs, a behavior-modification technique in which the children are removed from the possibility of getting attention. This action will be effective only if children actually stay the entire five minutes. School-age children often try to escape discipline.

Sibling rivalry may still exist, especially in young school-age children. Normally it becomes less intense as children grow and eventually disappears. Although siblings fight among themselves, they will often join together against an outside threat. Sometimes sibling rivalry remains unresolved. It can then continue throughout the life cycle, resulting in increased stress.

For children who have not attended nursery school, entry into school can represent the first prolonged absence from the security of the family. Children who have not developed trust, autonomy, and initiative in earlier stages can become fearful about attending school.

A fear becomes important when it is severe and persistent and when it interferes with the child's ability to function effectively. School phobia is a fairly common problem in the school-age child. The child who suffers from this phobia is often intelligent and achievement oriented but refuses to go to school. The child may give many excuses, present various physical complaints, and display anxiety.

School phobia occurs more often in the first five grades, but it also is seen in the adolescent. The phobia may result from traumatic experiences at school, a long illness, or academic failure, but the most frequent cause is thought to be separation anxiety. Many phobic children are immature and excessively dependent. They frequently have overprotective parents.

Encopresis. Encopresis is the inability to control bowel movements in a child who has previously gained control. Involuntary stooling may be due to chronic constipation, but most often it has an emotional cause. Generally the child is reacting to some type of stress such as felt rejection by a parent. The condition causes further stress because the child is unable to hide the problem from friends and classmates. He or she will certainly be ridiculed and teased unmercifully. The problem must be recognized and dealt with immediately. Because the child's inability to control his or her bowels causes embarrassment to the parents as well, they may not seek professional help. They may verbally chastise or even beat the child as a punishment. This only adds to his stress and increases the problem. The treatment of choice is behavior modification (see Chapter 4).

Adolescence (Twelve to Eighteen Years)

The goal of adolescence is the attainment of adult stature, privileges, and responsibilities. This means that adolescents must learn to give up their dependence and accept a more independent role. They have to provide for their own basic needs, select and prepare for a career, decide on a permanent lifestyle, and establish their own identities.

Adolescence is a period of vast changes. Teenagers must forge new biological and social roles while coping with strange new feelings and a widening cognitive sphere. The fact that everything seems to be changing at once increases adolescents' chances of experiencing stress. The growth spurt, coupled with secondary sex characteristics, often makes the teens feel awkward and self-conscious. Their bodies look, act, and feel differently. Moods change rapidly. One minute adolescents are up and the very next down. Boredom is prevalent. Young adolescents can be seen wandering aimlessly with their same-sex friends because they can think of nothing exciting to do. Because they are bored, because it represents a challenge, or simply to test their limits, teenagers may damage property, steal, or break other community rules.

Teens, especially young teens, are introspective and spend much time daydreaming. Their thoughts and ideas are then shared with friends. Because teenagers are trying to break away from dependence on the family, peers are used to clarify the adolescents' worth, their relationships with others, and their place in the world. Parental values that the child has internalized and previously followed are challenged. Values are individual rules that govern behavior. They form the basis for making life's decisions. Personal values are developed by comparing parental and social standards with one's own beliefs. Value clarification is a developmental task of adolescents. They test their beliefs and parental standards by screening them through peers.

The peer group is extremely important to young adolescents. Being different is the predominant fear. Teens dress, talk, and behave like their friends. Both boys and girls spend hours in front of the mirror to make their appearances acceptable. They are very choosy about clothing. Skin problems such as acne are a major embarrassment. Under the influence of peers, some teens may give up family religious beliefs, while others change church affiliations. Others may choose lifestyles objectionable to parents. In late adolescence, the identity emerges. Teens are clearer about their beliefs. They no longer are quite as dependent on the peer group as they were and have established their own individuality. Although parental values are questioned and even temporarily discarded, most children eventually incorporate many of the old values into their adult lives.

Erikson has assigned the task of *establishing identity* to this age group (Figure 3-6). Part of identity development centers around teens learning to relate to the opposite sex. If teenagers are unable to establish an identity, they will feel self-conscious and have many doubts about themselves and their roles. Although the shift away from the family is accelerated during this time, adolescents still need parental controls, which provide some security to teens' otherwise unstable world. Too much parental control, however, can stifle identity formation.

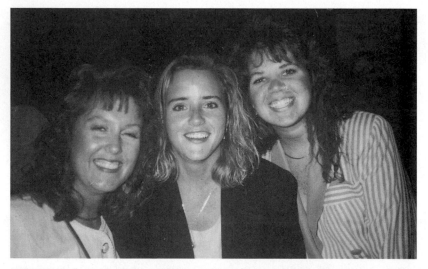

FIGURE 3-6 Part of an adolescent's search for identity can include involvement in a peer group. (Courtesy of Suzanne Fronk)

Adolescence is a stormy time for parents as well as for children. Teenagers may resent demands made by parents and refuse to accept their advice. At the same time, teens still expect the parents to pay the bills, feed them, and do their laundry. They want the privileges of adulthood, but not the responsibilities. Adolescents coin new words unfamiliar to the parents. This tends to interfere with the effectiveness of communication (see Chapter 8).

Parents fear the dangers and temptations adolescents may face such as accidents, alcohol, drugs, and early pregnancy. They are fearful of entrusting adolescents to their own judgment and want to protect them. Parents may be frightened because they see this as a test on the effectiveness of parenting. If teens succumb to one of the temptations, it may be interpreted by parents to mean that they have failed. Parents may also see this time as the last chance to influence their children's lives. In desperation, they push more demands and insist on obedience. Teens, feeling overwhelmed, may retaliate. Rather than changing the adolescents' behavior, parental demands tend to increase the rift.

Contrary to popular opinion, the rift only *seems* to be great. As the child grows to adulthood, it becomes evident that the distance between parent and child was, in most families, only superficial. Parents and children have disagreements, but they primarily disagree over things such as the use of the telephone and the car, curfews, appearance, and loud music.

Teens enjoy the music and, in fact, do not seem to be able to get along without it. They usually have the stereo blaring continuously. When out of the house, many teens can be seen with portable stereos. Television, movies, the VCR, computer games and video games are popular forms of entertainment. Teens particularly like adventure stories and stories of conflicts between generations.

Teens have a need for intimacy, which involves sharing confidences with friends. This sharing is often done on the telephone, with the child actually tying up the phone for hours (Figure 3-7). This is one of the points of contention between parent and child, but the parent must realize that the telephone is an important part of the child's growth process. This is true for three reasons: (1) talking on the phone takes up time and so lessens boredom; (2) things are constantly changing in the teen's life, and the need to share with friends is felt as urgent; and (3) the adolescent finds talking on the phone easier because the distance between the parties provides some safety when sharing intimacies.

Early and Late Maturing. Early and late maturing can cause stress for the teen. The adolescent whose body changes occur much earlier or much later than those of his or her peers is placed in the position of being different at the very time when differences are intolerable.

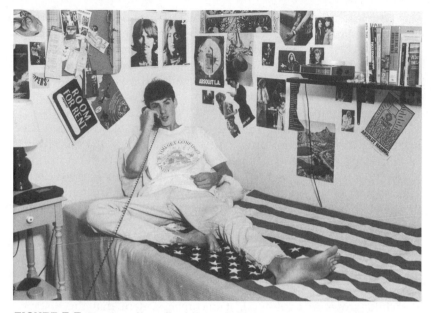

FIGURE 3-7 Teens often find it easier to talk on the telephone.

Early maturing girls may be given prestige by their classmates, but they also experience some difficulties. They usually associate with older teens who share their physical maturation. Unfortunately, they do not share the same interest or the same level of judgment as do their older friends. Adults seem to expect the early maturing girl to act more mature, which may frustrate her. She feels awkward dating prepubescent boys her own age, but she may find herself over her head if she dates older ones.

Early maturing boys seem to have the easiest time. They tend to be good at athletics and thus have the respect of both boys and girls. They tend to take leadership roles and retain them. Adults give them more freedom and responsibility.

Late maturing girls may be anxious about when their body changes will occur, but they often do not feel the stress that early maturing girls do. When puberty occurs, late maturing girls are more intellectually and emotionally ready for it.

The child that seems to suffer the most is the late maturing boy. He has to watch his classmates, both male and female, pass by him in height and maturation. His small stature and high-pitched voice can become the object of ridicule and teasing. Because of his size, he is unable to successfully compete in contact sports with his larger age-mates. Undressing in the locker room is often a source of great embarrassment for him. Many young boys are acutely concerned about their failure to develop and worry that something is drastically wrong with them. Both boys and girls need knowledge concerning puberty. They need to know that the time the changes occur has little effect on the degree of maturation. They also need to know that the normal age range for puberty is wide.

Young Adult (Eighteen to Thirty-Five Years)

Young adults continue the tasks of adolescence. They further clarify their values, continue to establish their identities, and choose lifestyles.

Intimacy is the main developmental task of this age group. If the person fails to establish close and sharing relationships, isolation results. Singles groups, computer dating services, and personal advertisements in newspapers attest to the fact that intimacy is not easily accomplished.

Many young adults postpone marriage and other responsibilities by continuing their schooling. Others combine college and marriage or a committed relationship. Still others enter the world of work following high school. Each has its own stressors.

The college student copes with studying for long hours, writing papers, meeting assignment deadlines, and passing exams (Figure 3-8). There is often little time or money to pursue special interests.

Marriage means a change in ideals, behaviors, and aspirations. Working requires finding a satisfactory job that provides status and

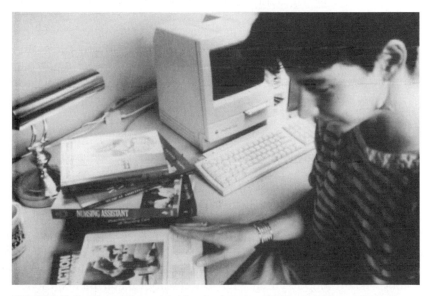

FIGURE 3-8 The college student copes with long hours of study.

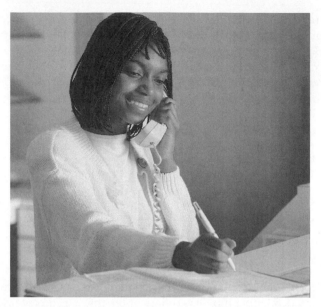

FIGURE 3-9 Working requires finding a satisfactory job that provides status and economic security.

economic security (Figure 3-9). This is often a difficult task that requires much effort on the part of young adults. They may change their minds several times and take many jobs before actually deciding on a career. If young adults have accomplished the developmental tasks of earlier stages, gained self-awareness and a good self-image, learned problem-solving techniques, established good interpersonal relationships, and taken the time to explore, they will find rewarding careers. Unfortunately, some adults spend their entire working lives in jobs that provide little satisfaction.

Middle Adult (Thirty-five to Sixty-five Years)

Erikson calls middle adult the stage of *generativity versus stagnation*. Society puts the greatest demands on middle-age adults. They are expected to be highly productive and financially secure. Many people at this age take time to assess their accomplishments. If they see them as worthwhile and productive and themselves as having improved life for future generations, they have successfully accomplished the developmental task. The task includes having a positive influence on children. Because of a rapidly changing society, more middle-age adults are finding their lives unworthwhile and have the feeling that they are stagnating. As a result, they may find it necessary to alter their lifestyles, marriage partners, or occupations.

Many physical changes occur during this period. Receding or graying hair begins to appear and eyesight becomes impaired. Metabolism slows, which results in weight gain if the diet remains the same. Menopause is another change with which the middle-age woman must cope. The change in hormonal levels sometimes results in hot and cold sensations, insomnia, mood swings, and anxiety symptoms.

This is also generally the time when children leave the home. Parents who have devoted themselves almost entirely to the children may find themselves alone and feeling useless. This can, however, be a time of freedom and creativity—a time to do things of interest that could not be done before because of family responsibilities (Figure 3-10).

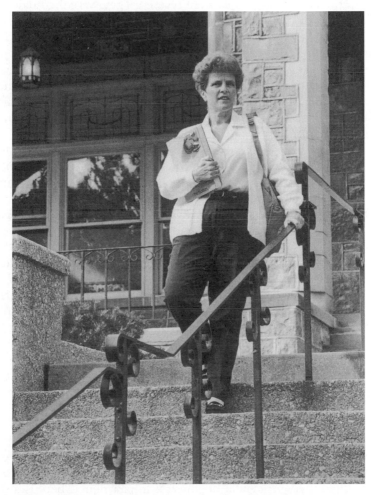

FIGURE 3-10 Many middle-age adults use their newly found free time to return to school.

Senescence (Sixty-five Years to Death)

Old age is arbitrarily set at sixty-five, the age of retirement. The people in this group are far less homogeneous than they were at any other time. Development depends on how well the individual has accomplished the tasks in earlier ages. There is also a vast difference between the young old (sixty-five to seventy-five) and the old old. The young old are more aligned with the middle adult, while the old old experience most of the losses attributed to this group. Special consideration must be given to cultural influences (African-American, Asian-American, Hispanic, and Native American) that affect one's perceptions and attitudes toward aging.

In the past, older people were revered. They were the holders of vast amounts of knowledge and the teachers of the young. Their advice was sought after and used by younger generations. In recent society, however, technological changes occurred so rapidly that the older person's knowledge and skills quickly became obsolete. Their values were no longer appreciated, and the computer has proved to be a more effective holder of information than the human brain. Although this is beginning to change, once a person has retired, he or she is seen by society as nonproductive and dependent.

Recently, though, there has been an increased interest in the feelings and needs of the aged. The term **senior citizen** was coined in an attempt to afford some status to them. In reality, it had little immediate effect. Nevertheless, things are now changing in both society in general and in the health care field. There are several lay and professional journals on the subject of aging. More books are appearing in the library, and senior citizen groups are visibly campaigning for their rights. There is an increased interest in geriatrics as a special field in both nursing, general medicine, and psychiatry.

Some people reach their prime in old age and enjoy this period of life. This is especially true if they have prepared for it by developing hobbies or special interests in earlier years. They then look forward to taking it easy. They no longer have to compete or engage in the day-to-day drudgery of some jobs. They are free to pursue their special interests, to think, and to take stock. Erikson says this is the time when people review their lives, accept their successes and failures, arrange matters, and get their lives in order.

Each age group has its stressors, but few suffer losses to the degree seen in old age. These losses make it more difficult to attain integrity, and despair may result. There is a drop in income, loss of useful employment, death of friends and family, and, because of chronic illness, there may be mental or physical impairment. There is also a change in the body image and a loss of independence to some degree.

The older person experiences changes in hearing and vision. Muscles become weaker and reaction time is slower. Even if the person does not have a chronic illness, it may still be more difficult to climb stairs, dress, maneuver on icy streets, get in and out of the tub, or drive a car. Even those who do not have debilitating chronic diseases may not be totally independent.

Retired people, including those capable of working, commonly find obstacles to obtaining employment. Although there are some older people who are rich and others who have adequate retirement incomes, some of the aged still live on incomes lower than poverty level. These people find themselves dependent on charity or their families for financial support.

Often individuals' identities are tied to their occupations. Retirement can then lead to a loss of identity. Retirement also can mean a loss of friends and associations, which leads to loneliness. Grief is another stress with which the older person must deal. The danger of death exists at any age, but the time element makes it more relevant for the older person. The death of a spouse or friends can lead to further isolation and loneliness.

Despite the obstacles, many aged are able to complete the developmental tasks identified by Erikson and to enjoy this period of life. They keep busy by volunteering for community service (Figure 3-11),

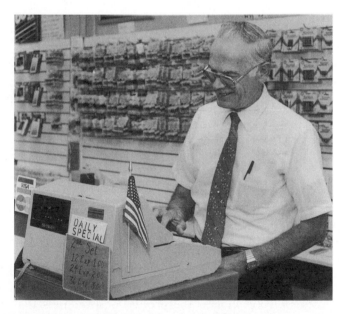

FIGURE 3-11 This senior citizen volunteers his time in a charitable thrift store.

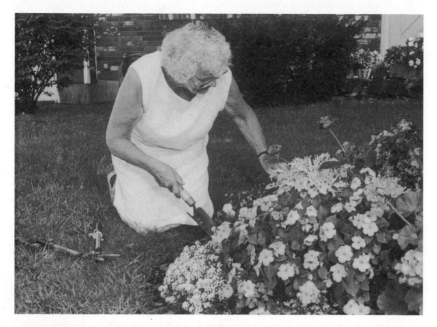

FIGURE 3-12 The older person may find some relaxing and enjoyable activity.

becoming foster grandparents, or offering their services as retired consultants. Many just enjoy relaxing and engaging in activities of special interest (Figure 3-12). Places or services such as retirement villages, senior citizen centers, day care for the aged, home-delivered meals, and homemaker home health aide services have helped the aged to overcome many stressors and to live the remaining years of their lives in comfort and dignity.

MASLOW'S HIERARCHY OF NEEDS

The ability to see things as they really are is probably the most difficult aspect of understanding others. Needs, beliefs, knowledge, and anxiety affect perception.

Stimuli in the environment are constantly bombarding the body. Since the brain cannot handle all of the stimuli, perception is a selective process. Only the strongest stimuli reach the brain, where they are interpreted in terms of past experiences, immediate needs, knowledge, and self-concept. Perception is the process of awareness that occurs between stimulus intake and thought. The way we perceive influences the impact of the stressors.

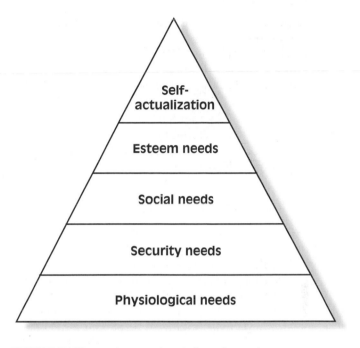

FIGURE 3-13 Maslow's Hierarchy of Needs.

Immediate needs are probably the most significant influence on perception. Abraham Maslow developed a theory of **motivation** based on needs (Figure 3-13). Maslow arranged needs in a hierarchy from basic physiological needs to self-actualizing needs. Satisfying the basic physical needs is necessary for survival. These basic needs include oxygen, fluids, food, and rest. Society does a fairly good job of helping people to meet basic needs, so their power as motivators is lessened.

Safety and security needs relate to protection. These needs include shelter, stability, and freedom from undue anxiety. If these needs are not met, the person experiences fear, panic, and physical danger. According to Maslow these lower needs must be met at least in part before the person can progress to the next higher level.

Loneliness and isolation are the result if the third need, that of love and belonging, is not met. This need is extremely important for mental health and seems to be more difficult to meet in a technological society. The need for esteem is dependent on feelings of being worthwhile. Meeting this need improves the self-concept. Failure to meet it leads to a lack of self-confidence.

The highest level of the hierarchy is that of **self-actualization**. Besides having the characteristics of the mentally healthy person, the self-actualizing person is confident, feels self-fulfilled, and sees beauty and harmony in even small things.

According to Maslow, the individual must meet the dominant lower needs, called *deficiency* needs, before attention can be paid to the higher, or *becoming*, needs. Progression does not occur at a steady rate. People may remain at one level for varying lengths of time, they may revert to a lower level, or they may simply remain at a particular level and never progress further. Collecting information about a client using the Maslow framework can provide pertinent data for enhancement or revision of the treatment plan.

DEFENSE MECHANISMS

Defense mechanisms are learned patterns of behavior. Freud believed they were used by all people to a certain extent. The defense mechanisms basically identified by Freud were once thought to be healthy ways of relieving stress. They were considered to be ways of avoiding failure and salvaging self-respect.

Although defense mechanisms are used by most people, humanistic psychologists do not believe they are essential to mental health. In fact, they are now seen as actually inhibiting personality growth. Since they interfere with awareness, defense mechanisms are a means of avoiding rather than solving problems. They help to temporarily avoid but do not change threatening conditions. Many mechanisms are costly in terms of adaptive energy. They may lead to less-than-desirable behavioral patterns, such as becoming class clown to gain recognition.

Defense mechanisms are either subconscious or unconscious. They are difficult to categorize because they are not clear-cut. It is not the behavior but the motive behind the behavior that distinguishes one mechanism from another. Common defense mechanisms include rationalization, repression, compensation, displacement, projection, conversion, regression, sublimation, identification, and reaction formation.

Rationalization

In rationalization, individuals deny their real thoughts and excuse their actions by presenting false but seemingly more acceptable reasons for behavior. Rationalization helps to save face when one feels guilty about an action or behavior. It is much easier to say "No one could get along with that client" than to accept responsibility by saying "I am not able to get along with that client." After failing a course, a student finds it more acceptable to say "I did not want to be a nurse anyway" rather than saying "I did not study and now I have given up my chance to be a nurse." Rationalization is not lying. The truth is repressed and the real motive is unconscious.

Repression

Repression is an involuntary exclusion of experiences or desires from awareness. The experience is forgotten, but it remains at the unconscious level and influences behavior. The repressed experience usually causes anxiety, but it may also result in physical defects and obsessions. Repression is different from suppression in that repression is on the unconscious level. A person who has experienced sexual trauma in childhood represses the painful memory.

Suppression

Suppressed experiences are at the conscious level and are more readily available to awareness. They are intentionally excluded from awareness since they are painful thoughts and desires. "I do not want to think about having a seizure disorder; I will think about it some other time."

Compensation

When a person uses extra energy to overcome a real or imagined defect, the person is compensating. For example, the student who feels unpopular may devote more time to achieving good grades. The neighborhood bully may be compensating for feelings of inferiority.

Displacement

Releasing pent-up feelings on a person or object that is less threatening than the person or object that caused the feeling is known as *displacement*. For example, a student may fear punishment if anger is displayed toward an instructor. To avoid a lower grade or some other form of discipline, the student vents the anger on an aide. The student has unconsciously substituted the aide for the teacher.

Projection

Blaming personal shortcomings on someone else is called *projection*. The student who is late explains that " My roommate was not ready." The truth is that the student started late. A student misses a question on a test and explains the mistake with "It was a trick question." Projection is transferring responsibility for unacceptable ideas, wishes, or thoughts to another. Projection is used more often by persons with mental illness than the healthy person.

Conversion Reaction

The term *conversion reaction* is used when an emotional conflict is repressed and appears as a physical symptom that has no physical cause. A person who has seen something overwhelming may repress it and then develop blindness. Another person may be unable to talk, while still another may become paralyzed. The internal conflict often relates to the physical disability, but not always.

Regression

When a person returns to an earlier pattern of behavior, he or she is regressing. It occurs when the person's usual means of coping have not been successful. The earlier behavior represents a time that was more secure.

Reaction Formation

Reaction formation is a defense mechanism through which a person acts in a way opposite of how he or she feels. The person is unable to cope with his or her real feelings because they are socially unacceptable. An employee who greatly dislikes his boss is extremely polite to his boss.

Sublimation

Substituting a socially acceptable behavior for behavior that is not socially acceptable is called *sublimation*. A person who is unmarried but desires to be a mother (or father) may sublimate by becoming a worker in a day-care center.

Identification

Consciously or unconsciously imitating the characteristics of another person is called *identification*. Identification is thought by psychoanalysts to be an important mechanism. They believe it is part of the personality development of children. It is also a way for adults to obtain satisfaction by participating in the success of people with whom they identify. Consciously internalizing the values and behaviors of an admired person is more growth producing than using identification as a defense mechanism.

As noted, it is not the behavior but the motive behind the behavior that distinguishes one defense mechanism from another (Table 3-4).

TABLE 3-4 Common Defense Mechanisms

DEFENSE MECHANISMS	DEFENSE EXAMPLE	POSSIBLE MEANING
Rationalization	"I am going to die of something anyway, so why quit smoking?"	"I am addicted to smoking and unable to quit."
Compensation	"I do not have time for dates. I am too busy with my ceramics."	"No one likes me enough to ask me out, but I can still feel important by excelling in art."
Displacement	"How many times have I told you to keep that bike out of the driveway?"	"The boss was really upset with me today."
Projection	"It is all your fault that I did not win the contest."	"I cannot accept that I am not the best, so my loss must be your fault."
Repression	"I cannot seem to remember my supervisor's name."	"I find my supervisor attractive. This feeling is unacceptable to me so my supervisor is blocked from my conscious level of thought."
Conversion reaction	"I am blind. I just suddenly went blind. The doctors cannot find out why."	"No one will know why, either. What I saw is so horrible I cannot even think about it."
Regression	"Since Jenny has been sick, she constantly cries for her mother."	"When Jenny was younger, things were more secure. She had her parents to take care of her and help when things went wrong."
Identification	"I have decided which shirt I want you to buy me. It is that one."	"That shirt is just like Uncle Joe's. I really admire Uncle Joe and want to be just like him."
Suppression	"I am really sorry I forgot. Now that you mention it, I do recall."	"I wish she had not reminded me. I really did not want to remember that."

(Continues)

TABLE 3-4 (Continued)

DEFENSE MECHANISMS	DEFENSE EXAMPLE	POSSIBLE MEANING
Sublimation	"I really love children, but I am not ready for marriage. I will get a job working with children in a day-care center."	"Working with children in a day-care center protects my ego because it is a more acceptable way for me to fulfill my desire of working with children than having my own children without being married."
Reaction formation	"Bill, I am going to pay your way to college. After all, you are my brother and I love you."	"You had everything. Mom and Dad loved you most. I got blamed for every-thing you did. I really hate you, but you are my brother, so I cannot hate you."

Defense mechanisms used for a short period of time can be helpful if the problem is dealt with and the outcome is effective. However, the nurse may note the client is excessively using defense mechanisms. When the client is calm and quiet, the nurse can approach a discussion with the client, noting his/her observable responses (defense mechanisms) and educating the client about defense mechanisms masking internal anxieties that contribute to conflict and stress.

SELF-AWARENESS

Self-awareness involves noticing how the self feels, thinks, behaves, and senses at any given time. It is only through awareness of how the self blocks messages and uses defense mechanisms that people can achieve self-understanding. Self-awareness differs from introspection in that awareness is simply observation of the way the self reacts. Introspection usually involves evaluation, or determining why the self reacts as it does. Awareness is a constant process, whereas introspection is an intermittent one.

Awareness is a way of focusing attention on the present, thereby strengthening the impact of life experiences. It is always available and, with practice, can be used successfully to enrich life. Awareness is not only the key to self-understanding, it is also the key to fullness of living. It is the first step in coping with stress. Fullness of living comes from the richness of experience. The more aware one is, the deeper one can experience feelings such as joy and pleasure.

People function at various levels of self-awareness. Those at low levels are not fully experiencing life. Awareness focuses on the present. It is only in the present that changes can be made and actions modified. Individuals without awareness are more apt to be governed by fears, anxieties and poor self-concepts. The nurse who is unaware is likely to make decisions in response to his or her own needs rather than the needs of clients. With self-awareness, behavior can be accepted or modified. For instance, many students are anxious about taking examinations. Anxiety is a vague feeling of impending danger. As long as the anxiety remains vague, little can be done to control it. With awareness, the anxiety becomes more concrete. Instead of vague feelings, the student is aware of tense muscles, a squeaky voice, and mild nausea. These are concrete symptoms that can be controlled. Students owe it to themselves and their clients to increase their self-awareness. They will find a fuller life in the process.

Improving Self-Awareness

Improving self-awareness requires concentration and practice. The following suggested guidelines can be used to develop self-awareness. Awareness should never be forced; it should simply be allowed to flow. Instant results should not be expected, because growth requires time.

1. Periodically stop and concentrate on what your body is feeling at the moment. At first, concentrate only on what the body senses. Later, include environmental awareness as well. Tell yourself what you are aware of.

2. Ask yourself what you are aware of when you are anxious, happy, joyous, frustrated. Concentrating on the bodily sensations that accompany these feelings will make them more concrete and therefore manageable.

3. Listen to what you say and how you speak. Persons often phrase sentences to avoid awareness, particularly awareness of responsibility. When responsibility for behavior is excluded from awareness, a person loses control over that behavior and is then unable to change it.

   ■ A sentence such as "It is scary" is an attempt to give up ownership of an emotion. Changing the ownership from *it* to *I* helps to increase awareness that it is really *I* who is scared, not *it* that is scary. Ownership is accepted and the emotion becomes controllable.

■ "You make me angry" is another example of giving up ownership of an emotion. Changing ownership from *you* to *I* increases awareness of who is responsible for the anger (e.g., "I am angry with you"). When individuals accept responsibility for their own anger, they become aware that no one else can cause it. Only they have control. Only they own the emotion and can accept or change it.

■ People often explain their own feelings by using the second or third person (*you* or *they*). For example, a person may say "You feel as if you are alone and no one really cares." This is again giving up ownership.

■ Saying *cannot* is another way of eliminating responsibility for an action. They are sometimes legitimate but the majority are really *will nots*. Saying "I will not" helps the individuals become aware of the fact that they also have rights.

4. Clarify vague feelings of dislike by a process called *exaggeration*. If you do not like something and do not really know why, you may be able to determine what you do not like through exaggeration. Pretend the disliked object (whether it be a dress, a classmate, or a piece of furniture) is directly in front of you. Tell it how you feel as if it were really there. Each time you repeat the statement, exaggerate. Allow yourself to say whatever comes to mind. At the same time, try to concentrate on the feelings.

5. Another way of increasing awareness is to handle disturbing experiences of the past by bringing them into the present. Relate the experience as if it were happening in the present. At the same time, try to sense the experiences and sensations. This procedure can be used when past experiences continue to disturb you and you do not know why. (For more information, see Chapter 5.)

SELF-ACCEPTANCE

Self-acceptance is a regard for oneself with a realistic concept of strengths and weaknesses. Behaviors of the self-accepting person include the following:

■ Persevering

■ Minimizing weaknesses

- Seeing reality
- Trusting and accepting others
- Continuing growth toward self-actualization
- Recognizing and accepting one's own behavior
- Reaching out to others
- Increasing strengths
- Learning from mistakes

The person who is self-accepting accepts others more easily. Therefore, it is important that the nurse work toward self-acceptance. The self-rejecting person is critical of others, more anxious, insecure, and depressed.

Whether a person is self-accepting depends on the self-concept. Self-concept depends on how a person thinks he or she is viewed by others. Since all experiences are filtered through the self-concept, people tend to behave in ways that reinforce the self-concept. People respond to other people in terms of their behavior. This reinforces the self-concept, thereby creating a vicious circle. This is called a **self-fulfilling prophecy**. Since the self-concept really depends on others, individuals must interact with others to improve it. However, the individual must first be self-aware. Without self-awareness there is no improvement.

Even though self-concept depends to a great extent on others, there are some things individuals can do to improve their own self-concept. Simply focusing awareness on personal strengths increases them and thus enhances the self-concept. A good self-concept leads to self-acceptance. Practicing potential strengths develops them into actual strengths. A strength is any interest, ability, talent, or characteristic that enhances worth.

SUMMARY

Understanding how personality develops and the ability to recognize behavior and motives as they exist in reality are essential to the helping relationship. Personality depends on heredity, nurturing, and environment. A personality continues to change throughout life as it is affected by stressors or developmental tasks at each stage of the life cycle. Needs, beliefs, knowledge, and anxiety affect reality perception.

Abraham Maslow developed a theory of motivation based on need. He arranged needs into a hierarchy. The lower needs of the hierarchy must be met before the individual can meet the higher needs.

Many people use defense mechanisms to avoid stress. Freud thought defense mechanisms were normal ways of saving the self. However, humanistic psychologists now believe they interfere with personality growth.

Self-awareness involves noting how the self behaves, feels, thinks and senses at any given time. Self-awareness is the first step to self-understanding and can be learned. Nurses owe it to themselves and their clients to increase self-awareness through observing their needs, beliefs, anxieties, and developmental tasks and initiating a personal self-care plan.

SUGGESTED ACTIVITIES

- Visit a day-care center and observe the actions of the children at various age levels.
- List at least five things you like about yourself.
- Identify two personal weaknesses and develop a plan for strengthening them.
- Observe people around you. Try to detect defense mechanisms they may be using.
- Which defense mechanisms do you use most frequently? Under what circumstances do you use them?
- Practice the self-awareness exercises described in this chapter.
- Think about the self-actualizing people you have met. Discuss with classmates why you think they are self-actualizing.
- In small groups, discuss a defense mechanism, develop a scenario and role-play the situation for the class to identify the defense mechanism used.

REVIEW

KNOW AND COMPREHEND
A. Multiple choice. Select the one best answer.

1. Satisfaction of needs during infancy has which of the following consequences?
   - ❑ A. It significantly influences subsequent stages of personality development.
   - ❑ B. There is no relationship to the development of the individual's personality.
   - ❑ C. It establishes all traits of an individual's personality in adulthood.
   - ❑ D. Personalities of siblings will follow the same patterns.

2. The self-concept is defined as
   - ❑ A. how others see an individual.
   - ❑ B. being aware of one's feelings.
   - ❑ C. the true self.
   - ❑ D. how people see themselves.

3. According to Erikson, the developmental task of the infant is the acquiring of
   - ❑ A. integrity.
   - ❑ B. identity.
   - ❑ C. initiative.
   - ❑ D. trust.

4. Which of the following factors has the greatest impact on personality?
   - ❑ A. temperament and heredity
   - ❑ B. heredity and environment
   - ❑ C. self-understanding
   - ❑ D. environment and nurturing

5. The developmental stage identified by Erikson for the toddler is the acquiring of
   - ❑ A. trust.
   - ❑ B. autonomy.
   - ❑ C. initiative.
   - ❑ D. integrity.

6. One developmental task of the toddler is
   - ❑ A. developing a conscience.
   - ❑ B. relating to peer groups.
   - ❑ C. beginning to develop a self-concept.
   - ❑ D. controlling bowel movements.

7. One developmental task of the young adult is
   - ❑ A. establishing an intimate relationship.
   - ❑ B. achieving economic security.
   - ❑ C. clarifying values.
   - ❑ D. adjusting to decreased health.

8. The stage of industry involves which age group?
   - ❑ A. middle adult
   - ❑ B. school-age child
   - ❑ C. adolescent
   - ❑ D. young adult

9. If adolescents do not accomplish the development tasks identified by Erikson, they suffer
   - ❑ A. despair.
   - ❑ B. role diffusion.
   - ❑ C. loneliness.
   - ❑ D. inferiority.

10. Daydreams of superheros are common to which of the following age groups?
    - ❑ A. adolescents
    - ❑ B. preschoolers
    - ❑ C. school-age children
    - ❑ D. toddlers

11. The adolescent who has the most difficulty adjusting is the
    - ❑ A. early developing girl.
    - ❑ B. early developing boy.
    - ❑ C. late developing girl.
    - ❑ D. late developing boy.

12. The peer group is most important to which of the following age groups?
    - ❑ A. young adult
    - ❑ B. adolescent
    - ❑ C. middle adult
    - ❑ D. school-age child

13. A psychiatric technician shows up late to work for the third time in a row and is questioned by the nurse supervisor. Later, the supervisor overhears the technician yelling at another nurse. The technician's behavior is an example of
    - ❑ A. projection.
    - ❑ B. rationalization.
    - ❑ C. identification.
    - ❑ D. displacement.

14. An infant cries incessantly, fails to gain weight, and has alterations in sleeping and eating. Which of the following problems should the nurse suspect?
    - ❏ A. failure to thrive
    - ❏ B. malnutrition
    - ❏ C. infectious illness
    - ❏ D. separation anxiety

15. Regression in an infant is most likely a result of
    - ❏ A. failure to thrive.
    - ❏ B. infectious disease.
    - ❏ C. separation anxiety.
    - ❏ D. ineffective parenting.

16. Rituals are characteristic of which age group?
    - ❏ A. toddler
    - ❏ B. infant
    - ❏ C. preschooler
    - ❏ D. adolescent

17. The toddler's frequent use of the word *no* indicates the child
    - ❏ A. will continue to be disobedient.
    - ❏ B. is not receiving sufficient nurturing.
    - ❏ C. needs additional support from caregivers.
    - ❏ D is trying to gain control over the environment.

18. The most common fear of the toddler is
    - ❏ A. animals.
    - ❏ B. darkness.
    - ❏ C. monsters.
    - ❏ D. separation.

19. The most common fear of the preschooler is
    - ❏ A. animals.
    - ❏ B. darkness.
    - ❏ C. monsters.
    - ❏ D. separation.

APPLY YOUR LEARNING

B. Multiple choice. Select the one best answer.

1. A nurse has worked in a peer's shift for 3 weekends so that the peer could have time off for recreational activities. The peer says to the nurse, "I need you to work for me next weekend too." Choose an assertive response for the nurse to give to the coworker.

   ❏ A. "I understand that you have plans for the weekend, but I have plans also. Since I've already worked 3 weekends for you, please ask someone else."

   ❏ B. "I had made plans for the weekend but realize it's important to help you. Sure, I'll work next weekend for you."

   ❏ C. "You're always asking me to work for you. You need to ask somebody else."

   ❏ D. "Why do you keep asking me to work for you? Don't you think I have a social life?"

2. The nurse gathers data from a new client admitted with Generalized Anxiety Disorder. Which statement by the client would indicate the client uses passive behaviors in interpersonal relationships?

   ❏ A. "I've been making my sister do my housework for me. She doesn't have a job and might as well help me."

   ❏ B. "I always put my children's and spouse's needs first, but it really tires me out and it's hard to keep up with what they want."

   ❏ C. "I think I take good care of myself. I'm proud of my professional work and have a rewarding relationship with my friends."

   ❏ D. "I've got to take care of myself because nobody else is going to do it. I always say, 'give them an inch, and they'll take a mile.' "

3. Consider the following dialogue.

   Client–"You're late bringing my medicine to me. Why can't you get it to me on time?"

   Nurse–"Getting your medicine to you is important to me. I have it for you now."

   Client–"Yea, you've got it now but I want it at 9:00 A.M. on the dot."

   What response by the nurse should come next?

❏ A. "Don't you think I have other clients? Here's your medicine. Take it."
❏ B. "The medicine was late from the pharmacy. It's not my fault."
❏ C. "You can't get everything when you want it. I'm doing the best I can."
❏ D. "Again, getting your medicine to you is important to me. I have it for you now."

4. A client experiences panic. Which nurse below is using the most helpful intervention? The nurse who:
   ❏ A. assists the client to use problem-solving techniques.
   ❏ B. gives simple directions and maintains the client's safety.
   ❏ C. offers the client choices for how to reduce the anxiety.
   ❏ D. encourages the client to think through the problem.

5. A client tells the nurse, "My car needs $947 in repairs. I don't have that kind of money. I'm going to lose my job if I can't drive to work." Which of the following strategies would the nurse use first to help the client solve this problem?
   ❏ A. Help the client to more clearly identify and define the problem.
   ❏ B. Suggest alternative means of transportation to and from work.
   ❏ C. Ask the client about public transportation availability.
   ❏ D. Refer the client to social services for financial assistance.

6. Ten minutes before a class is scheduled to begin, a nursing student says to the instructor, "I need you to answer some questions for me about how to do this term paper." Which response by the instructor best illustrates assertiveness?
   ❏ A. "Can't you see I'm trying to get ready to start this class on time?"
   ❏ B. "If I help you now, our class won't start on time. I can see you after class."
   ❏ C. "Ask one of your classmates to help you with these questions."
   ❏ D. "Sure, I'll be glad to help you. What are your questions?"

7. After receiving a poor grade on a test, a nursing student says to a peer, "I got a bad grade because other students were tapping their feet and smacking chewing gum during the test. I just couldn't concentrate." Which response by the peer would be most helpful?
   ❏ A. Ask the instructor to make an announcement about maintaining silence during testing.
   ❏ B. Talk to other students in the class about the importance of silence during testing.
   ❏ C. Help the complaining student recognize anxiety and explore ways to alleviate it.
   ❏ D. The peer should not respond. The problem belongs to the complaining student.

C. **Match the theorist in column I with his theoretical goal in column II.**

Column I	**Column II**
1. Erikson	a. Security
2. Maslow	b. Self-actualization
3. Sullivan	c. Task accomplishment

D. **Briefly answer the following.**

1. Give three reasons for ineffective parenting.

2. Name three things the adolescent is probably missing in development if he or she develops a mental health problem.

Effective Communication

OUTLINE

KEY TERMS

communication

abstraction

perception

cliché

self-disclosure

positive regard

rapport

genuine

attentiveness

clarification

empathy

validation

reflection

OBJECTIVES

After studying this chapter, the student should be able to:

■ List three goals of effective communication.

■ Give three reasons why communication can be ineffective.

■ Explain three ways to improve listening skills.

■ Identify responses that block communication.

■ Identify at least five effective communication statements according to category.

■ Name five ways to show caring.

■ Pair at least ten verbal responses with caring behaviors.

■ Name at least two ways of developing trust.

■ Describe two effective communication techniques and give examples.

EFFECTIVE COMMUNICATION

Effective communication adds to the client's psychological comfort; therefore, it is as necessary to recovery as diet, medication, or other treatments. Clients who experience psychological discomfort are often noncompliant, use poor coping mechanisms, and have less-effective problem-solving skills. This results in actions that increase physical distress and complications and slow recovery.

Communication is usually thought of as an exchange of words. In reality, it includes all methods used to relay messages between persons, including gestures, body movements, and tone of voice. Communication that does not involve the spoken word is referred to as nonverbal.

A sender and a receiver are necessary for communication to occur. To be effective, the message must be understood by the receiver in the way that the sender intended. Unfortunately, ineffective communication can occur (Figure 4-1).

> - Senders may not send the message they thought they were sending
> - Receivers may not hear the message the sender intended
> - Verbal and nonverbal messages may conflict
> - The message may be disguised by the sender
> - Many English words have multiple meanings
> - The message may be abstract and therefore confusing
> - The receiver may be prepared to hear another message

FIGURE 4-1 Some reasons for ineffective communication.

FACTORS THAT ALTER EFFECTIVE COMMUNICATION

Disguised Messages

Because clients may not trust the nurse's reactions to their feelings, they may disguise their messages before sending them. A client who says "No one is doing anything for me" may really be saying "I am afraid because I feel weaker and I do not think anything is going to help."

Conflicting Messages

Verbal messages have a nonverbal message attached to them. The tone of voice, the posture, and so forth can give the receiver a message that conflicts with the stated message. For example, clients who are sitting slumped over with their heads in their hands say in a low, dull voice, "There is nothing wrong, I am just fine." Although clients may be thinking, dozing, or meditating, the posture tends to communicate that things are not fine; thus the nonverbal message is different from the verbal message. When this happens, the receiver tends to believe the nonverbal message.

Unclear Meanings

Some English words have many meanings, and meanings change with use over the years. For this reason, statements may have one meaning for the sender and another for the receiver. *Gross* is an adjective that can be used to describe something terrible, something big, or something very noticeable. It can also refer to the amount, like twelve dozen, or the total amount, as in gross salary. A *bat* is a flying rodent, a stick for hitting balls, or a mean, old woman. *Gay* used to mean a state of happiness; now the word refers to a homosexual. *Bad* means one thing to a senior citizen and just the opposite to the modern teenager. If the young adult says "It's cool," the older person would probably expect him or her to be talking about the weather.

Abstractions

There is an even greater chance for misunderstanding when the terms used are **abstractions**. Young children have not developed the ability to think abstractly, and people under stress lose it. "The grass is always greener on the other side of the fence" and "a rolling stone gathers no moss" are common abstract proverbs that are difficult for some to interpret.

Perception

Perception is the means by which the receiver processes and interprets information and can be another source of misunderstanding. Each message is screened through past experiences, expectations, and self-concept. The receiver selectively tunes out messages that do not fit in with preconceived ideas. People hear what they are prepared to hear. Because their nurses are often receivers, it is most important that they increase their self-awareness. It is their responsibility to listen to messages and clarify possible misunderstandings. Communication is only effective if the message gets to the receiver the way the sender intended it to.

PURPOSE OF COMMUNICATION

Obtain Information

Effective communication is purposeful. The message is intended to accomplish a goal. As seen in Figure 4-2, there are many purposes for which the nurse can use communication. One is to obtain useful information about the client. Information is useful if it aids in developing nursing care plans. Before clients give information to the nurse, they have to feel secure with him or her. They have to trust the nurse. Communication is also used to help develop that trust.

To Show Caring

Trust is developed much more quickly if clients know that the nurse cares for them and accepts them as people. The little things a nurse does for clients, such as rearranging pillows or offering a drink of water, show caring. The idea of caring, though, is reinforced if the behavior is paired with verbal responses. This aspect will be explained later in the chapter.

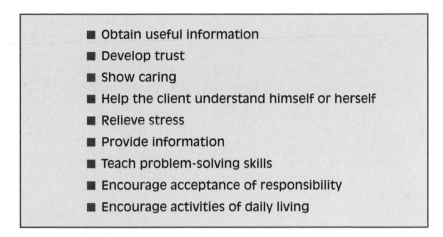

- Obtain useful information
- Develop trust
- Show caring
- Help the client understand himself or herself
- Relieve stress
- Provide information
- Teach problem-solving skills
- Encourage acceptance of responsibility
- Encourage activities of daily living

FIGURE 4-2 Goals of communication.

Provide Information

Clients often need information from the nurse. The nurse provides this information when he or she answers questions, teaches, and encourages. Vivid details of one's personal life need not be shared with clients.

The nurse helps clients understand their own communication patterns. Restating what the nurse hears the client saying sometimes makes the meaning clearer to the client. Sometimes, if the client can ventilate feelings to someone who accepts them, it will relieve stress. This makes listening and understanding therapeutic or helpful.

If the goal is to be met, communication must be received. Certain responses tend to close or block communication. When the receiver hears one of these messages, he or she usually stops sending, and further communication is stopped. The nurse needs to be aware of responses that block communication and work toward more effective responses.

BLOCKS TO COMMUNICATION AND ATTITUDES THAT AFFECT COMMUNICATION

Refer to Table 4-1 for a summary of blocks to communication.

Belittling

A client says "I have been looking forward to going to the senior prom since I was a freshman. Now with this broken leg, I will not be able to go." The nurse responds "If you had been more careful, this would not have happened" or "Do not get so upset over a silly prom. It is not that important." This communication does nothing to enhance the nurse-client relationship. It makes light of the client's feelings. The nurse is effectively telling the client that he or she is silly. Because the client sees that the nurse thinks so little of the problem, he or she will probably be afraid to talk further. The nurse will never know how the client really feels.

Disagreeing

A response such as "You do not have to stay home just because of a cast" may be just what the client wants to hear. However, the nurse does not know this, because he or she has not taken the time to find out. The nurse is responding to the client's verbal message only.

Defending

"We are doing the best we can to heal your leg" is a response that defends the nurse's ego, but it puts the client on the defensive. He or she is placed in a position of having to apologize for the nurse's misperception of the statement.

Stereotyped Statements

Nurses often use stereotyped comments such as "I know just how you feel" or "I understand." The nurse does not really understand because he or she has not taken the time to do so. The client recognizes this and feels there is no point in responding to such a comment.

Changing the Subject

If the nurse feels threatened by the client's statement or does not know how to respond, he or she may change the subject. "These are beautiful flowers. Did they come from your husband?" This is an effective way of telling the client "I do not want to hear about your problems." Changing the subject temporarily can be helpful if the client is having difficulty coping with the present topic, but it should be temporary and done to meet the client's need.

Reassuring Clichés

"Everything will be all right" is a reassuring **cliché**. Reassurance is important if it is real. False reassurance is easily detected and makes the receiver distrustful of the sender. The receiver may feel the statement means that his or her leg will be healed in time to go to the prom. The sender may mean that the client will probably get over not going to the prom. Even if believed, reassuring clichés are ambiguous.

TABLE 4-1 Blocks to Communication

TECHNIQUE	EXPLANATION	EXAMPLE
Belittling	Statement that tends to make light of the client's beliefs or fears	Client: "I will not leave here alive." Nurse: "That is ridiculous. You should not even think that way."
Disagreeing	Response that indicates that the nurse believes the client to be incorrect; it generally relates to the cognitive rather than the affective message	Client: "Why am I here? Nothing is being done for me and I am not getting any better." Nurse: "You are getting better."
Defending	Statement used to repel a verbal attack	Client: "I had my light on for fifteen minutes." Nurse: "I am doing the best I can. You are not the only client I have.
Stereotyped statement	Common statement made without sincerity	Client: "I am really worried about the children. I came to the hospital so quickly and I did not get to see them. They just will not understand. I wish I could have talked to them." Nurse. "I know exactly what you are going through."
Changing the subject	Different subject introduced to prevent talking about a topic that causes anxiety	Client: "They are doing a biopsy tomorrow. I hope it is not cancer." Nurse: "Are these your children? That is such a nice looking family."
Reassuring cliché	Reassuring statement that is not sincere	Client: "What will I do if it is malignant? Nurse: "Don't you worry. Everything will be all right."
Giving advice	Statement that tells the client what the nurse thinks the client should do	Client: "I broke my arm when I fell off a skateboard." Nurse: "At your age, I would suggest you give up skateboards."

(Continues)

TECHNIQUE	EXPLANATION	EXAMPLE
TABLE 4-1 (Continued)		
Agreeing	Statement that shows that the nurse believes the client's cognitive message is correct; it may not be the client's real concern	Client: "I am afraid the doctor will not discharge me tomorrow." Nurse: "I am sure you are correct. I doubt the doctor will let you go home so soon."

Giving Advice

"Now this is what you should do. Call your friend and explain about the accident. Your friend will understand" or "If I were you, I would forget all about the dance." This is giving advice, which is seldom effective. The client will accept it only when he or she is ready to accept it. Even if the client wants the nurse's advice, the nurse must take time to determine this before offering it.

Agreeing

A statement such as "That is right, you will not be able to go to the prom" closes communication. There is nothing left for the receiver to say so it belittles the client's concern. "That is the way it is, so accept it" shows no understanding of the client's strong feelings about the prom. Something that seems trivial to the nurse can be of extreme importance to the client.

Certain attitudes affect a nurse's ability to communicate effectively (Table 4-2).

Self-Disclosure

Whenever nurses interact with others, they make an impression. They cause some sort of reaction. It may be the reaction they intended or it may be just the opposite. The more nurses let people know them, the more likely they are to make the right impression. The process of letting people get to know one is called **self-disclosure**. To be effective, self-disclosure must be appropriate to the situation.

Self-disclosure means talking about oneself. It means opening up to another and discussing topics such as feelings, expectations, and ideas. It does not mean letting skeletons out of the closet, or discussing

TABLE 4-2 Attitudes Affecting Communication	
Self-disclosure	The process of letting people get to know one
Caring	Feeling that the client is important and caring for him or her is not just a job
Genuineness	Being oneself and not acting a role; being open and truthful
Warmth	Feeling of affection
Attentiveness	Demonstrating a concentration of time and attention on the client
Empathy	Understanding the client's feelings; seeing things as he or she sees them

one's date last night. It means letting the real self be known. In order to self-disclose, nurses must trust in themselves, in their feelings, and in others. They must see the worth of their feelings, ideas, and goals. They must also trust that the receiver will see their worth. Developing trust means taking risks. Unless nurses are willing to take a chance, communication will be ineffective. If, on the other hand, nurses are willing to risk opening themselves, the rewards can be great. Risking shows trust in the client. The more the client feels trusted, the more he or she will trust the nurse. The more the client trusts the nurse, the more apt he or she is to disclose fears, hopes, and expectations.

Risking is easier if nurses think positively about themselves and the person with whom they are attempting to communicate. Thinking positively about people and accepting them as they are is known as **positive regard** For nurses to self-disclose, they must trust the client. For the client to reveal himself or herself to nurses, he or she must trust them. The development of mutual trust is called establishing **rapport** It is fundamental to effective communication. Sometimes trust can be established quickly, but sometimes it can take days, weeks, or even months to develop. If the client sees by their verbal and non-verbal behavior that nurses really care, if he or she sees by their self-disclosure that they really trust the client, rapport will be established.

Caring

Nurses perform caring behaviors every day (Figure 4-3). In fact, all of their daily contacts with clients can show caring. Taking the time to do extra things for clients definitely shows caring (Figure 4-4). The idea of caring is even more effectively conveyed to clients if it is reinforced with verbal messages. For example, the nurse can say "Here is some

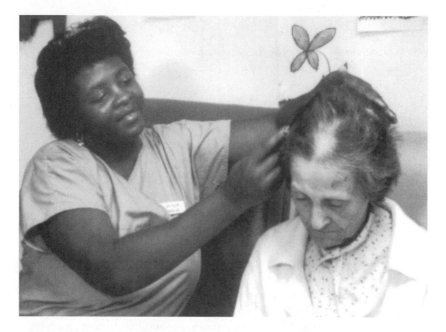

FIGURE 4-3 The nurse can show caring in everyday activities, such as combing the client's hair.

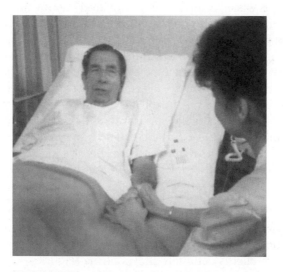

FIGURE 4-4 Spending quiet time listening to a client shows you care.

nice fresh water for you." when he or she offers a drink. "Let me help you be more comfortable" can be paired with rearranging a pillow (Table 4-3). It does not really matter what the nurse says as long as the message communicates the idea that the nurse is acting because he or she cares and not just because it is part of the job.

TABLE 4-3 Statements That Show Caring

ACTIVITY	EXAMPLES OF STATEMENTS TO PAIR WITH ACTIVITY
Bringing something for the client	"I brought you a book to read, It is one I thought you would like."
Covering the client with a blanket	"It feels chilly in here. Perhaps this blanket will help."
Assisting the client to dress	"I really like that robe. It brings out your color" or "I noticed you are having a little trouble getting your robe on. Perhaps I can help."
Feeding the client or serving a tray to the client	"It is time to eat. Your food arrangement is colorful."
Giving the client a drink of water	"Here is some fresh water for you" or "How would some cool water taste right now?"
Offering the client a chair	"You look tired. I'll help you with your chair."
Offering the client assistance	"Here, let me help you. Perhaps together we can arrange these flowers."
Leaving a room	"What else can I do for you before I go?" or "I am leaving now, but I will be back in twenty minutes."
Moving the client up in bed	"You look so uncomfortable. Let me move you up in bed."
Making the client's bed	"Now you have a nice fresh bed. I hope that will make you more comfortable."
Regulating the temperature of the environment	"It seems very warm in here. Perhaps if I turn the air conditioner up, it will help."
Rubbing the client's back	"A back rub sometimes helps to ease tension."
Turning the client in bed	"Changing position really makes a difference, doesn't it?"
Straightening a pillow	"Let me straighten your pillow for you" or "That ought to feel better now."

Another way nurses can show caring is to notice the client. First, they should make it a point to always greet the client by name. If nurses who have been caring for him or her walk by without even a glance, the client may feel ignored. Knocking on the door before entering shows respect, and a greeting each time nurses enter the room can help to make the client feel good. When talking to a coworker in the client's room, the nurse should:

- Include the client in the conversation
- Avoid colloquialisms that the client would not understand
- Refrain from topics that would not interest the client
- Speak in the client's native tongue if at all possible

Nurses can also choose something unique about the client and comment on it. For example, the nurse can say, "That is a lovely robe you are wearing. It is the right color for you" or "I really like the way you fixed your hair today."

Genuineness

No communication is effective unless it is **genuine**. Being genuine implies self-disclosure and means being honest with one's feelings and sharing them with clients.

> A student has taken care of Mrs. Jones for several days and has become attached to her. The student is in the room when the doctor tells Mrs. Jones that he has found a tumor and has scheduled a biopsy for the morning. All Mrs. Jones hears is "tumor," and to her, this is a death sentence. The student and the client are both very upset. Both want to cry, but neither does. The student can no longer control himself and leaves the room after a few minutes. The instructor visits Mrs. Jones later. Mrs. Jones reveals to the instructor that she had a very difficult time controlling herself, but she knew that if she cried, the student would cry, too. She knew the student had been trying hard not to cry.

Crying together would have allowed the client the needed release and would have demonstrated the care the student felt. It might have given Mrs. Jones the opportunity to talk about her fears, but instead she was forced to control herself. Perhaps one needs to differentiate between sharing tears with a client and crying by the nurse, which could get out of control.

Genuineness also means being truthful. Nurses should never attempt to answer questions when they do not know the answer.

Clients ask some very difficult questions. If nurses do not know the answers, they should say so. If the clients ask personal questions and nurses do not want to answer, again, they should be truthful. If nurses do not know how to respond, they should admit it.

> Mrs. Jamison had just attended the funeral of her two-year-old daughter when she was admitted to the labor room. The nurse who had cared for Mrs. Jamison two years before when her first child was born was on duty at the time of the second admission, so she knew the situation. She was anxious about meeting Mrs. Jamison this time because she did not know how to relate to the client. When Mrs. Jamison arrived, the nurse greeted her. During the examination, she simply said, "I am sorry about your daughter, but I honestly do not know how to handle the situation." Mrs. Jamison then told her that it was all right. Her daughter had been ill for a year. She had watched her suffer, and she was thankful that her child did not have to suffer any longer. They were then able to talk.

Another client might have said "I am not ready to talk about it." Nurses take their cues from the clients' responses to their disclosures.

Genuineness also means taking responsibility for one's own feelings rather than placing blame on someone else. "You make me angry" is not as helpful as "I am angry." Nurses should also direct feelings toward an object, behavior, or situation rather than a person. "I am upset with your behavior" is more effective and more genuine than "I am upset with you."

Warmth

Warmth is communicated primarily by nonverbal means. When appropriate, nurses should smile. Smiling shows that nurses care and demonstrates that they are paying attention to the client. Closely associated with smiling is a sense of humor. This does not mean that nurses must be stand-up comedians. It does mean that they should be able to see the humor in everyday situations. Humor can give the client just the reprieve he or she needs to cope with more serious news. Using humor to block unpleasant messages is inappropriate. As in everything else, nurses must take their cues from the client.

Touch is another way of showing warmth (Figure 4-5). Touch is important to people of all ages, but it is extremely important for the very young, the old, and others who are vulnerable because of physical or emotional problems. Touch is an extremely valuable tool, but it, too, must be used appropriately. A particular culture generally dictates

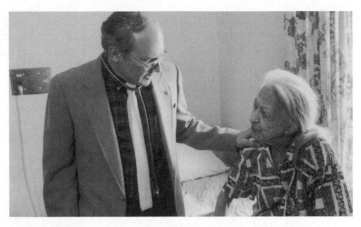

FIGURE 4-5 Touch is another way of showing warmth.

what touching action is proper in a particular situation. Holding or shaking a hand, stroking or touching an extremity, patting a shoulder, or even giving a hug can be therapeutic. Nurses may find the more intimate modes of touch helpful when caring for their more distressed or vulnerable clients.

Attentiveness

Posture and position indicate **attentiveness** and showing attention is necessary for effective communication (Figure 4-6). Leaning forward toward the client is better than leaning back or sitting up straight. An open body posture suggests the nurse is ready to give and receive.

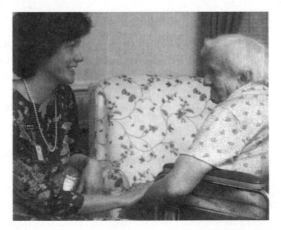

FIGURE 4-6 Attentiveness is necessary for therapeutic communication.

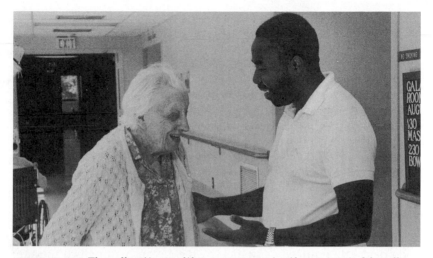

FIGURE 4-7 The client's positive response to the nurse's friendly touch shows that she feels her personal space has not been violated.

Folded arms are a closed body posture. Although tables and desks can give nurses some security, they do not help the communication process and should be avoided. There are exceptions, but generally it is best if nurses sit in front of the client as close as possible without violating the client's personal space (Figure 4-7). Personal space refers to the area that surrounds people or exists between them. Each person claims a specific territory around himself or herself as his own personal space. The amount of territory varies with individuals, but anxiety results if an unwanted person intrudes. When nurses sit so that they have eye contact, they not only communicate attention but also are in a better position to observe for nonverbal cues. Eye contact, positioning, and tone of voice are important considerations.

Listening is another way of showing attention. It is a very important aspect of communication. Unless nurses truly listen, they cannot hope to understand what the client is saying. The client needs to know that he or she has the nurse's undivided attention. Nurses should look at the client with whom they are communicating. Eye contact is essential.

Listening involves both verbal and nonverbal areas. It is an art and requires concentration. The following exchange demonstrates a lack of listening that results in ineffective communication.

Daughter: "Mom, I made an appointment to see a marriage counselor."

Mother: "That is nice, dear. Would you hold this for me?"

Daughter: "John and I are having problems. We just do not seem to understand each other."

Mother: "John is such a nice boy. I liked him the first time you brought him home to meet us."

Daughter: "Mom, you are not listening to me."

Mother: "Of course I am, dear. I heard every word you said."

Many times people are so concerned about what they are going to say when the other party stops talking that they fail to listen to the entire message. People often have difficulty avoiding distractions. They pay more attention to what is going on around them and therefore only partially listen. Listening is interrupted when the receiver starts judging what the sender is saying. Once people start judging, they are no longer listening attentively. Instead, they are focusing on their own judgment. Often nurses have their own concerns with which they are preoccupied. Listening totally to the client is impossible while nurses are thinking of all the work they have to do, the client down the hall, or the argument they had with a co-worker.

Listening takes total concentration. Fortunately, concentration is a skill that can be learned. Nurses should continuously practice giving clients their total attention.

Empathy

The ability to know and appreciate another is called **empathy**. It means seeing things in the way others do. It means putting away one's own values and taking on the values of another. It means literally walking in another's footsteps. It means really knowing what the other person feels and thinks.

Most messages have two parts: content and feeling. Paying attention and actively listening allow nurses to recognize each component. Effective communication requires that nurses respond to both parts.

I was really worried about that anatomy test. I never did well in school. I always had to work very hard. Anatomy is a difficult subject, too. I really needed to pass this test. I studied hard and I guess it paid off. I got an A. Imagine me getting an A. I still cannot believe it. Now I feel as if I can do anything.

The content of the message includes all the facts, "not expecting to do well," "anatomy is difficult," "had to work hard," "study paid off," and "I got an A." Besides the content message, there is a feeling message. The sender is amazed and thrilled. He or she has developed a great deal of confidence in the ability to learn. These feelings are revealed in the statements "imagine me getting an *A*," "I cannot believe it," and "I feel as if I can do anything."

The full meaning of the message cannot be understood without recognizing both parts. The full meaning of the message is that the sender is proud of himself or herself and has increased confidence in his or her ability to succeed. To get that meaning, the receiver must understand both the content and feeling messages. When the receiver understands the real message, he or she has empathy.

Acquiring empathy can seem like an impossible task, but nurses can learn it if they concentrate on listening, use caring responses, and are warm and genuine. All of the attitudes and behaviors previously mentioned help nurses to develop empathy. Empathy sets the stage for effective and helping communication.

EFFECTIVE HELPING COMMUNICATION

Empathy lays the foundation for effective communication. Only after the client feels trust in the nurse can he or she begin to assist with more helpful responses. Unless the nurse has first acquired the attitudes and mastered the behaviors previously mentioned, her attempts at helpful responses will be ineffective at best. The importance of building a firm foundation cannot be overemphasized.

Techniques of Helpful Communication

Reflection. Although both feelings and content give meaning to a message, either one can be more important at any given time. Some messages are predominantly content messages with very weak feelings. Others have strong feelings attached to them. To determine which kind of message is being sent, nurses must be able to recognize both so that they can determine which is prominent.

Reflection is a response that lets the client know the nurse understands both content and feeling messages. Nurses put into other words what the sender has communicated. They do not interpret the message in the Freudian sense. They restate the client's message and bring out both the content and feeling portions. They add nothing to it except their empathy. Nurses do not assume the client's feelings, but if they have established rapport, listened attentively, and developed empathetic understanding, they will have a good idea of what the person is experiencing.

Reflective responses usually start with such phrases as "you feel like," "sounds like you," "you mean," or "it seems like you." The beginning phrases can be implied or stated. If stated, phrases should be varied so they sound less mechanical. It is a better idea if nurses use their own words and phrases, ones that feel more comfortable to them.

Phrases such as "you feel guilty" or " you are depressed" should be avoided. Even if they are true, words such as *guilt, depressed, hostile,* and so on will probably be denied by the sender because of their strength.

> I just took over as head nurse and I am going through a lot of stress. It seems all the decisions are mine now. I worry that I have forgotten something or that I have made the wrong decision. I keep wondering if the clients are all right. I cannot eat or sleep. I am losing weight and I am tired and cranky all the time.

The content message includes taking a new job, experiencing a lot of stress, thinking too much about the job, losing weight, and not sleeping. The feeling message is more implied but includes being worried, overwhelmed, and depressed. The following are some possible reflective responses:

- "It seems to me that you are overwhelmed with your new responsibilities."
- "You feel like you have more responsibility than you might be ready for."
- "You are saying that the new position is really getting you down."

Reflective responses act like mirrors, allowing the sender to review the message. By restating the spoken message, including both content and feelings, the real meaning can be made clearer to the sender. This is the purpose of reflection.

Clarification. It is easy for nurses to have some difficulty in following what someone is saying, even if they are paying attention. As stated at the beginning of the chapter, there are several ways communication can be misunderstood. Regardless of the reason, nurses should never pretend they understand when they do not. This only leads to more misunderstanding. Nurses sometimes think they probably understand and that things will become clearer as the client goes on. This is generally not true. The misunderstood part needs to be clarified or it will lead to more misunderstanding.

Nurses ask the clients for **clarification** using several phrases. Statements such as "Let me see if I have this right," "If I am hearing you correctly," "I seem to have missed something," or "Do you mind going over it again?" are examples of good opening phrases (Table 4-4). The receiver's understanding of the sender's message follows the opening statement. The receiver's understanding is then matched by the sender

TABLE 4-4 Techniques of Helpful Communication

TECHNIQUE	EXPLANATION	EXAMPLE
Validation	A statement that attempts to verify the nurse's perception of the client's message in both content and feeling areas	"You really look distressed, like something is wrong."
Clarification	A statement used to clear up possible misunderstandings to seek information necessary to understanding	"If I understand you correctly, you are upset because your daughter has just told you she is getting married."
Reflection	Stating the nurse's perception of the client's message in both content and feeling areas	"You are afraid you will not be needed after your daughter marries."
Broad questions	Questions used to encourage the client to talk	"What would you like to talk about?"

to the actual message. The sender can then verify whether the receiver's understanding is correct.

I do not want to go to therapy. I am really tired and, besides, it is not helping anyway.

This statement can mean that the client does not want to go to therapy until after he or she has a nap; does not want to go today; or, because he or she says it does not help anyway, may be completely discouraged. Only through asking will the nurse be able to clear up any doubt and determine exactly what the client has said.

Validation. Validation is the process used to determine the meaning of nonverbal communication. Actions, posture, tone of voice, facial expressions, and so on always communicate a message (Figure 4-8). It can be different from the verbal message that is being communicated at the same time. The nonverbal message must be interpreted by the receiver and is often misinterpreted.

Specific gestures, postures, and so forth are often interpreted by the receiver in specific ways. For example, a gentle touch usually says "I care." A vigorous handshake conveys enthusiasm or confidence, whereas a limp one denotes shyness or a lack of interest. With a smile,

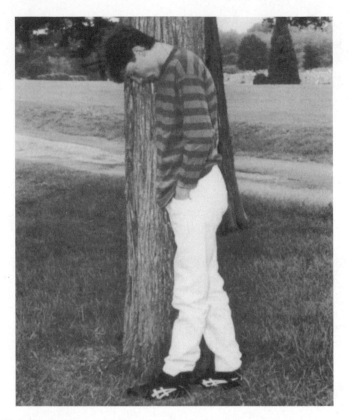

FIGURE 4-8 Posture can be a nonverbal cue.

one sends the message that everything is good, but a frown says something is wrong.

Raised eyebrows may indicate surprise, while lowered ones say "I am sorry" or "I am ashamed." Fear can be shown by hesitancy. Leaning or turning away says "I do not care," but leaning toward says "I am interested." Outstretched arms mean "come," but arms crossed on the chest mean "stay away" or "I do not want to talk." Facial expressions can show boredom, disinterest, anger, irritation, fear, love, compassion, or hate. These nonverbal cues are generally associated with the stated feelings, though they may not always be. As stated, nonverbal messages are often misinterpreted.

Perception of observations is based on past experiences, learning and the self-concept. Nonverbal messages have different meanings for different people. For example, a client is sitting on the edge of the chair, shaking. This action may indicate that the client is anxious, cold, excited, angry, or ill. Nurses cannot make the determination alone; they must check with the client. The process of checking with the client to determine whether perceptions are right is called validation.

First, nurses make a judgment, an educated guess, as to the meaning of the nonverbal message. To do this, they must know what the behavior could mean. They must listen carefully to the verbal message and then use their knowledge of people in general and knowledge of the client in particular to arrive at an appropriate assumption. Nurses can then ask the client whether they are correct by using validating statements.

Validating statements start with phrases such as "you look like," "I see you are," "you appear to be," or "I get the feeling you are." The validating phrase can appear at the beginning of the statement or at the end; for example, "You say everything is fine, but you appear to be very tense." As with reflective and clarifying statements, validating phrases can be implied. Instead of saying "You look lonely," the nurse can say "Being new around here is hard, isn't it?"

Questioning. Generally, questions should be avoided if possible. A constant barrage makes people feel that they are being interrogated. Probing just increases anxiety. The person under more than mild stress does not have the ability to think of answers to anything more complex than a simple concrete question. When questions are used, they should be interspersed with other types of responses.

Mrs. Smith is admitted to the orthopedic floor because of a fractured hip. The nurse goes in with the interview form to get information.

Nurse: "Mrs. Jones, I am Judy Goodheart and I will be taking care of you today. Now I need to ask you some questions."

Client: "All right."

Nurse: "Who is your doctor?"

Client: "Dr. Rafman."

Nurse: "Does he know you are here?"

Client: "Yes."

Nurse: "How did you break your hip?"

Client: "I fell."

Nurse: "Do you have pain?"

Client: "Yes."

Nurse: "Where is it?"

Client:	"Right here."
Nurse:	"Are you taking anything for it?"
Client:	"No."
Nurse:	"Are you allergic to anything?"

This type of interrogation is cold and does not demonstrate caring. Questions that can be answered with a *yes* or *no* tend to close communication. They provide little information. When questions are interspersed with other communication techniques, however, the conversation is warmer. For example, instead of the running barrage of questions, the nurse can begin as follows:

Nurse:	"Good morning, Mrs. Jones. I am Judy Goodheart and I will be taking care of you today."
Client:	"Good morning."
Nurse:	"You are a client of Dr. Rafman's right?"
Client:	"That is right. Do you know if he will be in today?"
Nurse:	"He usually comes in during the afternoon. Does he know you are here?"
Client:	"Yes, my daughter called him right after I fell, and after they looked at the x-rays in the emergency room, they called again."
Nurse:	"I am sure that breaking your hip and coming to the hospital today were not on your priority list. Can you tell me what happened?"
Client:	"Well, it was kind of dumb. I was working in my garden and stopped to admire my roses. I decided to pick some for the table and I stumbled over a rock. No one was home, so I laid outside for two hours before I could get help."
Nurse:	"That was quite an ordeal. Can you tell me more?"

This conversation is warmer and demonstrates caring. It also tends to produce more information. Questions should be stated clearly and concisely, and only one question should be asked at a time. If the answer can be obtained from some other source, the client should not be asked. For instance, the doctor's name can be easily obtained from the admission records. Give clients time to answer. Do not rush them.

Open-ended or broad questions are the most effective kind of questions. They are questions that cannot be answered with one or two words. Open questions allow the client to interpret and respond as he or she sees fit. These questions are good for getting the client to discuss feelings, fear, expectations, and so forth. "What do you think about. . . ?" "Would you explain further?" or simply "Will you go on?" are examples of open-ended questions.

Questions can be stated directly or indirectly. Indirect questions are statements that imply that the nurse is seeking information: "You look worried about something," "You must have a lot of questions on your mind," or "You must be tired after your long trip."

Although broad, open-ended questions are most effective, there are expectations. Questions that start with the word *why* are broad, but they tend to put the receiver on the defensive and should be avoided. Questions such as "Why didn't you take your medicine?" "Why didn't you keep your appointment?" or "Why did you get out of bed?" are examples of this type of question. They tend to close communication. A better way for nurses to state their concern would be, "I noticed you did not keep your appointment. Is there some reason?"

COMMUNICATING WITH DISTRESSED CLIENTS

It is difficult to establish rapport with distressed clients because they do not trust easily; therefore, the attitudes and caring behaviors become even more important. Nurses need to be patient but persistent. This does not mean that they should push their distressed clients to talk. It means that they should not get discouraged. Nurses should continue to show that they care. Sometimes just sitting quietly with a silent person is enough to help. Eventually, enough trust can be established for clients to feel they can communicate.

Probing and interrogating are to be avoided because these techniques add to the client's anxiety. Arguing and trying to reason with him or her are futile. The client under stress is less able to concentrate; therefore, he or she cannot be expected to remember. Directions may have to be repeated, or the nurse may have to take the client by the hand and guide him or her.

Clients under stress cannot process information well, and directions with more than one step can overwhelm them. For instance, the nurse should never say things such as "I am going to get you up now, Charlie." "Turn over, I am going to change your bed." or "I am going to lay out your clothes and I want you to get dressed." Such statements give clients too many things to think about. Consequently, they are unable to process the message and become confused. They may then retaliate with aggression.

Statements spoken to these clients need to be broken down into single steps. For example,

- "Sit up. That is right."
- "Bring your legs over. Good."
- "Now, turn toward me."

If this is done and clients are given time to process each step, they will be more cooperative. The more distressed the client is, the clearer and simpler the steps must be.

Nurses must always remain calm, even if clients become agitated. They must accept clients' anger and allow them to vent it. Some clients try to engage nurses in a power struggle. Nurses need to recognize this and avoid getting caught up in it.

SUMMARY

Effective communication adds to the client's psychological comfort, so it is necessary to physical and emotional recovery. Communication is not just an exchange of words. It includes all methods used to relay messages to another person, including body movements, posture, and tone of voice.

Communication can be ineffective if the sender sends disguised messages, when there are conflicting verbal and nonverbal messages, or when the receiver fails to listen. It can also occur if words with multiple meanings are used, if abstract messages are sent, or if the receiver's conditioning prepares him or her to misperceive the message.

Effective communication is purposeful. Gathering information, showing care, and developing trust are some of the goals. Many times, the nurse needs to provide information as well when encouraging or teaching good health habits.

Communication must remain open until the goal is reached. Certain responses tend to close communication; they include: belittling, disagreeing, defending, making stereotyped statements, changing the subject, falsely reassuring, giving advice, and agreeing.

Whenever nurses interact with other people, they make an impression. They cause some sort of reaction. The more nurses allow themselves to be known, the more apt they are to make the right impression. Allowing oneself to be known is called self-disclosure. To self-disclose, nurses must trust and work toward developing trust in clients. The development of mutual trust is called *estab-*

lishing rapport, and it is fundamental to the communication process.

Nurses must demonstrate certain attitudes if they are to effectively communicate. These include caring, genuineness, warmth, attentiveness, and empathy. Effective helping techniques include reflecting, clarifying, validating, questioning, and confronting.

Communication with distressed clients requires all of the nurses' skills. It is difficult to establish rapport because distressed clients do not trust easily. These clients need a calm, accepting atmosphere. Probing and interrogating should be avoided. Arguing and trying to reason with clients is futile. Nurses should establish eye contact so clients know they are talking to them. Statements are simple and concrete. Directions are broken down and given one step at a time.

SUGGESTED ACTIVITIES

- With a group, take turns communicating with nonverbal cues. See how many messages the group can correctly identify.

- Practice effective responses with classmates:
  Ask a classmate to say a few words or a phrase. Concentrate on the content of the message. Try to repeat it word for word. When this can be done, have the classmate gradually lengthen it to a sentence, then two sentences and so on. Keep going until an entire paragraph can be repeated verbatim.

- Make a list of all things you do for clients that show caring. Pair these with statements that reinforce your behavior.

- View 5 minutes of a television talk show. Pay attention to nonverbal cues and body language. What message is communicated? Make comparisons with classmates.

REVIEW

KNOW AND COMPREHEND
A. Multiple choice. Select the one best answer.

1. Communication is broadly defined as which of the following?
   - ❏ A. an exchange of words
   - ❏ B. a nonverbal message
   - ❏ C. the spoken and written word
   - ❏ D. all methods used to exchange messages

2. The nurse tells a client to "get out more and exercise" when the client confides that he is tired of being overweight. What block to communication is this an example of?
   - ❏ A. disagreeing
   - ❏ B. giving advice
   - ❏ C. changing the subject
   - ❏ C. reassuring clichés

3. The means by which the receiver processes or interprets information is
   - ❏ A. empathy.
   - ❏ B. perception.
   - ❏ C. reflection.
   - ❏ D. validation.

4. A nurse responds with what she perceives as the client's message. Which communication technique has been used?
   - ❏ A. confrontation
   - ❏ B. clarification
   - ❏ C. genuineness
   - ❏ D. reflection

5. When the nurse says, "I do not know how to answer that," the nurse has demonstrated which of the following?
   - ❏ A. genuineness
   - ❏ B. empathy
   - ❏ C. evasiveness
   - ❏ D. inattentiveness

6. Which technique should be used with distressed clients?
   - ❏ A. probing
   - ❏ B. confrontation
   - ❏ C. reality orientation
   - ❏ D. reasoning

7. When talking to a client, the nurse should sit facing the client because the position is better for
   - ❏ A. listening.
   - ❏ B. restraining.
   - ❏ C. intimidating.
   - ❏ D. observing.

APPLY YOUR LEARNING

A. Multiple choice. Select the one best answer.

1. A client says to the nurse, "I'm really upset about my son. He isn't doing well in school and he's been very worried recently." Which response by the nurse would be most helpful?
   - ❏ A. "Why do you think he's having so many problems?"
   - ❏ B. "Do you think his problems are your fault?"
   - ❏ C. "When did these problems really begin?"
   - ❏ D. "What do you mean when you say 'he's been worried'?"

2. A group of clients are stringing beads in an arts and crafts group. One client has stopped participating and has a sad facial appearance. Which of the following comments by the nurse would be most therapeutic?
   - ❏ A. "We only have 15 minutes more to finish our project."
   - ❏ B. "I noticed you have stopped stringing beads."
   - ❏ C. "Is something bothering you?"
   - ❏ D. "Why aren't you stringing beads anymore?"

3. The nurse seeks to build a relationship with a client readmitted to the hospital. The client has a diagnosis of end stage renal disease [ESRD]. Which of the following statements by the nurse would contribute to establishing trust?
   - ❏ A. "It must be frustrating to be readmitted to the hospital."
   - ❏ B. "Weren't you complying with your fluid restrictions?"
   - ❏ C. "You have to adhere to your diet unless you want to be rehospitalized."
   - ❏ D. "Everybody with ESRD ends up in the hospital from time to time."

4. The nurse discovers a client crying after learning that a malignant cancer has returned. Which behavior by the nurse is most likely to demonstrate caring?
   - ❏ A. Offer to take the client out of doors for some fresh air and change of scenery.
   - ❏ B. Research the cancer survival statistics and explain them to the client.
   - ❏ C. Reassure the client that successful treatment is available for this type of cancer.
   - ❏ D. Sit quietly with the client and say, "I'm here to listen if you want to talk."

5. A nurse assists a client with a meal tray. The client is experiencing moderate to severe anxiety. Which comment by the nurse would be most appropriate?

   ❏ A. "Here is your lunch tray. You can eat if you feel like it."
   ❏ B. "Do you feel like eating lunch today?"
   ❏ C. "First, put your napkin in your lap."
   ❏ D. "Eating lunch will help restore your strength."

6. A client says to the nurse, "I'm really worried about my relationships with my family." Which response by the nurse would be most therapeutic?

   ❏ A. Lean attentively toward the client and say "Go on..."
   ❏ B. "You're really worried about your family relationships?"
   ❏ C. "Family relationships are a frequent source of worry."
   ❏ D. "Why are you worrying about the relationships?"

7. A client says to his nurse, "Look how healthy I am. This tumor cannot possibly be malignant." The nurse responds, "I am sure everything will be all right. You just try to get a good night's sleep and do not worry." What are the consequences?

   ❏ A. The client will feel reassured.
   ❏ B. The conversation will stop.
   ❏ C. The client will think hospitalization is unnecessary.
   ❏ D. Communication channels will stay open.

8. A nurse tells a distressed client to get out of bed and get dressed. The client will probably

   ❏ A. get out of bed and get dressed.
   ❏ B. tell the nurse, "I cannot do that."
   ❏ C. scream.
   ❏ D. feel anxious.

C. Briefly answer the following.

1. List three goals of therapeutic communication.

2. Name three reasons for ineffective communication.

3. Name three attitudes essential for therapeutic communication.

4. List three techniques for effective listening.

5. Name the block to communication in each of the following responses, then formulate a helpful response.

a. Client to the nurse: "I am so fat I do not have any friends."
   Responses:
   - "Since you know what it is, why don't you do something about it?"
   - "Oh, you are not so fat."

   Helpful response: _____

b. One nurse talking to another nurse: "That Mrs. Jones is the most ungrateful client I have ever met."
   Responses:
   - "You should be more patient with her."
   - "Boy, I know exactly what you mean."

   Helpful response: _____

c. Disturbed client to the nurse: "Get out of my room. The next time you show your face, I will throw something at you."
   Responses:
   - "O.K., but if you do not get well, do not blame me."
   - "My, what pretty flowers."
   - "There now, you will feel better tomorrow."

   Helpful response: _____

CHAPTER 5

Relieving Anxiety

OUTLINE

KEY TERMS

stressors

anxiety

panic

systematic relaxation

desensitization

implosive therapy

modeling

role-playing

confrontation

behavior modification

operant conditioning

negative conditioning

positive conditioning

aggressive

passive

assertive

OBJECTIVES

After studying this chapter, the student should be able to:

- Differentiate the characteristics of anxiety, fear, panic, and aggression.
- List seven symptoms of severe anxiety.
- State four ways of reducing anxiety.
- Discuss nursing actions/interventions for the anxious client.
- Explain modeling, role-playing, confrontation, and behavior modification as techniques for changing behaviors.
- List three elements of passive, aggressive, and assertive behavior.

Stress is a nonspecific response to any demand made on the body. These demands are called stressors. People are constantly affected by physical and psychological **stressors** Adaptation usually goes unnoticed unless the stressors are severe or prolonged. How stress is perceived by the person determines whether the stress produces anxiety in that individual. It also determines the degree of anxiety produced. We have become a harried people with stressors rapidly accelerating and contributing to increased anxiety in our environment and daily life. Anxiety results from constant change. To live is to experience anxious moments, but anxiety can stimulate personal growth.

ANXIETY: MILD, MODERATE, SEVERE

Anxiety is a vague, uneasy feeling of discomfort. It is a term used to describe reaction to stress when the source is believed to be threatening but is not obvious. The source of anxiety is usually within the person's internal environment. Anxiety is different from fear in that fear is the reaction to a known and usually external threat. Everyone experiences anxiety at some point in their lives. In fact, some anxiety is necessary. Without it, people would be apathetic and disinterested in their surroundings.

Anxiety may occur at any time during the life cycle. It may be the result of a developmental or situational stressor. Situational stressors are disruptive changes in one's life such as divorce, serious illness, the death of a loved one, or loss of a job. Although anxiety is often acute and of short duration, there are people who consistently live with a certain level of anxiety. This is called chronic, or long-term, anxiety. People with chronic anxiety may additionally experience acute episodes of anxiety.

Anxiety can be mild, moderate, or severe. Mild anxiety warns the body to mobilize its forces to handle an impending threat. It increases the energy level and alertness. The individual is then better able to think, analyze, draw conclusions, and solve problems (Table 5-1).

Moderate anxiety decreases perception. The person focuses attention on the particular task or problem. This is called selective inattention. Other voices or events within the room may not be noticed. Physiological changes such as perspiration, muscle tension, and increased heart and respiratory rate may occur. Moderate anxiety, if not prolonged, may be useful for learning difficult tasks and for developing one's capabilities. If the anxiety is prolonged, discomfort such as fatigue, nausea, and diarrhea may result.

Severe anxiety decreases perception to an even greater extent. The person selects only part of an experience and focuses all attention on it. Abstract thinking is lost. Some concrete directions may be followed, but learning generally does not take place. Communication may be confused and the individual's speech may be difficult to understand. Physiological changes include profuse sweating; rapid, shallow pulse and respirations; a rise in blood pressure; dry mouth; speech impairments; increased muscle tension; rigid posture; and tremors or shivering (Figure 5-1).

Panic is a very high level of anxiety in which the person experiences intolerable stress. The physiological changes caused by anxiety are increased. Attention is focused on a minute detail that is often blown out of proportion. Speech is usually incoherent and communi-

TABLE 5-1 Characteristics of Mild, Moderate, and Severe Anxiety

ANXIETY	PERCEPTION	PHYSIOLOGICAL CHANGES	BEHAVIOR
Mild	Increased	Increased adrenal activity Increased energy	Alert Energetic
Moderate	Decreased; concentration on a single event	Perspiration Muscle tension Increased heart and respiratory rate Gastric distress	Concentration on particular problem Irritability Pacing
Severe	Focuses attention on only part of an experience	Dry mouth Profuse sweating Rapid, shallow pulse and respirations Rise in blood pressure Speech impairment Increased muscle tension Rigid posture Tremors or shivering Headache	Purposeless movements Concrete directions may be followed, but learning does not take place Crying Confused communication (speech impairments) Inability to think abstractly
Panic	Single detail blown out of proportion	Same as in severe anxiety but to an increased degree	Same as in severe anxiety but to an increased degree Unable to solve problems Fear of losing control

cation ineffective. A prolonged state of panic can have serious consequences. Death may even result.

Like stress, the degree of anxiety experienced depends on the individual's perception of the event and the degree of danger perceived. The level of anxiety also depends on the individual's immediate needs, belief about his or her ability to handle the situation, amount and quality of support available, and degree of accumulated and concurrent stress experienced.

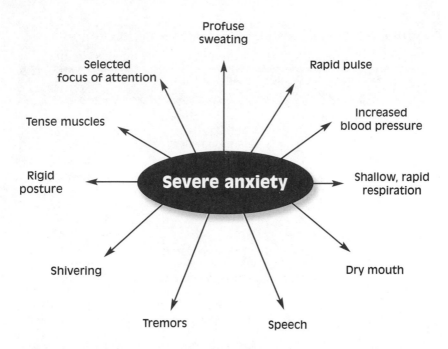

FIGURE 5-1 Physical and mental responses to severe anxiety.

ANXIETY-PRODUCING SITUATIONS

Anxiety-producing situations are not the same for all people. A situation that is unimportant to one person may cause anxiety in another (Figure 5-2). A situation that is seen as a challenge to one person may cause panic in another person. The following are examples of anxiety-producing situations.

> Joyce was brought up in a family that considered time very important. She was continually admonished to hurry and was punished for being late. She internalized this value of being on time and continued to function under its stress. Joyce coped with this stress by being fully aware of time, organizing her activities by the clock, and allowing added time for possible delays.
>
> One morning Joyce overslept. She handled this added stressor by hurrying. At the last minute, she discovered her car keys were missing. She felt overwhelmed and no longer able to rely on her usual coping mechanisms. Her muscles

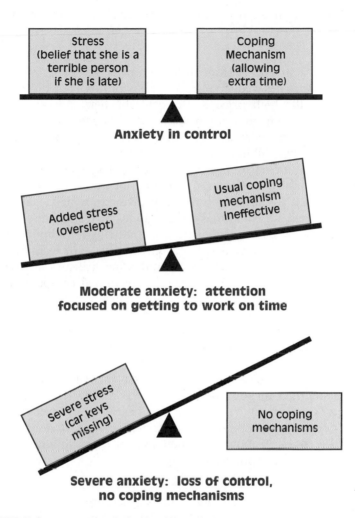

FIGURE 5-2 A seemingly insignificant situation can lead to severe anxiety if the person views the situation as a severe threat.

became tense, her thinking was disorganized, and she felt helpless. Having excess energy and not knowing what to do, she moved from place to place, becoming less aware of her environment. She felt like screaming or crying. She looked at her keys several times but did not see them. As her anxiety grew, there was a greater disruption in processing stimuli from her senses. When someone else found the keys and handed them to her, the severe anxiety ended. By this time, Joyce had already spent a great deal of adaptive energy.

■ ■ ■

Karen, a straight *A* student, was known as a "brain." Her classmates believed studies were easy for her. They did not realize the high price Karen paid for her achievement. Karen came from a family that prized success. Her father was a pathologist and her mother a college professor. When other children were praised for good work, she was criticized for not doing more. Nothing less than the best was tolerated. She began to feel inferior to others but was still under the stress of constantly having to achieve. Karen discovered she could make good grades by reading lessons over and over. Consequently, she spent many extra hours in study and many anxiety-filled days before each examination. Without time for friends and other activities, Karen was left alone. To protect her self-esteem and compensate for her lack of friends, Karen achieved high grades.

Karen's tactic is an example of domination. Many times domination is a façade; the person using it is often insecure. The dominant person must project an image of strength and competence. Karen dominated in the classroom, but others may project dominance in general. The dominant person must make all of the rules. Dependency causes anxiety because trust in others has never developed. Forced into a dependency position, the dominant person may defy the rules, complain about incompetence, and discredit others in order to remain superior.

■ ■ ■

John, too, functioned under stress. Because of his background, he viewed all clients with mental illness not as they were but as he expected them to be. He reacted to the expectations that had been established in his youth. From the time John could remember, his family frequently talked about "crazy" Aunt Suzy: "She should be locked up. She can not be trusted. You never know what she is going to do." Even though John never met his Aunt Suzy or any other person with mental illness, he formed opinions about them. These opinions lay dormant beneath his awareness. John went into nursing from high school. He was well liked by his classmates and faculty.

During the first semester, John achieved scholastic success without difficulty. During the second semester, he was scheduled to take a class on the care of clients with mental illness. His conditioned opinions were forced to awareness; he could no longer suppress them. As a result, he frequently argued with his classmates about what the instructor had said. He did not realize it, but he was filtering the instructor's words through his previously formed opinion. He heard only what he wanted to and was prepared to hear. When assigned to care for a psychotic client, John's anxiety turned into physical symptoms. He felt uneasy, had headaches, and became sick to his stomach. He dropped out of school because the anxiety of facing one of those "crazy, distrustful lunatics" was overwhelming.

Withdrawal is the way John coped. He ran away from something he wanted. When withdrawal is temporary, it can be helpful. It removes the person from the stressful event, allowing time to resolve a problem. If carried to extremes or if it interferes with the person's goals, withdrawal is detrimental. People who use withdrawal excessively have not learned to trust others and are threatened by the world around them. They progressively move away from other people and become indifferent to them. This leads to loneliness and isolation, as shown in the following poem.

ISOLATION

I keep my real self
>   deep inside somewhere
Hidden from a threatening world.
>   I feel protected there.
I learned quite early not to trust
>   life to treat me well,
And so I formed within myself
>   a safer place to dwell.
What I think and what I feel,
>   these things cannot be shared.
Too often I'm beset by fears
>   and turn from those who've cared.
Unable to reach out, to touch,
>   I'll always be alone.
Isolation precludes love.
>   I reap what has been sown.

>   —L.F.E.

■ ■ ■

One evening, Jack was driving his car along a dangerous mountain road. His eight-year-old son was sitting next to him. Traffic was heavy in the opposite direction and most of the drivers failed to dim their headlights. Jack was driving slowly, but the drivers behind him seemed to be in a hurry. They followed closely behind and honked their horns. Jack began calling the other drivers names. He purposefully turned on his bright lights whenever a car approached. When his young son remarked that his dad seemed awfully tense, the father responded by shouting, "Don't you dare say a word. If it was not for you, I would not be on this road, so you just keep quiet."

Common ways in which people tend to handle a stressful situation and lessen anxiety include dependence, domination, withdrawal, and aggression. Joyce was dependent on time. More commonly, one depends on other people. In a time of stress this is helpful, but it becomes a problem when the dependence persists and is extreme. Dependent people are insecure and cannot accept that they have capabilities. They are highly sensitive to criticism, neglect, or anything that may be viewed as rejection. For this reason, dependent people generally follow the demands of others, even if those demands conflict with their own wishes.

Joyce, John and Jack were in a crisis. A *crisis* occurs when the problem that produced the anxiety is overwhelming and the usual coping mechanisms are not effective. Helping a person resolve a crisis means helping the person solve problems. For problem solving to occur, anxiety must be lowered to a level at which learning can take place. Attempting to help Joyce, John or Jack problem solve in their state of severe anxiety would have been fruitless.

RELIEVING ANXIETY

Systematic Relaxation

Systematic relaxation is one method developed by behavioral psychologists to relieve anxiety. It is based on the fact that anxiety and relaxation cannot coexist. Relaxation exercises stem from the idea that awareness of a tense muscle enables one to relax that muscle. This is not easy to do and conscious effort must be used. Although the level of anxiety may begin to lower immediately, total relaxation may take several weeks.

A comfortable position, either sitting or lying down, is assumed. Muscles are consecutively tightened and relaxed. To begin, the fists are tightened slowly. It might be helpful to count slowly to six while the muscles are being tensed. Concentrating on the tension is essential. The fists are then relaxed just as slowly, to concentrate on how the muscle feels when it is relaxed. This process is continued with other muscle groups: arms, feet, shoulders, legs, chest, pelvis, and face.

Each muscle group is tightened and relaxed separately while concentrating on how it feels. Practice sessions last for twenty to thirty minutes a day. Some muscle groups—such as those across the back of the shoulders—may be more difficult to relax. Once muscle relaxation is learned, it can be used to relieve anxiety at any time.

Desensitization

Another method used by therapists to relieve anxiety is called desensitization. **Desensitization** is a way of conditioning a client to be non-responsive to a stimulus. This technique is usually done by counselors, nurse clinicians, and psychologists, but other health care workers should be familiar with the method. Clients are first trained in muscle relaxation. They are then asked to identify (1) the anxiety-producing situation; (2) a place (usually home) in which they feel safe and secure; and (3) another place or situation that is relaxing, such as lying on the beach. Clients are then asked to imagine the anxiety-producing situation while the therapist describes it in some detail. When clients feel the first sign of anxiety, they give a prearranged signal, such as moving a finger. The description of the stressful event is stopped and the therapist begins describing the safe haven. When clients feel secure, they are taken, through imagination, to the relaxing situation. When clients are fully relaxed, the entire process is repeated.

Suppose Karen undergoes desensitization. The therapist might ask Karen to imagine herself in a specific situation as he talks. He might begin by saying "You are now sitting in the classroom. Your desk is cleared. Your pencil is out. You are ready to take the exam. The professor walks in the room. He has papers under his arm. He asks everyone to clear their desks. The test papers are passed out. You receive your paper and look it over. There are some questions you do not remember ever discussing. You are trying to think of the answer but it will not come."

Karen might raise her finger at this point. The therapist immediately responds with, "O.K., you are now out of the classroom. You are at home with your family. You are sitting at the piano. Your mother is sewing and your father is smoking his favorite pipe. The dog lies nearby. There is a fire in the fireplace and the warmth from it feels good. Your father smiles as he listens to you play."

When Karen appears more relaxed, the therapist might continue with. "Now you are lying on the beach. The white sand is warm against your skin. You can hear the quiet splashing of the waves against the shore. The sun is warm. You can feel your muscles relaxing as the sun's rays warm each part."

The therapist then takes Karen back to the classroom when she appears relaxed. "You have now handed in the test paper. You have to wait for the grade. You have no idea how you did, but you are worried about the questions you did not recognize. . ."

The entire process is repeated over and over, until Karen no longer experiences anxiety while thinking about the stressful event.

Implosive Therapy

Implosive therapy is in direct contrast to desensitization. **Implosive therapy** attempts to arouse as much anxiety in the individual as possible. Relaxation is sometimes used but only at the very end of the session.

Caution: This technique requires a professionally trained therapist.

Relaxation and desensitization are not the only means of reducing anxiety. In working with others, the nurse will find that a calm attitude and quiet music can have a soothing effect. Warm baths or hot drinks sometimes help. Diversional activities have also been used successfully to relieve anxiety. Once anxiety is lowered to a manageable level, the problem that caused the anxiety must be solved.

PROBLEM SOLVING

Solving a problem may involve selecting other options, changing beliefs about an event, changing behavior, or finding a more effective coping mechanism. Problem solving involves a change. Before a problem can be solved, the person must recognize the need for change and know that he or she has the ability to change.

Very few problems have clear-cut solutions. In making a decision, it is necessary to weigh possible satisfactions against possible risks and costs. Since all things that affect an action cannot be controlled, it is impossible to know whether the chosen decision will actually produce the planned result. However, a decision must be made. It will be a more effective solution if the entire health team, as well as the client, is involved in the process.

The first step in problem solving is to clarify the problem and assess the situation. This is not easy. Often the real problem is hidden from awareness. Time is wasted on superficial difficulties while the real problem goes unsolved. If Joyce were asked what her problem was, she probably would answer, "I cannot find my keys" or "If I could find my keys, I would not have a problem." Karen would no doubt say "I have to make an *A* on this test," even if she could not explain why. John could be expected to complain of physical distress. Even if Joyce finds her keys, Karen gets her *A*, and John's abdominal discomfort is relieved, the underlying problems—the ones that cause the anxiety in the first place—are still there. These are underlying problems that need to be identified.

The following information about Karen might help the team discover the problem and assess the situation.

- How does Karen view the problem?

- Has Karen ever received less than an *A* on an exam? What coping mechanisms did she use at that time? Were they effective?

- Has Karen ever felt overwhelmed by anything before? If she did, what was the situation? What coping mechanisms did she use then? Were they effective?

- What are Karen's future goals?

- What is her relationship with her family?

- On whom does she call for help? Did she ask this person's help at the time of the problem? Did the person respond?

- In whom does Karen confide?

- What is Karen's developmental level?

Answers to these questions will help the team reach some conclusions about Karen. Some of the conclusions they might reach are

- Karen has a poor self-concept.

- She is unable to function effectively when things do not go as she planned.

- She has poor problem-solving skills.

- She does not use adaptive coping mechanisms.

- Her present situation is making excessive demands on her.

- She does not utilize her family as a support system.

- She has not clarified her goals for the future.

Once the problem or problems have been identified and the situation assessed, the team can prepare the plan. Planning involves setting goals and determining possible actions to reach these goals. Goals are extremely important in this process, because they set priorities and give direction to the nursing care Karen will receive. Possible goals for Karen might be

▓ Help Karen become more aware of her situation.

▓ Teach Karen problem-solving skills.

▓ Teach her more adaptive coping measures.

▓ Assist her in setting more realistic goals for herself.

▓ Teach her assertive skills.

▓ Help Karen improve her relationship with her family.

▧ Nursing Care Plan: ▧
The Client with Anxiety and Stress

Chris, a thirty-nine-year-old lawyer, presents in an emergency medical facility stating that he has been vomiting small amounts of blood for the past few days. He relates to the nurse practitioner that he has been experiencing symptoms of heartburn and epigastric pain for the past month. Vital signs are temperature 98.6, pulse 90, respiratory rate 24, and blood pressure 134/80. During the initial assessment interview, he relates that his wife asked for a divorce six weeks ago because of his long working hours and time away from the family. He states that he also is in the middle of a difficult criminal lawsuit. He has a medical history of asthmatic attacks.

A complete blood count and an upper gastrointestinal exam are ordered for the next morning. The nurse practitioner recommends that Chris see a clinical specialist in psychiatric nursing to discuss the stresses in his life. The initial screening reveals that he is experiencing symptoms of moderate to severe anxiety. Chris has agreed to an extended evaluation after the initial interview. Chris relates that he has been experiencing frequent headaches and is finding it difficult to concentrate on his court case.

NURSING DIAGNOSIS 1

Anxiety related to possible loss of wife and family secondary to divorce as manifested by concern of impending divorce, vomiting blood, frequent headaches, inability to concentrate, and history of epigastric pain and asthmatic attacks.

Outcome Identification

1. Chris will identify stresses in his life after three counseling sessions.
2. Chris will list effective methods to cope with stress by the end of treatment.

Nursing Interventions	Rationales
1a. Provide a supportive nurse-client relationship in which Chris will feel free to vent feelings of anxiety and identify etiology.	1a. Providing a supportive relationship gives Chris the sense of security to share life situations and stresses.
1b. Encourage keeping a log of headaches, decreased concentration, epigastric pain, and circumstances occurring when symptoms develop.	1b. Listing symptoms and circumstances helps Chris identify stressful situation in his life.
1c. Review log at each counseling session.	1c. Reviewing the log during counseling sessions gives Chris an opportunity to process stressful situations.
2a. Provide opportunities for Chris to relieve feelings of anxiety during counseling sessions.	2a. Chris will have an opportunity to vent and process feelings of anxiety.
2b. Teach problem-solving techniques during counseling sessions.	2b. Learning problem-solving techniques encourages Chris to see possible options and decreases anxiety.
2c. Encourage Chris to keep a daily journal of stresses and methods of solving difficult situations.	2c. Journal writing provides an opportunity for Chris to process life situations.
2d. Teach methods of relieving stress (e.g., exercise, yoga, or relaxation techniques).	2d. Stress-relieving techniques reduce anxiety.

Evaluation

Chris is exercising three times a week and practices relaxation techniques when he becomes tense. He is applying some problem-solving techniques in his daily life.

NURSING DIAGNOSIS 2

Decisional conflict related to risk of losing family at the expense of occupational responsibilities secondary to possible divorce as manifested by statement of wife requesting divorce due to Chris's occupational responsibilities and medical symptoms (frequent headaches, inability to concentrate, and epigastric pain).

Outcome Identification

Chris will evaluate potential outcomes of divorce and occupational responsibilities and prioritize results within one week.

Nursing Interventions	Rationales
Discuss Chris's expectations of marriage and occupation.	Discussing personal marital and occupational expectations assists in clarifying values and roles.
Role-play interactions with family and work associates.	Role-playing provides opportunity to identify with others' feelings and thoughts.
Discuss possible behavior changes as needed.	Discussion assists Chris in identifying rewards of present and potential behavior changes.

Evaluation

Chris made a list of positive and negative consequences of marriage and divorce as they relate to his occupation. He is beginning to mentally prioritize the list.

TECHNIQUES FOR CHANGING BEHAVIOR

Behavioral psychologists have developed several techniques designed to change behavior. One or more of these might be chosen to help Karen reach her new goals. Some of these techniques are modeling, role-playing, confrontation, behavior modification, and assertiveness training. These techniques can be included in the interdisciplinary plan of care.

Modeling

Modeling is a method used to improve interpersonal communication skills. The nurse, acting as the teacher, demonstrates how Karen might handle a particular problem.

Role-Playing

Role-playing is another technique useful in improving interpersonal relations. Its primary purpose is to identify and understand the feelings and attitudes of others. Karen might be asked to play the part of her father as the therapist plays Karen. As Karen plays the part of her father, she begins to get some feeling or understanding of her father's attitudes. Usually, role-playing is done in a group setting. It is a fairly structured technique and is divided into several steps:

- **Preparation.** The participating group is made aware of the problem. Each character is described briefly, and the group is helped to identify with each character. The players are given a few minutes to discuss the situation together. Questions are asked of the actors in an attempt to give them the feel of the roles they are playing.
- **Enacting the Situation.** The players then act through the situation. There is no prepared script or specified length of time. The players act and speak as they feel.
- **Discussion.** Following the role-playing episode, the group is asked to identify (1) feelings demonstrated in each character and (2) responses that seemed to elicit effective or ineffective responses in the other players. The actors are also asked how they felt in each instance.
- **Reenacting the Situation.** It may be helpful to reenact the situation a second time. In the reenactment, Karen may be asked to play herself or she may observe others in the role.
- **Drawing Conclusions.** Conclusions and suggestions for problem solving are then discussed by the entire group.

Confrontation

Confrontation is a method of communication that forces the client to look at inconsistencies in feeling and vocalizations. It is a means of helping the person validate reality. The nurse might confront Karen with the following: "You told me your father expects you to get all *A*s. Can you relate one incidence in which your father told you this?"

Behavior Modification

Behavior modification is a technique based on the theory that behavior must be rewarded or reinforced to continue. This technique has been used frequently with children but is effective with all age groups. Behavior is determined by the reinforcement pattern the individual has learned throughout his or her life. This is known as **operant conditioning.** Rewarding an undesirable behavior is known as **negative conditioning;** reinforcing a desirable behavior is called **positive conditioning.** Behavior, whether socially acceptable or not, is continued for a reason. The individual exhibiting the behavior sees this reason as good, no matter how distressing it may seem to others.

To change an undesirable behavior, the reward for the behavior is removed. To strengthen an acceptable behavior, the behavior is rewarded. It sounds simple, but in actual practice it is not easy. Not all behaviors are continued by the same reinforcement and not all people respond to the same reward.

If a behavior is to be changed, it must first be specifically identified. The behavior must be stated in concrete terms. A baseline is then established by observing the behavior to be changed and recording the number of times it occurs. This provides a basis for determining the effectiveness of modification attempts.

One of the most difficult aspects of behavior modification is to discover the reward the individual is receiving from the behavior. During the baseline observations, events before and after their behavior are recorded. This may give a clue to the reward the individual is receiving from the behavior. In the following example, it is evident that the reward an individual receives from a behavior is not always obvious.

> On several occasions, Billy hit Annie while playing in the playroom. After each occurrence, the nurse reprimanded Billy and took him out to the nurse's station where she could watch him. Even though the nurse punished Billy by cutting short his playtime, the behavior continued. Although the nurse thought she was punishing Billy, she was actually rewarding him with her attention. Behavioral

scientists have discovered that attention is a very powerful reward. When the nurse began ignoring Billy's action and taking Annie out to the desk with her, Billy's aggressive behavior stopped.

Sometimes a written contract is used in behavior modification. The client and nurse agree in writing on the desired behavior change and the reward to be received when the behavior is achieved. The contract is dated and signed by both the client and the nurse (Figure 5-3).

Assertiveness Training

People may respond to situations in an **aggressive**, passive, or assertive manner. Aggression implies meeting one's own needs without regard for others. The passive person suppresses his or her own desires in favor of others. Assertive behavior implies meeting one's own needs, but unlike aggression, it also involves considering the other person's needs.

Traditionally, women were conditioned to be **passive**. This means they were taught to suppress their needs. The passive person is often taken advantage of. Passive people can be counted on to do what

August 28, 2XXX

During the week of September 7 through September 14, we, the undersigned, agree to the following:
1. Each evening that Jamie completes all her homework, she will be rewarded with one hour of free time at her Playstation.
2. If Jamie completes all her homework every evening, she will receive an extra hour of free time at her Playstation on September 14.

Signed,

_____

_____

FIGURE 5-3 Example of a contract used in behavior modification.

is asked of them, but they may resent it. They can become very angry, but the anger is seldom expressed openly. If they do express anger, they feel guilty and must make amends. Passive people have a great need to be liked. Their self-concept is vulnerable to the comments of others. Consequently, they are not self-directing and have difficulty feeling good about themselves.

Men in our society have traditionally been taught to be openly aggressive. Women have been encouraged to be aggressive only in a passive sense. Passive aggression refers to a manipulative type of behavior. The manipulator attempts to get his or her way by inflicting guilt on the receiver. The following is an example of manipulative behavior.

> It is all right if you want to go to your party and leave me all alone. Enjoy yourself and do not give a thought to your poor mother in this big house with nothing to do. I stayed home with you when you were small because I loved you, but I do not want you to feel obligated. You go to your party and have a good time.

This kind of statement is effective for getting what is desired by inflicting guilt feelings.

Assertive requests are made in a normal tone of voice. They are specific and reasonable and include three elements:

- Consideration of the other person's feelings

   (I understand how you feel.)

- A statement of one's own feelings

   (This is the way I feel.)

- The request itself

   (This is what I would like.)

The following example illustrates the difference between aggressive, passive, and assertive responses.

Situation: Jane is a nurse working in a twenty-bed complete care unit. There is a head nurse, a staff RN, and an aide. Jane has been assigned eight clients, the RN has five clients, and the aide has seven. Jane feels she cannot give adequate care to eight and that the assignment is unfair since she has taken the heaviest assignment all week. She decides to talk to the head nurse about the situation. The head nurse responds, "I am sorry. There is nothing I can do. The

	floor is understaffed and we all have to do the best we can."
AGGRESSIVE:	(loud, stern, angry voice) "I have been given the majority of clients for a week now. It is not fair. The RN could do more. Why am I the one who has to do all the work?"
PASSIVE:	(low, calm, quiet tone) "It is all right. I understand. I will do the best I can."
ASSERTIVE: (I understand)	(normal tone of voice) "I realize we are shorthanded and you are trying to do the best you can under the circumstances, but I do not feel I can give the care these clients need when my assignment is so heavy. Since I have taken the heaviest assignment all week, I would like to have one or two of my clients reassigned.
(This is how I feel)	
(This is what I want)	

Assertive requests may need to be repeated. Assertiveness is a skill and, like all skills, needs to be practiced. Assertiveness helps people cope with interpersonal conflicts. It enhances the self-concept and is necessary in overcoming passive behavior (Table 5-2).

When the chosen intervention has been carried out, the nurse evaluates the situation to determine whether the intervention has been successful in changing behavior. If it has not, the nurse goes back to step one in the problem-solving process.

TABLE 5-2 Mental Health as Affected by Passive, Assertive, and Aggressive Behavior

PASSIVE BEHAVIOR	ASSERTIVE BEHAVIOR	AGGRESSIVE BEHAVIOR
Lowered self-esteem	Increased self-esteem	Lowered self-esteem
Lack of self-direction	Self-directing	Vulnerable to criticism
Resentment	Controls the situation	Easily exhausted
Vulnerable to criticism	Has own needs met	because of increased
Increased stress	Limits stressors	use of adaptive energy
Susceptible to	Meets needs of	Guilt feelings
colitis, ulcers, and	others	Increased stressors
coronary disease		May be feared but not
Depression		liked

SUMMARY

Anxiety is a vague feeling of impending danger. It is a term used to describe reactions to stress when the source is believed to be threatening and when it is not obvious to the person involved. Anxiety is different from fear, which is a reaction to a known threat.

Everyone experiences anxiety at some point in their lives. Anxiety can be mild, moderate, or severe. Extreme anxiety is called panic. Some anxiety is necessary, but as anxiety increases, perception and the ability to learn and think lessen. Anxiety produces physical and emotional symptoms.

Anxiety-producing situations are individual. What is stressful for one person may be unimportant to another. When a person encounters anxiety, he or she attempts to lessen it with usual coping mechanisms. Common methods of lessening anxiety include dependence, domination, withdrawal, and aggression. Dependence and withdrawal can be helpful if not carried to extremes.

A crisis occurs when the problem producing the anxiety is overwhelming and the usual coping mechanisms are not effective. Helping a person resolve a crisis requires problem solving. Since anxiety interferes with problem solving, stress must be lowered before crisis resolution can begin. Some ways of relieving anxiety include relaxation, desensitization, and implosion.

Problem solving involves assessing the situation and defining the problem, deciding on an appropriate goal, implementing techniques to meet the goal, and evaluating. Modeling, role-playing, confrontation, assertiveness training, and behavior modification are ways of changing behavior.

SUGGESTED ACTIVITIES

- Consider the circumstances under which you become anxious. Do you usually respond by becoming dependent, withdrawn, aggressive, or dominant?

- Try to recall the feelings evoked in you when you are around someone who is experiencing moderate or severe anxiety.

- Practice the relaxation exercises described in this chapter for twenty to thirty minutes a day.

- Make a conscious effort to relax before your next examination. During the exam, try to detect your feelings. Were they different from your usual feelings during an examination?

■ Make a list of behaviors you would like to change in yourself.
Think about possible reinforcers that are sustaining each behavior.

REVIEW

KNOW AND COMPREHEND
A. Multiple choice. Select the one best answer.

1. Anxiety is different from fear in that anxiety
   ❏ A. usually results from an external threat.
   ❏ B. only occurs when the personality is unhealthy.
   ❏ C. is due to an obvious external threat.
   ❏ D. results from vague or unknown stimuli.

2. When interpersonal skills are demonstrated, what technique
   is the nurse using?
   ❏ A. role modeling
   ❏ B. behavior modification
   ❏ C. confrontation
   ❏ D. assertiveness training

3. In order to change an undesirable behavior by behavior
   modification, the nurse
   ❏ A. confronts the client.
   ❏ B. removes the reward for the behavior.
   ❏ C. sets limits.
   ❏ D. reprimands the client.

4. A crisis occurs when a person experiences
   ❏ A. stress associated with developmental tasks.
   ❏ B. passive or aggressive behavior.
   ❏ C. a need to depend on significant others.
   ❏ D. overwhelming anxiety and coping mechanisms are
      ineffective.

5. The ultimate aim of crisis resolution is
   ❏ A. relieving stress and anxiety.
   ❏ B. teaching problem-solving skills to clients.
   ❏ C. solving problems for the client.
   ❏ D. giving support during the crisis.

6. Which of the following is a major premise of behavior
   modification?
   ❏ A. Tension and relaxation cannot coexist.
   ❏ B. Behavior must be reinforced to continue.
   ❏ C. People create their own crises.
   ❏ D. Awareness of a behavior leads to its modifications.

7. The behavior displayed by a hospitalized client who constantly complains and defies rules is
   - ❏ A. dependence.
   - ❏ B. withdrawal.
   - ❏ C. domination.
   - ❏ D. aggression.

APPLY YOUR LEARNING

A. Multiple choice. Select the one best answer.

1. A nurse has worked a peer's shift for three weekends so that the peer could have time off for recreational activities. The peer says to the nurse, "I need you to work for me next weekend, too." Choose an assertive response for the nurse to give to the co-worker.
   - ❏ A. "I understand that you have plans for the weekend, but I have plans also. Since I've already worked three weekends for you, please ask someone else."
   - ❏ B. "I had made plans for the weekend but realize it's important to help you. Sure, I'll work next weekend for you."
   - ❏ C. "You're always asking me to work for you. You need to ask somebody else."
   - ❏ D. "Why do you keep asking me to work for you? Don't you think I have a social life?"

2. The nurse gathers data from a new client admitted with Generalized Anxiety Disorder. Which statement by the client would indicate the client uses passive behaviors in interpersonal relationships?
   - ❏ A. "I've been making my sister do my housework for me. She doesn't have a job and might as well help me."
   - ❏ B. "I always put my children's and spouse's needs first, but it really tires me out and it's hard to keep up with what they want."
   - ❏ C. "I think I take good care of myself. I'm proud of my professional work and have a rewarding relationship with my friends."
   - ❏ D. "I've got to take care of myself because nobody else is going to do it. I always say, 'give them an inch, and they'll take a mile.'"

3. Consider the following dialogue.

   Client–"You're late bringing my medicine to me. Why can't you get it to me on time?"

   Nurse–"Getting your medicine to you is important to me. I have it for you now."

   Client–"Yea, you've got it now but I want it at 9:00 A.M. on the dot."

   What response by the nurse should come next?
   - ❏ A. "Don't you think I have other clients? Here's your medicine. Take it."
   - ❏ B. "The medicine was late from the pharmacy. It's not my fault."
   - ❏ C. "You can't get everything when you want it. I'm doing the best I can."
   - ❏ D. "Again, getting your medicine to you is important to me. I have it for you now."

4. A client experiences panic. Which nurse below is using the most helpful intervention?

   The nurse who:
   - ❏ A. Assists the client to use problem-solving techniques.
   - ❏ B. Gives simple directions and maintains the client's safety
   - ❏ C. Offers the client choices for how to reduce the anxiety.
   - ❏ D. Encourages the client to think through the problem.

5. A client tells the nurse, "My car needs $947 in repairs. I don't have that kind of money. I'm going to lose my job if I can't drive to work." Which of the following strategies would the nurse use first to help the client solve this problem?
   - ❏ A. Help the client to more clearly identify and define the problem.
   - ❏ B. Suggest alternative means of transportation to and from work.
   - ❏ C. Ask the client about public transportation availability.
   - ❏ D. Refer the client to social services for financial assistance.

6. Ten minutes before a class is scheduled to begin, a nursing student says to the instructor, "I need you to answer some questions for me about how to do this term paper." Which response by the instructor best illustrates assertiveness?
   - ❏ A. "Can't you see I'm trying to get ready to start this class on time?"
   - ❏ B. "If I help you now, our class won't start on time. I can see you after class."

❏ C. "Ask one of your classmates to help you with these questions."

❏ D. "Sure, I'll be glad to help you. What are your questions?"

7. After receiving a poor grade on a test, a nursing student says to a peer, "I got a bad grade because other students were tapping their feet and smacking chewing gum during the test. I just couldn't concentrate." Which response by the peer would be most helpful?

❏ A. Ask the instructor to make an announcement about maintaining silence during testing.

❏ B. Talk to other students in the class about the important of silence during testing.

❏ C. Help the complaining student recognize anxiety and explore ways to alleviate it.

❏ D. The peer should not respond. The problem belongs to the complaining student.

C. Define the following.

1. anxiety

2. panic

3. fear

4. aggression

D. Briefly answer the following.

1. Create a table listing each level of anxiety and an example of how you have experienced each level. What symptoms did you experience with each event?

2. What are four ways to relieve anxiety?

Psychotherapies

OUTLINE

KEY TERMS

somatic therapy   instincts

milieu therapy   drives

id   ego

superego

libido

free association

catharsis

hypnosis

dream analysis

resistance

transference

incongruent

empathy

behaviorism

catastrophizing

cognitive-behavioral therapy (CBT)

natural consequences

script

OBJECTIVES

After studying this chapter, the student should be able to:

- Identify the theories of three psychotherapies.
- Identify techniques used by each type of psychotherapist.
- Define terms frequently used in psychotherapy.
- State the function and level of consciousness of the id, ego, and superego.
- Name three essential attributes of the client-centered therapist.
- Explain how self-awareness helps to solve mental problems.

There are many methods used to treat mental health problems. Methods used directly on the body are called **somatic therapies**. When the environment is changed or controlled, the treatment is referred to as **milieu therapy**. Psychotherapy uses verbal and expressive techniques to help clients resolve inner conflicts and modify behavior.

Freud, Rogers, and Perls are just a few of the people who have developed psychotherapies. Each of these men has contributed information useful in understanding and treating human behavior problems.

The nurse needs to have some knowledge of the techniques employed, the terminology used, and the basic beliefs underlying each psychotherapy (Table 6-1). Although the LPN is not a psychotherapist, the LVN interacts with clients who are being treated by psychotherapy and, therefore, should understand the principles of the psychotherapy involved.

TABLE 6-1 Psychotherapies

THERAPY	CONCEPT	PURPOSE	TECHNIQUES
Behaviorism	Behaviorism is a result of conditioned reflexes caused by previous events; it can be unlearned and replaced by new, more appropriate behavior	Determine stimulus for current behavior and then help person change that behavior by removing the stimulus	Behavior modification Modeling Desensitization Muscle relaxation Assertiveness training Role-playing
Client-centered therapy	Every person wants to achieve self-actualization and this drive is the person's motive for action	Help the person become self-aware so that he or she can change his or her own behavior and improve self-concept	Reduce anxiety, tension, and defensiveness by providing a nonjudgmental environment Reflect feelings Accept person as is Restate person's thoughts and feelings
Gestalt therapy	The mind conceives experiences as a whole; when an experience is incomplete, a problem may result	Help the person become more aware so he or she completes experiences, accepts responsibility for his or her life, and solves problems	Dream experiences Learning self-awareness Relaxation Presentizing Fantasizing Exaggeration
Psycho-analysis	Abnormal behavior is a result of experiences that have been repressed into the person's unconscious mind	Bring repressed experiences to the conscious mind where they can be resolved	Therapist interpretation of statements Free association Catharsis Hypnosis Dream analysis
Rational emotive therapy	Behavior is due to what people believe about an event and not the event itself	Help the person to achieve a more realistic belief system and to know that he or she has the ability to cope with events	Behavior modification Desensitization Muscle relaxation Problem solving Assigned readings and activities

(Continues)

TABLE 6-1 (Continued)

THERAPY	CONCEPT	PURPOSE	TECHNIQUES
Reality therapy	People have limited control over their feelings so only behavior can be changed; people must take responsibility for changing their behavior	Help the person see himself or herself accurately, face reality, and fulfill his or her own needs by becoming responsible for his or her behavior	Self-evaluation of behavior Decision making Development of plan for change Commitment to change
Transactional analysis	People act according to a script and counterscript based on parental influences and the decisions they make about themselves and others	Help the person to analyze his or her transactions with others and have a positive feeling about self and others	Analysis of transactions with others Improving self-concept through positive feedback

PSYCHOANALYSIS

Psychoanalysis is a commonly used form of therapy in which the therapist obtains information about past and present experiences that have been repressed to the client's unconscious mind. By learning the source of the problem, it can be brought to the conscious mind and then changed or eliminated. Psychoanalysis is based on the work of Sigmund Freud.

The mind is divided into three levels—the conscious, the subconscious, and the unconscious. The conscious or upper lever contains all the things of which a person is aware. Thoughts in the subconscious or second level are not in the person's present awareness. However, they can easily be moved to the conscious level at any time. The unconscious contains all thoughts, experiences, and beliefs that cannot be easily moved to the conscious level. The aim of psychotherapy is to move troublesome thoughts in the unconscious to the conscious level where they can be explored.

The id, ego, and superego balance each other to check behavior. The **id** controls the physical needs and instincts of the individual. The id is thought to be the first part of the personality to develop and is responsible for the survival instinct. Freud used the term **instincts**, whereas modern psychoanalysts use the term **drives**. Two major drives are aggression and sex. The id operates at the unconscious level and is ruled by the pleasure principle. There is no sense of right or wrong in the id, only the seeking or demanding of immediate satisfaction.

The **ego** is the conscious self. It is through the ego that thoughts, feelings, sensations, and compromises are formed. The ego serves to control the pleasure principle of the id by substituting the reality principle. This means that the ego seeks to delay the drives of the id until they can be released through appropriate behavior.

The ego serves to control and to guide the actions of an individual. It is a mediator between the instinctive drives of the id and the demands of society. It develops through interaction with the environment. Development of the ego begins during the first six to eight months of life. At about the age of two years, it is usually fairly well developed.

The superego develops later, usually around the age of three or four. It is generally fairly well developed at the age of ten years. The **superego** is the internalized parental value system called the conscience. It is concerned with the demands of society and therefore controls impulses that would endanger society. It is responsible for helping the individual to distinguish right from wrong. The superego works at both the conscious and unconscious levels but primarily at the unconscious level.

STAGES OF PSYCHOSEXUAL DEVELOPMENT

Libido refers to the sexual drive. Freud proposed that the libido begins to develop at birth and goes through characteristic stages in the life of the individual (Table 6-2). The first stage of libido development is from birth to eighteen months. This is known as the oral stage because the infant receives all of his or her pleasure through the mouth. The second stage is the anal stage, which occurs between the ages of one and three. It is in this period that toilet training becomes very important. The third stage is the phallic stage. Here the child begins to develop a sexual identity and becomes aware of his or her body, especially genitalia.

During the third stage, the child develops strong feelings toward the parent of the opposite sex. The boy falls in love with his mother and becomes jealous of his father. The girl grows closer to her father and becomes jealous of her mother. This behavior, necessary for normal development, is called the Oedipus complex in males and the Electra complex in females. The Oedipus complex is named after the mythical king, Oedipus Rex, who killed his father and married his mother.

TABLE 6-2 Freud's Stages of Psychosexual Development	
Oral stage	The chief source of need gratification is through the mouth in the form of sucking, eating, and chewing.
Anal stage	Need gratification is obtained through ability to control elimination or retention of feces.
Phallic stage	Sexual identity begins to develop. The pleasure zone is the genital area. The child develops intense feelings for the parent of the opposite sex and wants that person all to himself. The stage ends when the child starts to identify with the parent of the same sex.
Latency stage	Between the ages of six and eleven, sexual urgings are dormant. The child participates in more socially approved activities. Group interaction is very important.
Genital stage	This is the final phase and is a reawakening of sexual urges. The stage begins with adolescence and moves toward sexual maturation and sexual relationships.

It should be noted that some experts do not believe that all children experience Freud's stages of libido development. Furthermore, these stages are not accepted by all authorities.

According to Freud, psychological problems may occur because of arrested development of the libido. The therapist attempts to discover where the libido stopped developing and why. It is believed that this information is in the unconscious. Through psychoanalysis, this information is raised to conscious level where it can be dealt with.

Free association, catharsis, hypnosis, and dream analysis are techniques used in psychoanalysis. **Free association** refers to a process of counseling in which the person says aloud whatever comes to mind. The therapist listens and interprets the person's statements. **Catharsis** is a method of recalling to memory an experience that is causing a problem and helping the person to express it. **Hypnosis** is an artificially induced state in which there is increased responsiveness to suggestion. In **dream analysis**, the therapist interprets the imagery that occurs during sleep.

Resistance and transference are also terms frequently used in psychoanalysis. **Resistance** occurs when the person tries to prevent the moving of information from the unconscious to the conscious level. Unless the person is able to work through this resistance, progress will not continue. **Transference** occurs when the person gives the therapist characteristics of significant others in the person's past life. This process is thought to be necessary for recovery.

Psychoanalysis is a very slow process. Recovery may require from one to many years of intensive treatment.

CLIENT-CENTERED THERAPY

Client-centered or nondirective therapy was developed by Carl Rogers, a contemporary psychologist. According to Rogers, the actualizing tendency is the person's motive for action. He believes that under the proper conditions, people have a natural tendency to progress to self-actualization.

Rogers does not use terms such as *subconscious* or *libido*. He does not believe it is helpful to interpret past experiences. Instead he uses terms such as *self-awareness* and *actualization tendencies*. Rogers believes that attention should be centered on the person's personality and feelings at the present.

A poor self-concept can prevent self actualization. When people see themselves as different from what they are actually experiencing, they become **incongruent** (lacking internal harmony). They distort and deny anything that is not consistent with their self-concept. Incongruence causes them to become anxious. The purpose of client-centered therapy is to help people increase their self-awareness and thus improve their self-concept. By becoming self-aware, people can view their problems more realistically. This enables them to begin to accept themselves and their environments.

Techniques used by the therapist are based on the belief that the person has a strong drive for self-actualization. The therapist tries to help the person reduce anxiety, tension, and defensiveness that block this drive by providing a nonjudgmental environment in which the person actually helps himself or herself. A nonjudgmental environment helps the person to feel safe and understood. When defenses are relaxed, a more realistic concept of self and the environment can develop. The therapist accepts the person as he or she is and does not try to change him or her. The therapist promotes an environment in which the person can change himself or herself. The client is encouraged to express his or her feelings. The therapist listens, tries to understand, and then restates the person's thoughts and feelings. In this way, the person is able to hear his or her own feelings expressed. This leads to increased self-awareness. Once a person is aware of how he or she feels and what makes the person feel that way, he or she can begin to improve the behavior. Rogers' approach to psychology is humanistic and hopeful.

The attitude of the therapist is of primary concern to Rogers. Rogers believes that the therapist must have three basic qualities to bring about behavioral change: empathy, positive regard, and genuineness. The most important of these is empathy. **Empathy** is the quality of fully understanding the person, knowing his or her experiences, and trying to see the world as the client sees it. Empathy is understanding the person's feelings, even those below awareness. The second quality, positive regard, means that the therapist must accept the person as he or she is. The therapist never judges, interprets, or probes. The client is trusted to make the changes necessary for himself or herself. Genuineness is the third quality. For change to occur, the therapist must communicate sincerity to the person.

BEHAVIORISM

Behaviorism is a type of therapy that examines normal and abnormal behavior as a result of conditioned reflexes. It is primarily used for people in anxiety states or with affective disorders. It is seldom used with a thought-disordered person. Joseph Wolpe has done much work in behaviorism.

Behaviorism is based on the belief that all action (*response*) is caused by a previous event (*stimulus*). Responses are learned during life processes. When a stimulus occurs, a person responds in a way that gives pleasure or prevents hurt. For example, each time a child goes near a glass vase, the mother says *no* with a threat of punishment. This is the stimulus. The child stops to save himself or herself from hurt. This is the response. When the child learns that stopping is the safest behavior, this behavior continues each time the stimulus occurs. Eventually the response becomes automatic. The child is then said to be *conditioned.* All responses have both positive and negative aspects. The child's response saves him or her from punishment, but it denies the pleasure of touching the vase. If a response has more positive than negative aspects, it is said to be *adaptive.*

Children may respond to stimulus with temper tantrums. If the tantrums result in them getting what they want (in this case, handling the vase), they will continue using this behavior. However, a tantrum is costly in terms of energy, so it is considered a maladaptive response.

Once a behavior has been learned, it may result from a stimulus similar to or associated with the original one. This is called *generalization.* For example, a man develops a fear of plane trips because of an accident. Eventually, this fear may generalize to other things. The man may feel anxiety when he goes to the airport to meet a friend. The sight and sound of a plane may bring distress. Even tall buildings may cause him to feel uneasy.

Some terms common in behaviorism are *extinction, displacement, reinforcement,* and *conflict. Extinction* occurs when a conditioned response is stopped. To Freud, displacement meant taking out hostility on someone other than the one for whom it is intended. To behaviorists, *displacement* is the act of engaging in substitute behavior. *Reinforcement* is the satisfaction one gets from a particular response. It is why the behavior continues. *Conflict,* as used by the behaviorist, refers to a situation in which two conditioned responses oppose each other. For example, Jane's boyfriend has requested that she wear a particular dress on a special date. Unfortunately, Jane has gained weight and the dress no longer fits. Jane has been conditioned to please her boyfriend, so she goes on a diet. She also has been conditioned to satisfy frustration by eating. If Jane becomes frustrated while dieting, she is faced with conflict because she must give up one conditioned response to satisfy another.

Maladaptive responses result from earlier events, but the behavioral therapist is not interested in exploring the client's past. It is the current behavior and its current stimulus that interest the therapist. Behavior continues only as long as it is reinforced. The stimulus or reinforcer must be determined and stopped, an aversive consequence added, or a different behavior reinforced for change to occur.

During the first session, the therapist takes a detailed history. The history includes such items as the client's age, marital status, education, and occupation as well as his or her relationships with others. Usual behaviors, activities, and likes and dislikes also are discussed at this time. The focus is on the behavior the client wishes to change. The therapist may ask the client to keep a diary. The history and diary help the therapist determine the maladaptive behavior, the extent of the behavior, and the stimulus for and consequences of the behavior.

The behaviorist is primarily a teacher of new behaviors. Actions are oriented toward a goal that is stated in specific, measurable terms. Helping a person to improve his or her personality is not a measurable goal, because it is too vague. Success of the therapy cannot be determined by a vague goal. Goals must be specific. An example of a specific goal is "Teach the client muscle relaxation exercises she can use to relieve anxiety before examinations."

The technique used by the behaviorist depends on the situation and the consent of the client. Techniques may include

- Modeling to demonstrate appropriate behavior.

- Desensitization.

- Muscle relaxation.

- Assertiveness training.

- Role playing.

- Behavior modification.

RATIONAL EMOTIVE THERAPY

Rational emotive therapy, known as RET, is related to behaviorism. Rational refers to the person's ability to think; to emote is to express feelings. Its founder, Albert Ellis, was convinced that a person's behavior is due to his or her own thinking. Problems are not caused by specific events but are a direct result of what the person believes about the events.

For example, Karen expects all *A*s but receives a *B* on a test. As a result, Karen becomes depressed and leaves school. Superficially, it seems that the grade caused the depression. Ellis, however, would take the position that it was not the grade but how Karen viewed the event that caused the depression. To Karen, the *B* meant failure. She tells herself that she is an awful person because she did not get an *A*. This makes the event a disaster that Karen cannot handle. If the grade had not been all-important, the depression would not have occurred. Ellis calls this type of thinking *masturbatory* and says it is the cause of all mental health problems.

In RET there are no *musts* or *shoulds*. There is only the reality of the situation. One should not demand but only desire. It is not rational to believe that one must get all *A*s. It is irrational to demand that others respond in a certain way. Some events are important, but none are all-important. Some events are undesirable or inconvenient, but none are disastrous.

To Ellis, when a person sees an event as awful or terrible, he or she is *awfulizing* or **catastrophizing**. Catastrophizing results in a loss of control over behavior. Without control, there is no problem solving. The consequences may be self-defeating or maladaptive. The philosophy of rational emotive therapy is expressed in the phrase "If the world gives you a lemon, make lemonade." It is not what happens to a person but what the person does about the event that counts.

Since problems are a result of masturbatory thinking, the therapist verbally attacks the client's thinking or belief system. Though other techniques are used, this confrontation or attack is the one true, basic RET technique. The therapist might say something such as "Where is the law that says you must always get an *A*?" "Show me the proof that you are an awful student." Through this technique, the therapist teaches the person to think realistically. Realistic thinking leads to problem solving or to the ability to cope with situations that cannot be changed. Many RET therapists encourage their clients to live by the following prayer:

> God grant me the serenity to accept the things I cannot change, the courage to change the things I can, and the wisdom to know the difference.

COGNITIVE-BEHAVIORAL THERAPY

Today, **cognitive-behavioral therapy (CBT)**, adapted from the work of Aaron Beck, is a current, successful form of psychotherapy, especially in outpatient settings for both individual and group therapy. In CBT, the client is confronted with irrational, negative beliefs and attitudes that drive faulty, negative thinking and emotions. The goal is to recognize the connection between precipitating events, thoughts, and actions. The "I should/could/would/ought to/might have/ if only" thoughts are reframed into "I will" (a positive thought producing a position action). The result is an increased ability to adjust and function effectively, which leads to more satisfaction with life.

Styles of disordered thinking include catastrophizing, overgeneralization, and all-or-nothing thinking.

- Catastrophizing: exaggerating the importance of negative aspects and playing down the importance of positive things.
  - Negative thought: I am alone in the world.
  - Positive thought: I know and love many people.

- Overgeneralization: making a general rule from one instance.
  - Negative thought: I am a total idiot at math.
  - Positive thought: I'm having a difficult time right now; however, I am improving my math scores now that I have a tutor.

- All-or-nothing thinking: things are black or white, good or bad, there is no middle ground.
  - Negative thought: I am not perfect; I am a total failure.
  - Positive thought: I have imperfections, so does everyone. I am making an effort to feel good about myself.

Adapted from Burns, D. (1980). *Feeling good.* New York: Signet.

GESTALT THERAPY

Gestalt therapy was developed by Fritz Perls. It is a very complex system based on the theory that the mind conceives experiences as a whole. When an experience is incomplete, a problem may result. The goal of the Gestalt therapist is to help the person complete the experience and increase awareness. A completed experience is called a *gestalt.*

To the Gestalt therapist, homeostatic balance between the person and his or her environment is important to health. The healthy person is in balance with the environment and motivated by an awareness of needs, resources, and restrictions. This awareness makes choices available and allows the person to take control of his or her life. Problems result from a disturbance in homeostasis. Symptoms arise as a result of the body's attempt to maintain the status quo.

Experience and awareness are the two most important aspects of Gestalt therapy. Only the present exists because only the present can be experienced. Gestalts that were incomplete in the past must be brought to the present in order to be completed. Each person has the ability to complete his or her experience and relieve the problem. The therapist acts as a guide in helping the person become more aware.

Gestalt therapy is used to treat people in anxiety states and those with somatic and affective disorders. It can also be used to enhance living for the mentally healthy person. Three common techniques in Gestalt therapy are exaggeration, fantasizing, and presentizing.

Exaggeration is a technique used to help the person become aware of his or her body language, verbal language, or feelings. For example, the student just bought herself a new dress. She spent a great deal of money on it, but now she does not like it. The problem is that she does not know why. The student is told to look at the dress and tell the dress she does not like it. She may be asked to repeat the words several times, each time saying them louder and more forcefully. Soon awareness will occur if the student is listening to her feelings instead of just her words.

Exaggeration is also used when a person is unaware of his or her body language. If the client waves his hand while talking, the therapist might ask him to exaggerate the movement by waving his arm in an ever-widening arc. Since the movement is exaggerated, awareness of the movement increases. When a person is aware of behavior, he or she can control it.

When *fantasizing,* the client is asked to bring the future to the here and now. The student wants to buy a new car and has to choose between two possibilities. One is a brightly colored sporty car and the other is a much less expensive compact. She continually vacillates between the two and just cannot make up her mind. To help her, the therapist asks the student to fantasize that she has each of the cars, one at a time. She is asked to pretend that she is sitting in them, driving them and meeting her friends. When she tries on each situation, she is asked to concentrate on how each feels.

Presentizing is a means of bringing a past event into the present as shown in the following example.

A student comes to the therapist because she feels guilty. She had been invited to visit her great aunt but went out with her friends. The aunt died suddenly and the student cannot forgive herself. The therapist encourages a dialogue between the aunt and the student. An empty chair is placed in front of the student. The student pretends the aunt is seated in the chair. She is then asked to converse with the aunt. The student alternately takes the part of her aunt and herself, changing chairs when appropriate. She is encouraged to say whatever comes to her mind while playing each part. She is also encouraged to be aware of her feelings while playing each part. This dialogue is a fantasy, but it helps to increase awareness. Through the experience, she is able to become aware of her feelings toward her great aunt. Awareness is usually sudden, as if a light has been turned on. With awareness comes control. The student is then able to rid herself of her guilt feelings.

For Gestalt therapy to be effective, the person cannot think during presentizing, fantasizing, or exaggerations, he or she is just to experience feelings. Feelings are the major concern. For the person to experience feelings, it is necessary to be self-aware. A great deal of time may be spent by the therapist in helping the client increase his or her self-awareness. The therapist may draw attention to the client's posture or tone of voice. The therapist's own feelings, doubts, faults, and strengths may also be expressed.

Dreams are a dramatization of an incomplete experience. Unlike Freud, the Gestaltist does not attempt to understand or analyze dreams. The therapist helps the client experience the dream and increase awareness. Experiences are taken at face value. The Gestalt therapist feels that meanings emerge by themselves with time. The therapist uses varied and personalized techniques. All techniques are geared to help the person increase his or her self-awareness, experience feelings, and complete previously incomplete experiences.

REALITY THERAPY

William Glasser's reality therapy is one of the newest psychotherapies. Its purpose is to help people see themselves accurately, face reality, and fulfill their own needs. Glasser believes that each person has a responsibility for his or her own behavior. A person's present behavior cannot be blamed on what occurred in the past. Reality therapy has been used extensively in the rehabilitation of juvenile delinquents and with children who have failed in school. It has also successfully been used to enhance the lives of people during marital conflicts, crises, and in treatment for chemical dependency. Reality therapy has been successfully applied by parents, teachers, and other laypeople.

The reality therapist must be a warm, concerned person who is real and genuine. When appropriate, therapists discuss their own experiences, admit personal faults, and are willing to have their views challenged. Most importantly, the therapist truly cares about the client.

The reality therapist is concerned about behavior, rather than feelings or thoughts. Glasser believes that people have limited control over their feelings and that only behavior can be changed. If the person complains of guilt feelings, the therapist might ask what the person is doing to make himself or herself feel guilty. This changes the complaint from a feeling to a behavior. It also focuses responsibility for the guilt on the person. Only the present is important; the past is gone and cannot be changed. If the past is discussed at all, it is to discover the person's strengths. The strengths are then related to current behavior.

Each person has a responsibility to evaluate his or her own behavior. This evaluation is essential because behavior cannot be changed unless the person is convinced that the behavior is harmful to him or her. The therapist may express personal values but does not attempt to impose them on the other person.

After behavior is evaluated and a decision is made to change a specific behavior, a plan is developed for changing that behavior. Much of the therapist's time is spent in helping the person make plans for this change. The next step is for the client to commit himself or herself to carrying out the plan. Essential to reality therapy, the commitment may be verbal or in the form of a written contract. It is usually made to someone other than the client. Glasser believes people fail because they cannot make commitments to themselves.

If a plan fails, no excuse is accepted. Sometimes the person is asked whether he or she intended to fulfill the commitment. Sometimes the client may be asked when he or she intends to do what was promised. At other times, the plan may require revision. Absolutely no excuse is acceptable, not even a disaster. This is extremely important to reality therapy. An excuse takes responsibility from the person and emphasizes failure. Reality therapy aims at providing success.

Verbal or physical punishment is never used by the reality therapist. Glasser employs what he terms the **natural consequences** of an act. For example, a child may commit himself or herself to practice the drum every day in exchange for playtime. If the child fails to practice, he or she does not get to play. This is the natural consequence because it was mutually agreed on before the act. Reality therapists believe that responsibility is the same as mental health. If people act in a responsible way, they attain growth, happiness, and success.

TRANSACTIONAL ANALYSIS

Transactional analysis was developed by Eric Berne in the 1950s. The aim of transactional analysis is to help people improve their lives. It has been successful with mentally healthy people as well as those in anxiety states and with affective disorders. Unlike the other therapies, transactional analysis is primarily concerned with groups.

Berne believes that each person acts according to a **script** or counterscript. The counterscript comes from parental influences. The script is written by the individual at a very early age and is based on a decision the individual makes about self and others. According to transactional analysis, a person can make one of four decisions:

- ▨ "I'm O.K., you're O.K."
- ▨ "I'm O.K., you're not O.K."
- ▨ "I'm not O.K., you're O.K."
- ▨ "I'm not O.K., you're not O.K."

The actual script is patterned on the life of a significant other. At first, it is an outline, but gradually it is modified and detailed. Eventually, it becomes the script that influences the person's life.

A person ensures the outcome of his or her script through game playing. A *game* is a series of interpersonal relationships that leads to desired results for each game player. A script based on "I'm not O.K." may call for the individual to get hurt. If people do not automatically hurt him or her, the person engages in behavior that will force them to do so. This behavior is what Berne calls *game playing*. The end result of a game is the reinforcement of the person's feeling about self.

Transactional analysis recognizes three ego states: the parent, the child, and the adult. These three ego states exist simultaneously in all people; however, only one is dominant at a time. Behaviors belonging to the three ego states are learned by children from their significant others. Parents contain all the rules and admonitions children have heard; the looks of love and the disapproval seen on the mother's face, the tender hugs and the severe spankings the child has received. Parents can be either nurturing or critical.

Children hold all the feelings and may be natural or adaptive, joyful, sad, or mischievous. Natural children behave by laughing, smiling, playing, and crying. They are impulsive and spontaneous. They feel joy, sorrow, guilt, and fear. Natural children are creative, whereas adaptive children are involved with rituals and conformity.

The adult processes and analyzes stimuli. It is the adult who asks questions, reasons, plans, and makes decisions (Table 6-3).

People respond in any interaction through one of these ego states. A husband comes home from work and asks in his "adult" "When will dinner be ready?" His wife may respond by saying "Is that all you think I have to do? You could do some things around here to help. Then maybe you would have your dinner on time." She would be responding in her "critical parent." Had she replied, "It will be ready

TABLE 6-3 Various Ego States

EGO STATE	CHARACTERISTICS	EXAMPLE
Critical parent	Critical Holds all rules and admonitions	"What do you have to do all day? I would think you could at least have my dinner ready on time." "Your hands are dirty. You had better go wash them." "I do not approve of that kind of behavior."
Nurturing parent	Sympathetic Caring Solicitous	"You look tired. You just sit down and I will take care of everything." "Oh you poor darling, you fell down. Does it hurt much?" "So you did not get that job. You need something better than that, anyway."
Adult	Information keeper Computer	"Dinner will be ready in an hour." "It looks like rain today." "The price of beef is rising."
Adaptive child	Conformity Rituals	"I cannot do this. My mom said no." "That is not right. It has to be this way."
Natural child	Spontaneous Creative Impulsive	"I have a great idea. Let's go out to dinner tonight." "Oh, come on. It will be great fun." "I just love surprises."

in a few minutes. You just sit down there and put your feet up. Gee, honey, you look so tired," she would be responding in her "nurturing parent." Her "child ego" might have said "Let's go out and eat tonight" or "Is that all you expect from me?" Her "adult" would have simply said "Dinner will be ready in a half hour."

In any transaction, one cannot predict the ego state in which another person will respond. If the response is in the same ego state as

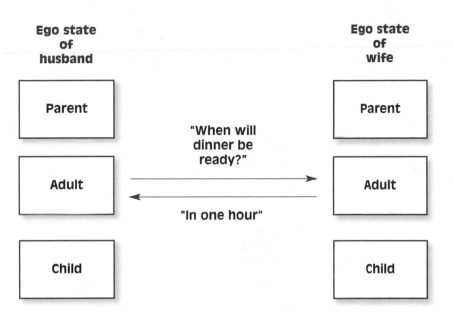

FIGURE 6-1 A simple uncrossed transaction. Three ego states exist in all people simultaneously. People respond in any interaction through one of these ego states. If the response is in the same ego state as addressed, a simple uncrossed transaction occurs and communication continues.

addressed, a simple uncrossed transaction occurs and communication continues freely (Figure 6-1). A crossed transaction occurs when the response comes from an ego state that was not addressed. When transactions become crossed, communication ceases or becomes destructive. Often, one or both parties are hurt (Figure 6-2). Transactional therapy helps people to

- Analyze their transactions with others
- Keep their "adult" in control at all times
- Allow the other ego states to be used in constructive ways

Clients are helped to recognize the games they play and are guided to the conclusion of "I'm O.K., you're O.K." Berne believes that if people are aware of transactional principles, they can make a decision to be mentally healthy and to rewrite their scripts.

Many therapists follow a specific school of psychology; that is, they are Freudians, Gestaltists, transactional analysts, rational emotive therapists, or behaviorists, and so forth. They use exclusively the techniques of their chosen philosophy.

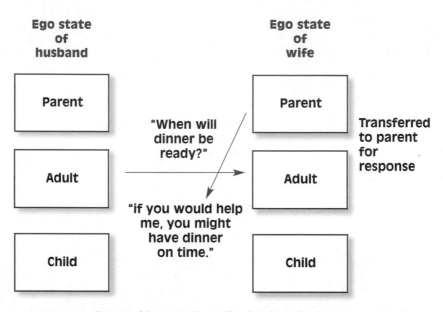

FIGURE 6-2 Crossed transaction. The husband asks a question in his adult ego state, but the wife responds in her critical parent. The critical parent directs her statement to the child; thus, the transaction is crossed. Crossed transactions are often destructive.

Others, though, feel that the various schools of psychology have something to offer, but none has the entire answer. These therapists are known as eclectics. They pick and choose techniques from any school that seems to fit the situation. They might analyze relationships with one client and use fantasy with another. They may confront one client and use the word association with another. Many times these therapists have two or three favorite therapies that they use most often, but they use none exclusively.

SUMMARY

Psychotherapy is a method of treating mental illness in which verbal and expressive techniques are used to help the person resolve inner conflicts and modify behavior. Many techniques are used, including psychoanalysis, client-centered therapy, behaviorism, rational emotive therapy, Gestalt therapy, and transactional analysis.

Psychoanalysis is based on the work of Sigmund Freud. The therapist obtains information about past and present experiences that have been repressed in the client's subconscious mind. By learning the source of the problem, the problem can be brought to the conscious mind where it can be dealt with. The id, ego, and superego balance each other to check behavior. Psychoanalysis is a very long process, sometimes taking many years.

Client-centered therapy is based on the belief that people naturally grow toward self-actualization under the right conditions. It is the purpose of the therapist to provide these conditions. The therapist provides an accepting, nonjudgmental environment aimed at reducing the client's anxiety and defenses that block this drive. Clients are encouraged to express their feelings and increase their self-awareness. When people are aware of how they feel and what makes them feel that way, they can work on improving behavior. Empathy, positive regard, and genuineness are characteristics that the client-oriented therapist must show the client.

Behaviorism is a school of therapy that believes actions are caused by past events. Behaviors continue only if they are accompanied by a reward. When a learned response becomes automatic, people are said to be conditioned to the response. Therapists are primarily teachers of new behaviors. They use a variety of techniques to eliminate rewards for undesirable behavior or increase rewards for desirable behavior.

Rational emotive therapy is related to behaviorism. Its founder, Albert Ellis, was convinced that a person's behavior is due to his or her own thinking. Problems are not caused by events that happen but are a direct result of what the person believes about the events. Therapy is aimed at changing the person's belief system and teaching the person that he or she has the ability to cope with any event.

Cognitive-behavioral therapy is adapted from the work of Aaron Beck. It is a current and successful form of therapy in outpatient settings. Clients are confronted with irrational, negative beliefs and attitudes and learn how their beliefs influence their thoughts, feelings, and actions.

Gestalt therapy is based on the theory that the mind conceives experiences as a whole. When an experience is incomplete, a problem may result. The goal of the Gestalt therapist is to help the client complete the experience through awareness. Experiencing and awareness are the two most important aspects of therapy. With awareness, the person can change his or her own behavior. The therapist spends much time helping people become more aware.

Reality therapy aims to assist people to see themselves accurately, to face reality, and to fulfill personal needs. Individuals are responsible for their own behavior; present behavior cannot be blamed on past events. The reality therapist is concerned with behavior, rather than feelings. Clients are encouraged to evaluate their behavior and commit to changing maladaptive behavior. The therapist helps clients to make plans for that change. Reality therapists believe that responsibility is the same as mental health.

Transactional analysis is a group therapy method. It helps people to analyze their transactions with others and guides them to the conclusion, "I'm O.K., you're O.K."

The eclectic therapist uses techniques from more than one school of psychology.

Since nurses work with clients under treatment, they need to understand the basis of the therapy clients may be receiving. They should be familiar with the terms commonly used and the goals of the therapies nurses might encounter.

SUGGESTED ACTIVITIES

- With a small group, make and play word bingo. Make several bingo cards with definitions of psychotherapy terms. A caller calls out the terms. Each player tries to find the definition on his or her card. The first player to cover the definitions correctly wins.

- Make a card file for the various psychotherapies. List the psychotherapy, its intended goal, and the techniques used to accomplish this goal.

REVIEW

KNOW AND COMPREHEND

A. Multiple choice. Select the one best answer.

1. *Conditioned reflexes* is a term associated with which of the following psychotherapies?
   - ❏ A. behaviorism
   - ❏ B. Gestalt psychology
   - ❏ C. client-centered therapy
   - ❏ D. reality therapy

2. According to Freud, which of the following controls and guides the actions of a person?
   - ❏ A. ego   ❏ C. libido
   - ❏ B. id   ❏ D. superego

3. A Gestalt therapist assists a client in acting out a memory of a traumatic childhood experience with an abusive family member. Which technique is the therapist using?
   - ❏ A. fantasizing
   - ❏ B. presentizing
   - ❏ C. resistance
   - ❏ D. awareness

4. Freud defined the *Oedipus complex* as which of the following?
   - ❏ A. an abnormal behavior in developing girls
   - ❏ B. a feeling of inferiority associated with family relationships
   - ❏ C. a strong feeling of closeness a child has for the parent of the opposite sex
   - ❏ D. a strong feeling of closeness a child has for the parent of the same sex

5. The term *libido* refers to which of the following?
   - ❏ A. conscience
   - ❏ B. self-concept
   - ❏ C. available sexual energy
   - ❏ D. conditioned response

6. Which phrase correctly defines *transference*?
   - ❏ A. moving unconscious thoughts to the conscious level
   - ❏ B. attributing characteristics of a significant other to the therapist
   - ❏ C. substituting one behavior for another
   - ❏ D. verbalizing feelings of guilt and anxiety

7. Which situation accurately identifies incongruence? Clients:
   - ❏ A. see themselves as different from what they are experiencing.
   - ❏ B. play manipulative games to satisfy internal drives.
   - ❏ C. respond to a message in a child-like manner.
   - ❏ D. change their behavior in response to a repeated stimulus.

8. Which therapist would use desensitization and relaxation techniques?
   - ❏ A. behaviorist
   - ❏ B. client-centered therapist
   - ❏ C. psychoanalyst
   - ❏ D. reality therapist

9. Which therapist would use presentizing and fantasizing techniques?
   - ❏ A. client-centered therapist
   - ❏ B. Gestalt therapist
   - ❏ C. transactional analyst
   - ❏ D. behaviorist

10. According to Freud's stages of libido development, which stage develops first?
   - ❏ A. anal
   - ❏ B. phallic
   - ❏ C. superego
   - ❏ D. oral

APPLY YOUR LEARNING

B. Multiple choice. Select the one best answer.

1. The nurse is assigned to care for a newly admitted adult client on the psychiatric unit. The nurse's physical features and mannerisms are similar to those of the client's mother, who was physically abusive during the client's childhood. Which factor below is most likely to affect the nurse-client relationship?
   - ❏ A. transference
   - ❏ B. displacement
   - ❏ C. game playing
   - ❏ D. catharsis

2. A client diagnosed with an anxiety disorder is involved in Gestalt psychotherapy. The client attends sessions twice a week with the psychotherapist. In which of the following ways would the practical nurse most appropriately support the psychotherapy?
   - ❏ A. Have the client describe the discussion from each session with the psychotherapist.
   - ❏ B. Use exaggeration, fantasizing, and presentizing techniques in the nurse-client interactions.
   - ❏ C. Ask the client to describe dreams and help the client interpret the dreams' meanings.
   - ❏ D. Assist the client to attend the psychotherapy sessions regularly and to be on time.

3. A client says to the nurse, "My doctor recommended that I attend psychotherapy sessions to help me with my problems, but I'm not going. I've seen examples of psychoanalysis in movies and that's not for me." Which response by the nurse would be most appropriate?
   - ❏ A. "Psychoanalysis would be very effective for your problems. You should follow your doctor's recommendation."
   - ❏ B. "Psychoanalysis is just one type of psychotherapy. You and your therapist can decide which approach is best for you."
   - ❏ C. "You have the right to decide whether or not to follow your doctor's recommendations."
   - ❏ D. "It doesn't sound like your doctor is offering helpful recommendations. Perhaps you should change doctors."

4. The nurse assists a client during an arts and crafts group. The client says, "I'm just no good at this stuff. I don't know why I keep coming to these groups." The client's plan of care also includes cognitive-behavioral therapy sessions twice a week. Which comment by the nurse would be supportive of the plan of care?
   - ❏ A. "I noticed you stayed for the entire arts and crafts group and were encouraging to others."
   - ❏ B. "What types of activities would appeal to you more than arts and crafts?"
   - ❏ C. "You should try harder to finish the craft projects you start. You give up too easily."
   - ❏ D. "Go easier on yourself. Arts and crafts is just a simple recreational activity."

5. A client in a psychiatric unit, who is also a successful investment analyst, says to the nurse "I'm never going to become a partner at my company. I just can't predict financial trends like other analysts." The hospital uses problem-oriented progress notes. Beside which of the following problem statements would the nurse document the client's comment?
   - ❏ A. defensive coping
   - ❏ B. impaired adjustment
   - ❏ C. altered role performance
   - ❏ D. self-esteem disturbance

C. Match the psychotherapy in column II with the correct statement in column I.

Column I	Column II
1. Bringing experiences repressed in the unconscious to the conscious level	a. Behaviorism
	b. Client-centered therapy
2. Providing an accepting, nonjudgmental environment aimed at reducing the client's anxiety and defenses that block self-actualization tendencies	c. Gestalt therapy
	d. Psychoanalysis
	e. Rational emotive therapy
3. Removing or increasing a reward to change conditioned responses	f. Reality therapy
	g. Transactional analysis
4. Irrational beliefs are reframed into a positive thought producing a positive action	h. Cognitive-behavioral therapy

5. Therapy based on the belief that problems are caused by what a person believes about an event and not the event itself

6. Helping the client to complete an incomplete experience

7. Helping the client to see himself or herself accurately, to face reality, and to make plans to change maladaptive behavior

8. Group therapy in which clients are helped to analyze their transactions with others

D. Briefly answer the following.

1. Define psychotherapy.

2. State the function of the id, ego, and superego. Indicate the level of consciousness at which each operates.

3. Name three essential attributes of the client-centered therapist.

4. How does self-awareness help a person to solve a mental problem?

5. Describe the practical/vocational nurse's role regarding psychotherapy.

Group Process

OUTLINE

KEY TERMS

group work	tangential
cohesion	blocking
explicit norms	scapegoating
implicit norms	confidentiality
content	theory base
group process	social skills
role	

OBJECTIVES

After studying this chapter, the student should be able to:

- Define group and group work.
- Differentiate between explicit and implicit group norms.
- Differentiate between group content and group process.
- Discuss the role of group leader.
- Identify task versus maintenance group functions.
- Compare and contrast at least two stages of the group.
- List three curative group factors.
- Describe group psychotherapy.

People have a need for social interaction. Human needs can be met within a group. Belonging, acceptance, and validation are some of the needs that a group has the potential to provide and are important needs in Maslow's Hierarchy of Needs. A group can offer an opportunity to work with others on common tasks or to share common experiences with one another. Some groups form and have a particular, clearly spoken objective that is set within a specific time frame; other groups form with a more diffuse goal but have other supportive, enduring elements. In a group, boundaries can be tested and experiences can be taken from the group and generalized to other relationships outside of the group. The quality of one's life can be improved through cooperation and coordination learned within a group. Group members can begin to explore and understand why they do what they do and learn to accept help willingly and wait patiently. Group participation can increase communication and observational skills, problem-solving abilities, and emotional expressiveness. Nurses work in both formal and informal groups throughout their nursing experiences: inpatient unit conferences, staff meetings, family meetings, and psychiatric unit community meetings.

It is important to note that groups have become the psychotherapy setting of the millennium due to drastic financial cutbacks by third-party reimbursements.

GROUP WORK

The primary work of a group is to build trust. As people become more trusting and accepting, the effectiveness and productivity of the group increase. In **group work**, members are able to listen to others and recognize the importance of developing openness. Group learning occurs, and the following accomplishments are seen:

- Improved eye contact
- Increased listening skills
- Increased use of open-ended questions
- Giving and receiving of feedback
- Self-disclosure

In contrast, the development of fear in a group member can lead to extreme politeness, horsing-around behavior, or resistance. Resistance occurs when a group member works against the group's goals or purposes or deliberately withholds active participation in the group. Sometimes people fear being part of a group and worry that the group will reject them if they speak out.

As the group becomes more mature, the following characteristics are observed:

- **Cohesion**—a mode of sticking or hanging together
- Clear communication
- Goals accepted by group members
- Feedback mechanism
- Decision-making method

Norms are standards or ground rules adhered to by the group. Assumptions or expectations held by the group members can be helpful to the group or create group barriers. For instance, a person's beliefs may be that he or she is able to speak only when spoken to; therefore, as a group member the person remains silent, waiting to be singled out by the group leader to comment.

All people have beliefs concerning what kind of behavior fits into the following categories:

right	wrong
good	bad
allowed	not allowed
appropriate	inappropriate

Key sources of norms are our past experiences. Norms can be explicit or implicit. **Explicit norms** are overt and are openly verbalized and clearly stated. **Implicit norms** are covert and unspoken. They are sensed but are not immediately obvious and below the individual's level of awareness. Implicit norms can lead to hidden agendas by group members. The group cannot resolve a problem until the problem is brought forward by the group, recognized, and discussed.

PROCESS VERSUS CONTENT

Two major components of an interaction are content and process. **Content** is the subject matter on which the group is working. It is the group's basic material or what the group is talking about. However, the major dynamic of the group is called group process. **Group process** is what is happening to the group (i.e., morale, feeling, tone, and atmosphere) and what is happening among the group members (i.e., influence, participation, cooperation, competition, and styles of leadership). If one pays attention to group process, one gains the ability to assess group problems, look at the norms developing in the group, and determine major causes of ineffective group action.

ROLES

Group participation gives one an opportunity to look at personal communication styles and behavioral patterns. A **role** is the position one undertakes in the group. Four components of one's role are

- Expectation—what others desire
- Conception—what others think their jobs are
- Acceptance—what you are willing to do
- Behavior—what you actually do

Many roles may be observed in a group (Table 7-1).

TABLE 7-1 Group Participation Roles

GROUP BEHAVIOR	DESCRIPTION	STATEMENT
Harmonizer	Agrees, understands, accepts	"O.K., that is understandable."
Clarifier	Restates an issue	"Sally, when you said _____, did you mean _____?"
Dominator	Interrupts	"I would just like to add that I believe the way we used to do things was better, and furthermore _____."
Self-discloser	Shares a personal feeling or experience with others	"I experienced something similar when I got divorced."
Gatekeeper	Invites other group members to talk; looks at nonverbal cues	"John, did you have something to add to that _____?
Summarizer	Restates discussion	"Today this group has been _____."
Compromiser	Yields his or her position	"After what you just said, Jane, I will change my mind about_____."
Consensus validator	Determines whether group is reaching an agreement	"Does everyone agree with Mary's statement?"

ROLE OF THE GROUP LEADER

The group leader can be considered a facilitator, trainer, or therapist. The leader models effective communication and assists the group members in achieving their goals. Behaviors of the leader include the following: understanding, flexibility, tolerance, encouragement, sensitivity, and caring.

Yalom states that the leader demonstrates liking, valuing, noticing, and reinforcing of a member's strengths. It has been noted that group members pattern their behaviors after the leaders. The group leader observes, assesses, and analyzes the group while encouraging interaction, exploring problems, focusing, and offering support to all members on group progress. Yalom states that the group member's trust and understanding is enhanced by the leader's self-disclosure. Self-disclosure is the exposing of one's feelings or point of view on a particular subject matter or personal experience. The group leader needs to be attuned to verbal and nonverbal communication. The group leader may have to encourage or steer to improve communication.

- "I believe we have gotten off the subject."
- "Maggie, I am not sure you heard John correctly."
- "John, could you restate what you just said?"

Cotherapy or coleadership of a group can occur. Cotherapy consists of two or more designated leaders. This style allows for peer feedback and personal growth. Time needs to be scheduled for cotherapists to share feelings and opinions so that the therapists can feel comfortable with each other's leadership styles.

The leader can appoint a group observer. The observer does not actively participate in the group but observes the group for some of the following behaviors:

- Was the group purpose attended to?
- Was clear communication established?
- Did the group stay with the topic or get tangential?

    (**Tangential**—going off the subject being discussed and talking about another topic.)

- Did all group members talk?
- Was conflict open or hidden?
- What was the general atmosphere and morale?

GROUP STRUCTURE

Structural patterns are networks that develop and come forth as group members work together. Argyle divided structure into four pattern areas: task, power, communication, and sociometric.

Task structure refers to the patterns of individual role performance in the group. Look at interactions as they relate to the talk or work of the group—who suggests, initiates, summarizes, or pushes for group decision making.

Power structure refers to the identification of patterns of influence. Influence is the power to indirectly affect a person or events in the group. Look at who communicates to whom, who is listened to, and who makes decisions.

Communication structure refers to the exchange of thoughts and messages. Look at who talks to whom, who listens to whom, and who responds to whom. Also be aware of who does not participate in the communication structure.

Sociometric structure refers to preference and interpersonal intimacy. Look at who refers to whom in the group and who sits next to whom; carefully observe physical proximity, facial expression, tone of voice, and eye contact.

The environment influences the growth and development of the group. Group environment includes room size, physical location, type of furniture (i.e., comfortable chairs), seating arrangements, and educational resources (i.e., blackboard, video). Observation of the group atmosphere is important. Is the group congenial and friendly? Are unpleasant feelings expressed? Do group members disagree? Are members spontaneous or withdrawn?

FUNCTIONS OF GROUPS

There are two basic functions of groups: task and maintenance. The task function keeps the group on target and gets the job done. Some behaviors that occur during task are initiating activity, seeking information, giving or asking for feedback, coordinating, summarizing, and evaluating. Task function can be slow moving, may be defined or need to be defined, and pertains to content.

The maintenance function is to strengthen the group spirit and satisfy the needs of group members. Some behaviors during maintenance are standard setting, consensus testing, encouraging, energizing, and expressing a group feeling. Maintenance functions create an effective group atmosphere among group members so they can attempt to work together in a smooth and effective manner. If maintenance functions are inadequate, nonfunctional behaviors such as the following usually occur:

- **Blocking**–resisting contributions of other group members or going off on a tangent with unrelated information

- Dominating–manipulating, controlling

- Clowning–horsing around, disrupting the group, mimicking another group member

- Self-confessing–telling all, using the group as a sounding board

- Withdrawing–pulling away from the group although remaining physically in the group; sometimes whispering to others or wandering from the subject

- **Scapegoating**–someone bearing the blame for others

Silence, hostility, and humor can be considered either functional or nonfunctional behaviors. Silence in the group can prove to be awkward, tense, and anxiety producing. Nonverbal cues need to be carefully observed, because sometimes silence can be reflective and the group members can be relaxed in posture. Group members verbalizing hostile feelings can actually contribute to the group's growth. Humor at any appropriate moment can be tension reducing; however, joking and horsing around can block group and personal growth experiences.

Another group function is to develop a basic operating agreement or group contract. A group contract includes the following: general expectations, purposes, goals, time for group meeting, rules (i.c., tardiness versus punctuality, meeting begins promptly at 10 A.M.; no one can enter the group after the meeting has started), attendance (i.e., after three consecutive absences, you will no longer be considered a group member), and group **confidentiality** (i.e., what we talk about in these group meetings is not to be discussed outside the group).

STAGES OF GROUP DEVELOPMENT

There are four stages of group development (Table 7-2). The stages are distinct but can overlap. Regression to an earlier stage can occur at any time during group development.

During the orientation task (stage 1), affirmation and emotional skills are being demonstrated and can provide valuable cues for the group and group leader. Affirmation skills can include being aware of each individual's rights, verbalizing appreciation, praising, showing interest per verbal reaching out, or nonverbal affirming of an individual in the group through observable nodding in agreement or leaning forward to listen attentively. Assessing individual emotional skills is important during this orientation stage. How is a feeling expressed to another? Who is openly sarcastic or humorous? Do people disagree openly? Who continues to remain silent and on the fringe? How are conflict, anger, silence, and compliments handled?

During the organizational stage (stage 2) it becomes important to define the ground rules and time elements. Ground rules include expectations: all members will participate in each session, members will listen with openness, confidentiality will be maintained, and each member will give and receive positive feedback. Creating a colorful poster stating the rules is helpful so it can be visible at each session. Define how many sessions the group will have and length of each session (e.g., one and a half hours) and include information about a break (e.g., one fifteen-minute break will be provided). If applicable, there will

TABLE 7-2 Stages of Group Development

STAGE	PERSONAL RELATIONS	BEHAVIOR	TASK
1	Dependency	Insecurity Lack of trust/support	Orientation
2	Conflict	Frustration Resistance	Organization
3	Cohesion	Fitting into new roles Groupness	Group work
4	Collaborating	Working together Summarizing Evaluating	Creative problem solving

be no break and everyone is expected to remain in the room during the session. Starting and finishing the session on time will contribute to an organized group style.

Reserve time at the end of the session for summarizing. At first, the group leader can summarize by clarifying the issue or problem discussed and focus on ideas that emerged from the group and any goals or actions decided on. Later, as the group's cohesiveness and collaborating spirit is in place, the group leader can ask for a group member to volunteer to summarize for the group what happened at the session.

GROUP PHASES

The group phases can be divided into the following categories: initial or orientation, working, termination, and evaluation. In orientation phase, the group settles down to work. The members size each other up and look for approval, acceptance, and respect. Questions the group might ask are the following: Why are we here? What are we going to set as our goals and how are we going to get this done? There is usually a polite atmosphere with dependency needs being expressed toward the group leader. The group discusses its purpose, and group rules are discussed to arrive at a group contract. Conflict will surface as group members become preoccupied with control and power. During the conflict phase, the group may even insist that the leader "fix it" for them. Carl Rogers describes this first stage as milling around, with group members demonstrating a resistance to expressing past personal experiences. Finally, a cohesive state emerges. The suspicious, guarded behavior of the group members decreases and trust and self-disclosure increase.

During the working phase, group identification increases, and the group begins to realize that conflict can be useful. One need not hide feelings or remain silent in a group. Similarities and differences in the group members are recognized, and mutual acceptance begins. Cooperation, compromise, and collaboration are key words that describe this working phase. Feedback is given and requested by the group members. The group begins to look forward to the completion of the task.

The termination phase usually occurs when goals have been met. This phase can be difficult because the group will be ending and the individual members will lose the group support. Separation anxiety may be evident. The work of this phase is putting the group into perspective, evaluating what has been significant or important for each group member, and sharing feelings. This increases awareness that coping strategies learned in the group must be applied to other situations.

During the evaluation phase, the group takes time to observe and comment on the changes that are observable in each group member. The effectiveness of the group in meeting its goals and abiding by the group contract can be discussed.

To visualize a group database, see Figure 7-1.

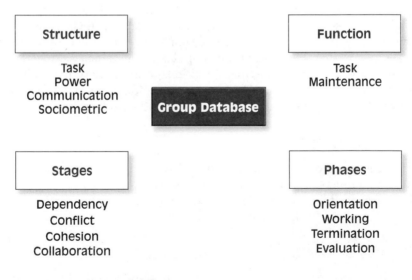

FIGURE 7-1 Group database.

Yalom has described curative factors that occur in the group. Some of Yalom's curative factors include the following:

- Installation and maintenance of hope

  "Others have the same problems as I do."

- Universality

  "We are people—all in the same boat."

- Altruism

  "I am now putting the needs of others above my own self."

- Self-understanding

  "I am learning why I think and feel the way I do.

  I have some hang-ups from long ago."

- Group cohesiveness

  "I belong to a group now, and I am being accepted by others."

- Catharsis

  "I am beginning to express my positive and negative feelings toward other group members. I like being able to say what bothers me."

TYPES OF GROUPS

Nurses may encounter many types of groups. The primary purpose of a group is to be therapeutic to the group members through supporting, educating, motivating, and problem solving with them. A group needs a purpose statement, length of time to meet, and date, time, and place of meeting. Becoming more popular in outpatient settings are closed groups with specific membership, specific time frames, and a set number of sessions. See Figure 7-2 for a typical announcement of a specialized group meeting. Following are some sample groups.

Teaching Group

The teaching group presents specific information. Active participation by the members is encouraged (e.g., a four-week nutritional group led by the dietician for cardiac clients, a medication group co-led by a nurse and pharmacist for inpatient psychiatric clients).

Discussion Group

The discussion group encourages communication and the building of the individual's self-esteem. It usually has an educational and motiva-

---

COPING WITH CHRONIC PAIN

GOAL: Empower you and address your needs to deal with the mental, emotional, behavioral, and spiritual dimensions of your chronic physical condition. This group is aimed at helping you learn how your health status is influenced by thoughts, feelings, coping skills, and social support.

DATE: June 20 – September 12
            (12 weeks, every Wednesday)
TIME: 10:00 – 11:30 A.M.
            (1 1/2 hours)
PLACE: Room C-12087

NOTE: After completion of this group, members can shift to a monthly pain support group facilitated by a health care professional.

FIGURE 7-2 Notice of regularly scheduled group meetings for a specific health problem.

tional component (e.g., a discharge planning group on a psychiatric unit, a coping-with-diabetes group for newly diagnosed diabetic clients, an assertiveness training group). It creates a friendly, informal atmosphere. Understanding the purpose of the discussion group helps the members stay focused and increases participation in the group. At each session, summarize and arrive at a decision. What have we said here today? How does all of this relate to your individual problems? Specific assignments or homework can be appropriate enhancement.

Self-Help Group

The self-help group meets to share mutual concerns and goals and to offer supportive help (e.g., Weight Watchers, Ostomy Club, Alcoholics Anonymous). Since group members are coping with a common problem, important curative group factors can occur: instillation of hope, universality, catharsis, and group cohesiveness. Frisch (2002) describes online computer self-help groups that are advantageous to homebound clients who can connect with others who have a similar disorder. By interacting with the group members, these clients receive supportive empathy and diminishing loneliness. In most cases, clients must have a reading ability suitable for navigating in cyberspace and hand coordination to operate a computer mouse.

Focused Task Groups

Group dynamics occur in a wide variety of situations in our work environment: task groups, team meetings, and committees. We are assigned themes or problems to solve through working with others. If a committee is not functioning at an optimum level, observe low work behaviors: socializing, playfulness, casual conversing, attitude (boring, not interested, wasting my time), and leadership style (no direction). A group task must look at the time available and what decisions need to be made. Allocating five minutes to agenda setting can save time and make certain that each member understands the problems to be discussed and the resources needed. Setting priorities and time limits allows the group to be flexible yet have a sense of organization. List problems on a chalkboard or flip chart and then number according to importance per group consensus—Why are we here? What are we supposed to do? How are we going to get it all done? What is our time frame? What are our goals? (e.g., protocol for the suicidal patient, documentation guidelines for a mental status exam, a standard of care that meets JCAHO criteria)? Task groups are clear, concise, and accomplished provide consistency and continuity for the patient care and increase team-unit efficiency and overall satisfaction.

Psychotherapy Group

Another type of group is a psychotherapy group led by a therapist. Group therapists can be psychiatrists, psychologist, social workers, or advanced practice nurses. It is important that the group therapist have expert knowledge and experience in the dynamics of human behavior and psychopathology. The group is approached from the therapist's theory base. A **theory base** is a systematic, organized knowledge base that helps one analyze, predict, or explain a phenomenon (e.g., what is happening in the group, to the group members). This theory base serves as a guide for the therapist when leading the group interactions: therefore, utilizing a theory base is quite different from experimenting, practicing, or "doing therapy by the seat of your pants."

The following are examples of theoretical approaches:

Dialectical Behavioral Therapy. Dialectical behavioral therapy (DBT) is cognitive-behavioral therapy with the addition of psychosocial skills. DBT was developed by Marsha Linehan for a specific diagnosis:

borderline personality disorder. Therapy plus skills training assists clients' emotional regulation and modulation. Looking at the interrelatedness of behavioral patterns contributes to interpersonal effectiveness.

Gestalt. The group focus is on the individual within the group. Roleplaying is used to help the individual group member explore his or her feelings. Some therapists use the hot seat approach. A person concentrates on his or her problems as the group observes.

Transactional Analysis. Group members' behaviors and communication patterns are observed and analyzed according to the adult-child-parent transaction model.

Communication Theory. The group is observed for ineffective communication patterns. Patterns are identified and problems solved through the establishment of feedback channels. The therapist models good communication styles to diminish dysfunctional communication by the group members.

In psychotherapy groups, the group members are selected for a group through an interviewing process, and personalities and behaviors are considered. The group experience will facilitate behavioral changes and allow for reality testing and risk-taking in a safe environment. The goal is that the group members will experience an increase in caring and belonging and a decrease in loneliness and isolation.

Psychodrama. A group member dramatically acts out or relives a stressful life event as the group provides a safe environment for the client to deal with difficult unresolved issues in the here and now. The other group members act as an interactional audience. Morena (1970) originated psychodrama and today it is frequently used with hospitalized client groups.

Social Skills Building Group

Clients with chronic mental illnesses are frequently isolated and need to develop and assess their **social skills**. The main goal of this group is to decrease the amount of anxiety experienced by clients in social interactions and provide a safe environment where they can be social and friendly. For a group of elderly, a reminiscing group may be appropriate. Persons with mental illnesses may enjoy planning a barbecue with outdoor games and activities. Day-hospital clients may enjoy a shopping excursion for food for their designated menu and then returning to their facility and participating in the meal preparation. Gatherings with holiday themes and decorations can be enjoyable for clients and staff.

SUMMARY

Groups provide people with the basic human need of social interaction. The primary work of a group is to build trust. All groups adhere to certain explicit and implicit norms. Two major components of an interaction are the content and the process. Each group member undertakes a role in the group. The group leader models communication and assists the group members in achieving their goals. Group structural patterns can be divided into task, power, communication, and sociometric. Two basic functions of groups are concerned with task and maintenance. Functional and nonfunctional behaviors can occur. Groups experience four stages: dependency, conflict, cohesion, and interdependence. Group phases can be categorized as the initial or orientation, working, termination, and evaluation phases. Many curative factors emerge during the group process. Groups can support, educate, motivate, or assist with problem solving. Group work can be growth promoting because the group leader and group members have an opportunity to explore their interpersonal styles and behavior patterns within a group.

SUGGESTED ACTIVITIES

- Select one of your leadership qualities that you can identify and would like to improve. Focus on specific ways of improving this quality.
- Identify one area of communication in a group (e.g., listening, clarifying, or asserting) for which you are not assuming responsibility and state how you are going to change this behavior.
- Assess a group of which you are a member for individual roles in relation to

  A. Task structure—how does the work get done?

  B. Power structure—who influences whom?

  C. Communication structure—who talks to whom?

  D. Sociometric structure—who likes whom?

REVIEW

KNOW AND COMPREHEND

A. Multiple choice. Select the one best answer.

1. Which factor is most important in enhancing the effectiveness and productivity of a group?
   - ❏ A. listening skills
   - ❏ B. clear communication
   - ❏ C. trust and acceptance
   - ❏ D. eye contact

2. A major component of a group interaction is the process. Select the best definition of process.
   - ❏ A. what the group desires to do
   - ❏ B. the group's subject matter
   - ❏ C. what the group is talking about
   - ❏ D. what is happening among group members

3. Select the term that refers to a group's structural patterns regarding personal preference and interpersonal intimacy.
   - ❏ A. sociometric
   - ❏ B. communication
   - ❏ C. power
   - ❏ D. task

4. Select the term that means exposing one's feelings or point of view on a particular subject matter or personal experience.
   - ❏ A. clarifying
   - ❏ B. gate-keeping
   - ❏ C. self-disclosing
   - ❏ D. dominating

5. Groups develop in phases. In which phase would the nurse expect milling-around and resistance to expressing past personal experiences?
   - ❏ A. orientation
   - ❏ B. working
   - ❏ C. evaluation
   - ❏ D. termination

6. Which comment by a group member best illustrates universality?
   - ❏ A. "I belong to the group now."
   - ❏ B. "I am beginning to express my positive feelings."
   - ❏ C. "I am now putting the needs of others above my own."
   - ❏ D. "We are people—all in the same boat."

APPLY YOUR LEARNING

B. Multiple choice. Select the one best answer.

1. These statements are made by participants in a group. Which speaker is contributing to the group's effectiveness?
   - ❏ A. "I want to explain to everyone how my problems developed."
   - ❏ B. "We're not making progress because our group leader is ineffective."
   - ❏ C. "I don't want to hear anything else about your relationship with your stepchildren."
   - ❏ D. "We began by talking about parenting, but it seems like we've gotten off the subject."

2. A leader speaks at the first meeting of a new group. Which comment would be appropriate?
   - ❏ A. "Let's begin by asking each person to define their main problem."
   - ❏ B. "Let's first establish the ground rules for our group's operation."
   - ❏ C. "Would each person explain why you are attending this group?"
   - ❏ D. "Bringing visitors to our group is a great way to expand our vision."

3. A practical nurse wants to help clients by co-leading a group. Which type of group would this nurse be qualified to co-lead?
   - ❏ A. transactional analysis
   - ❏ B. dialectical behavioral
   - ❏ C. psychodrama
   - ❏ D. medication education

4. A registered nurse and a practical nurse plan a group for clients with serious and persistent mental illness. Which group topic would be most appropriate?
   - ❏ A. giving and receiving compliments
   - ❏ B. emotional regulation and modulation
   - ❏ C. exploring feelings of loneliness
   - ❏ D. relationship analysis

5. A home health nurse visits a client one month after bilateral amputations of the lower extremities. The plan of care has the following nursing diagnosis: Social isolation related to changes in mobility as evidenced by sitting alone at home for the past 3 weeks. The nurse wants to recommend an on-line

self-help group for the client. What information would the nurse gather prior to making this recommendation?

❑ A. What grade of education the client finished.

❑ B. Characteristics of the client's neighborhood.

❑ C. The client's reading ability and hand coordination.

❑ D. The client's ability to perform independent transfers.

C. Define the following.

1. Content

2. Harmonizer

3. Power structure

4. Group contract

5. Catharsis

D. Briefly answer the following.

1. Define *norm* as it pertains to group and give examples of an explicit and implicit norm.

2. List and define the two functions of a group.

3. Differentiate between two functional and nonfunctional aspects of silence in a group.

4. Describe three of Yalom's curative factors that occur in group therapy.

CHAPTER 8

Emotional Aspects of Maternal and Child Care

OUTLINE

KEY TERMS

stressors of pregnancy

primary bonding

quickening

postpartum depression

teratogenic

regression

OBJECTIVES

After studying this chapter, the student should be able to:

■ Compare the normal developmental stressors of pregnancy with the stressors faced by the pregnant teenager.

■ Briefly explain the emotional nursing care needs of the pregnant teenager.

■ List three ways in which primary bonding is enhanced.

■ Explain the effects of bonding on the infant.

■ Describe the mechanisms used by parents to cope with a malformed child.

■ List the emotional needs of the mother with a malformed infant.

■ Briefly explain postpartum depression.

■ List three education/information areas requested by mothers with serious mental illness.

■ Contrast the emotional reactions of children of each age level to hospitalization.

■ Describe the general nursing needs of hospitalized children.

■ Describe emotional therapeutic nursing interventions for hospitalized children.

Emotional care in maternal and child health is a vast subject. Though every pregnant woman and every child has emotional needs to be met by the nurse, this chapter is limited to the teenaged unwed mother; fostering the bonding process; assisting parents to cope with a malformed or stillborn infant; and the general emotional needs of the hospitalized child.

PREGNANCY AS A DEVELOPMENTAL STRESSOR

Too often, nurses caring for pregnant women concern themselves primarily with physical care. Testing urine, checking vital signs, and making relevant observations are important to a safe delivery and a healthy child. However, it is also important to recognize that psychological factors affect physical status.

Pregnancy is a developmental stressor. Many of the emotional manifestations in pregnancy are thought to be due to normal physiological changes. Childbearing women often become progressively

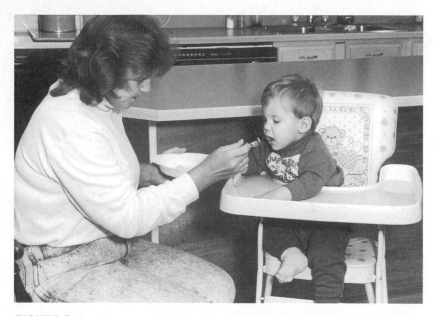

FIGURE 8-1 This young mother's education has been put on hold until her son is old enough for school.

more introspective. They become primarily concerned with themselves and their infants as thinking turns inward. Pregnant women experience frequent and exaggerated mood swings that may disturb them and their families. They may become more passive and dependent. This may result in increased sensitivity to anything that might be interpreted as inattention or lack of concern.

Pregnancy is often thought of as being joyous, but all families may not be happy about it. A child means extra expenses, added responsibility, and a change in lifestyle for the couple. A baby may interfere with future educational or career plans (Figure 8-1). Parents may fear the pain of labor or birth of a malformed infant. Even in families that are pleased, practically every woman encounters anxiety to some extent at some point during her pregnancy. Most women, even those who sincerely desire children, experience some negative feelings.

Some women are better able to cope with the **stressors of pregnancy**. These include women who have accomplished previous developmental tasks; women who have their physiological, safety, love, and belonging needs met; and women who have the support of their loved ones/significant others. The unwed teenager may have her physiological, safety, love and belonging needs threatened and may also be missing the support of the baby's father.

STRESSORS IN ADULT AND TEENAGE PREGNANCY

The pregnant teenager has a more difficult time adapting to the stressors of pregnancy (Table 8-1). She must face the normal hormonal, physical, and metabolic changes of pregnancy before she has had time to adjust to the changes of adolescence. She must adapt to the role of parenthood while still facing the role change to adulthood. She must accomplish Erikson's stage of identity and at the same time accomplish the stage of intimacy versus isolation. She must discover who she is as a mother before she discovers who she is as a person. Her search for independence is often blocked by the financial and emotional demands of pregnancy. Even in this sophisticated society, teenagers have a lack of knowledge about pregnancy and parenthood. This lack of knowledge gives rise to exaggerated and unrealistic fears. The young teenager's reasoning skill is still developing and she has not yet acquired the ability to look at things apart from the particular instance. Without this ability, she has difficulty recognizing the future consequences of her actions.

While she has more stressors to face, the adolescent has less coping ability. She is still growing, clarifying her values, and developing her self-concept. If her sexual partner refuses to acknowledge his participation or role, the girl's self-concept is lowered. Her family may also

TABLE 8-1 Stressors in Adult and Teenage Pregnancy

ADULT PREGNANCY	TEENAGE PREGNANCY
Cope with hormonal changes brought on by pregnancy	Cope with hormonal changes brought on by adolescence and hormonal changes brought on by pregnancy
Adjust to the role of parent	Adjust to the role of adult and adjust to the role of parent
Accomplish the stage of intimacy and begin the stage of generativity	Accomplish the stage of identity and the stage of intimacy, and simultaneously cope with the stage of generativity
	Develop independence while increasing dependency caused by pregnancy
	Develop cognitive abilities while often being forced to quit school
Take on responsibility for another person	Clarify own values and take on responsibility for a child
	Improve the self-concept in spite of a pregnancy, which tends to lessen it

reject her, which further lowers her self-worth as well as giving her added financial burdens.

Teenagers are categorized according to young, middle, and late adolescence. Pregnancy has been increasing in the youngest group. This young adolescent thinks in the present. She gives little thought to the possible effects of coitus. Knowledge of her body, pregnancy, and contraception is limited and what knowledge she does have is often incorrect. There is usually no lasting relationship between the young teen and her boyfriend. She often becomes pregnant following the first sexual experience. Denial is a common defense mechanism and she may deny the pregnancy even when it is evident to others. If she accepts the pregnancy, she often denies responsibility. This blame is placed on her sexual partner, who is then despised. Adoption is seldom considered. More often, the baby is turned over to the grandparents to raise as the mother's sibling.

The middle adolescent is a little more sophisticated in her knowledge. She is aware of the possible effects of coitus. She knows about contraceptives but many times fails to use them. There are many theories to explain this. If the girl uses contraceptives, she is obviously planning on having sexual relationships, which goes against her parentally instilled values and makes her a "bad" girl. If coitus is not planned, she can save her self-concept by blaming "the moment" or passion. Pregnancy is actually sought by some middle teens because it means maturity and independence to them. It may also be a rebellious act against her parents. In some groups, it is simply the "in" thing to do. Whatever the reason, the middle adolescent usually denies responsibility for the pregnancy. She often blames her parents.

The middle teen rarely has a desire to marry her boyfriend, but she does need his support. Without his support, she experiences increased anxiety. Even though she may have consciously or unconsciously sought the pregnancy, she often has unrealistic fantasies and ambivalent feelings about motherhood. The pregnant teen demonstrates her extreme anxiety through rebellion, anger, disinterest, and boredom, as well as numerous somatic complaints. She is usually very frightened of medical care and seeks care late, if at all. Because of anxiety and distrust of authority, she may be uncooperative during examinations and may not follow through on directions. The baby may be raised by the grandparents. In other cases, the teen is forced to assume complete care to the detriment of her education and social life.

The late adolescent girl frequently views her relationship with her sexual partner as meaningful and often has planned to marry him at some time in the future. Even if marriage is not sought when pregnancy is discovered, recognition and support from the sexual partner seems to be important. Although older adolescent males tend to accept responsibility for paternity more often than younger adolescents, the vast majority still reject the girl. Unfortunately, the older adolescent is also the one most often rejected by the family. This girl is able to recognize the financial, social, and emotional problems to be faced as a single mother. Without the needed support, she is apt to become depressed and to feel that no one cares. Although schools are now more lenient, the older adolescent is often forced to quit school because of financial and time constraints. Most pregnant adolescents keep their infants, but abortion and adoption are acceptable alternatives for some.

Nursing Care of the Unwed Pregnant Teenager

It is easy to stereotype all unwed pregnant adolescents, but they do not fit neatly into one category. Although there are many problems, some teenagers are proud of the pregnancy and look forward to the experience of motherhood. As with any other client, it is important that the nurse get to know the teenager.

> Mary Ann is fifteen years old. She presents herself at the clinic because she has missed some periods. She is not certain how many. She sits quietly while her blood pressure is taken and submits reluctantly to a weight check. She rebels at the vaginal examination, pushing the doctor away and screaming "Do not do that."

Mary Ann acted as she did because she was frightened of certain things that she did not understand. She was embarrassed, self-conscious, and distrustful of all the new people around her.

Before the nurse can effectively help Mary Ann, he or she must develop a trusting relationship. Trust takes time; several visits may be needed. It would be ideal if one nurse saw Mary Ann each time she came to the clinic. To develop trust, the nurse needs to explain all procedures before they are done in terms that the teenager understands. Mary Ann is still developing her ability to think in general rather than specific terms. Since she is experiencing stress, explanations should be in simple terms, using visual materials whenever possible. Developing trust also involves continuity, accepting Mary Ann without criticism, and providing understanding and concern.

Communicating with the adolescent is not easy. The nurse should not expect to discuss Mary Ann's needs on the first visit. Mary Ann, as other teenagers, is more apt to talk to a person with whom she has established trust. The average teenager communicates more with nonverbal methods. Therefore, the nurse can often be more effective with a smile or a look (Figure 8-2). Generally something that bothers

> Uses more nonverbal communications
>
> Responds literally to questions
>
> May have different meaning for words or use neologisms
>
> May not be aware of feelings or have words to express feelings
>
> Frequently repeats because of fear of being misunderstood

FIGURE 8-2 Characteristics of the Adolescent Communication Pattern.

the teenager will surface nonverbally. However, few adolescents will offer information without direct questioning. Young and middle teenagers think in specific terms and respond literally to questions. If the nurse asks "Can you tell me about it?" the answer is likely to be simply "Yeah." To get the right answer, the nurse should say "Tell me about it." Teens also use the language differently.

Nurse:	"I hear you have a new motorbike."
Client:	"Oh yeah, it's cosmo."
Nurse:	"It's cosmo! What does that mean?"
Client:	"You're really a squid. It's qual, real bad."
Nurse:	"You mean it's cool?"
Client:	"Right. It's a b-a-a-d bike."

To express confusion, a teen may say, "I don't have my head on straight" or "I'm hung over." A "bummer" means things are not good.

Young and middle adolescents may not be aware of their feelings or they may not have the words to express their feelings. When an adolescent describes an experience, she may start over several times because she has a fear of not being understood. It takes good observation and timing to initiate therapeutic communication with the adolescent.

Nurse:	"You look like you have lost your last friend. Bad news, Mary Ann?"
Client:	"Nah, piece of cake."
Nurse:	"But I see you have a sad face. What did the doctor tell you?"
Client:	"Oh, nothing."
Nurse:	"He confirmed the pregnancy, didn't he?"
Client:	"It's a real bummer."

Sometimes the nurse must take the initiative, such as "Mary Ann, there are some things we need to discuss." This is less effective because the adolescent may or may not comply.

To determine Mary Ann's needs, the nurse should gather information about:

- What pregnancy and parenthood mean to her
- Her level of anxiety
- What effect the pregnancy has on her relationship with her family and her boyfriend
- With what other developmental stressors she is dealing
- The level of her need for fulfillment according to Maslow (Are her physiological, safety, love, and belonging needs being met?)
- How she sees her situation
- What plans she has for herself and her baby
- What she feels she needs from the nurse

The nursing team may then determine that she has the following strengths and weaknesses:

Strengths	Weaknesses
She accepts responsibility for the pregnancy	She has not told her family and fears rejection
She has continued support from her boyfriend	Her future plans are vague
The school has a program for pregnant teens	She has an unrealistic view of pregnancy and parenthood
She feels she needs preparation for labor and delivery and parenthood	Her physical, safety, love and belonging needs are threatened
She has the support of her boyfriend's parents	

Mary Ann, like all teenagers, needs the support of her family. She may need help in gaining it. A referral to social services or a visiting nurse might provide support when she tells her parents. Mary Ann also may benefit from modeling. Modeling would demonstrate how she might talk to her family. If the family rejects her, she will need a referral for financial assistance and shelter.

Since Mary Ann expressed the need for education, this should be given priority. This need can be met in a group with other teenagers or individually during her clinic visits. Preparation for labor should include relaxation exercises and some type of breathing techniques to lessen anxiety during labor. Probably the most important thing the nurse can do for Mary Ann, and teenagers like her, is to provide support and be there when she needs someone.

During labor, Mary Ann has the same needs as any other mother: relief of pain, information, and emotional support. She needs to have the person she trusts, whether it be her mother, her boyfriend, or both, with her.

To help the young mother after birth, the nurse should manipulate the environment to provide success experiences for her. She should provide compliments and gently correct mistakes. If the girl decides to keep her baby, rooming-in should be encouraged so that the mother can learn to care for her infant with the nurse's help. If she is planning on putting the baby up for adoption, she may want to see the child and care for it while the baby is in the hospital. When the baby is adopted, she will face separation anxiety, but not seeing the baby often causes lasting anxiety. Since the young mother is in the hospital for such a short time, referral for home health nursing service is usually indicated.

PRIMARY BONDING

Primary bonding is the process of establishing an intimate interdependent attachment among mother, father, and infant (Figure 8-3). Research on bonding, which began to surface in the 1960s indicates that bonding is important to the child's future interpersonal relationships. It also shows that infants not bonded to their mothers in the critical immediate postpartum period were more apt to be abused and neglected. Children who were not bonded experienced more anxiety and were less able to cope with stress. The bonded person is the child's primary support.

Bonding normally begins in the prenatal period when the mother feels **quickening** (the first movements of the baby.) The mother then can be seen massaging her growing abdomen, delighting in fetal movements, and talking to the fetus. The immediate postpartum period seems to be most crucial. Some mothers who have had negative feelings about being pregnant have effectively bonded to the infant during the time just after birth. Although bonding may occur late, it seems to be more difficult and intervention is usually essential.

Natural bonding is initiated by either the parent or the infant through behavior to which the other person responds. The baby cries and the mother picks the baby up and cuddles him or her. The baby stops crying and molds himself or herself to the mother's body. The

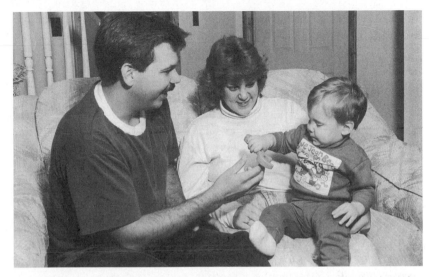

FIGURE 8-3 Some bonding behaviors are eye-to-eye contact and holding the baby no more than 17 inches from the parent's face.

mother further responds by smiling. Eye contact, skin-to-skin contact, and touching seem to be essential to the process (Figure 8-4). If not interfered with, bonding occurs automatically. The process can be enhanced prenatally and postnatally.

Bonding is encouraged prenatally by allowing parents to listen to fetal heart tones, teaching them to massage the mother's abdomen, and showing them how to feel and recognize fetal parts. In the post-natal period, the parent is taught to hold the infant no more than seventeen inches from the face. The infant cannot see clearly beyond seventeen inches. Eye-to-eye contact is important. Talking to the infant should be encouraged. Some mothers feel uncomfortable talking to an infant. They may feel as if they are talking to a doll or a wall. The nurse can help by pointing out the baby's responses.

Eye-to-eye contact at no more than 17 inches distance

Skin-to-skin contact

Touching and stroking

Speech in high-pitched voice

Cuddling

Baby care

FIGURE 8-4 Factors that enhance bonding.

Allowing the mother to care for the baby, including feeding, changing diapers, and bathing, also encourages bonding. The young mother in particular should be encouraged to provide physical care for her infant. Rooming-in helps the bonding process. The nurse supervising the infant's care should compliment the mother and minimize corrections. If the mother is having difficulty with the baby's care and becomes upset, it is important that the nurse not take over. The mother sometimes believes the baby evaluates her against the more skilled nurse and her self-concept is lowered. Of course this is not true, but it is nonetheless a real concern to the mother. Instead of taking over, the nurse should help the mother to relax and then assist her with suggestions. If the environment is manipulated to give the mother success, her self-concept is enhanced.

The unwed teenager sometimes opts to turn her baby over to her mother to raise, hoping to later assume the mothering role. This may be impossible. The infant who has bonded to the grandmother may refuse to relate to the teen as a mother.

COPING WITH A STILLBORN OR MALFORMED INFANT

Whenever a problem in delivery occurs or is anticipated, at times the father is banned or banished from the scene. The infant is then taken quickly to the nursery, and bonding with both parents is interrupted. If the mother is awake, she quickly becomes aware that something is wrong and anxiety results. If she is anesthetized, anxiety is only delayed.

Parents dream of having a perfect child. When a malformed or seriously ill infant is born, the parents must grieve for the loss of the dream child before they can even begin to accept the real child. Denial is often the mechanism used. Denial is manifested by a refusal to name the baby, by refusing to see, touch, or talk to the baby. The parents may withdraw. They may accuse the hospital of changing babies or of not doing what they could to save the infant. The parents often feel guilty about malformations and wonder what they have done to cause it. They are embarrassed and feel inadequate as people. Having a malformed child can be a blow to the self-concept.

Sometimes the mother is given a tranquilizer to help calm her. Rather than delay the grief process, it is better to handle it with the support of the nursing staff. Denial may lessen anxiety, but the problem still remains. The parents should see the child as early as possible. No matter how deformed the child is, reality is usually less disturbing than the parents' imagination.

The mother should be the one to make the choice of moving to a private room or off the floor. If she decides to leave the maternity floor, she should be allowed to return whenever desired. The maternity nurse should at least visit her and keep her informed of the baby's progress.

Parents have the right to truthful information. Though it is generally the doctor's responsibility to keep them informed, the nurse should be prepared to answer questions. The parents need to be encouraged to talk together and share their feelings. Though talking may seem difficult and the parents may cry or become angry, it must be remembered that it is the event that is disturbing, not the talking about it. Talking brings out the hurt, but it also allows the event to be faced. Denial only delays problem solving.

Nurses often neglect the mother with a malformed child because they experience anxiety themselves and do not know what to say. The nurse's withdrawal only adds to the parent's anxiety. The nurse can best help by letting the parents know it is all right to talk about their feelings if they desire (Figure 8-5). Many times parents feel they must maintain a facade for nurses and visitors. The nurse can give the parents permission to talk by saying "Would you like to talk about it?" or "I will be here if you would like to talk," or "Getting it out sometimes helps." The nurse can then take cues from the parents. "What can I do to help you?" "Would it help if I called your minister?" "Would you like to see the baby?" or "Would you feel better if I limited your visitors?" False reassurances such as "Your baby is going to be all right" are never helpful. The parent is not ready to hear statements such as "At least you have a healthy child at home" or "You are still young, you may have other children."

- ■ To be given continuous and truthful information about the baby's progress
- ■ To be encouraged to discuss feelings with spouse
- ■ To have nonjudgmental acceptance of behavior
- ■ To be given the chance to ventilate feelings if desired
- ■ To be given emotional support
- ■ To have periodic visits from the nursing staff if transferred off the maternity floor
- ■ To see and touch the baby
- ■ To be able to withdraw, if necessary, without being labeled a rejecting parent

FIGURE 8-5 Needs of the parents of a malformed infant.

The nurse should point out the baby's healthy aspects. If the child has a name, it should be used and the child should always be referred to by the correct sex. As they care for the child, nurses should be alert for signs of anxiety in the mother and allow her to withdraw from the child if the mother feels the need.

If the infant dies or was born dead, allowing the parents to see the child prevents denial. The infant may have been severely deformed and the death anticipated, but the event is still stressful. This parent, too, needs to have time with the baby to complete the grief process. Crying should be encouraged. Nurses may also feel like crying. By doing so, they share the sadness with the parents.

POSTPARTUM DEPRESSION

As previously stated, pregnancy is a significant stressor with normal mood fluctuations. Depressive symptoms may occur or, if already present, may worsen. The continuing stigma of mental illness contributes to the underreporting of depressive symptoms by pregnant and lactating women. Some contributing factors to depression during pregnancy and lactation are:

- Chronic financial strain
- Everyday life hassles
- Disrupted or abusive relationships
- Unstable housing arrangements
- Social isolation
- Hormonal influences and fluctuations
- History of depression or medical problems
- Lack of community resources

Postdelivery, some women may have a brief period of the "blues," while other women are clinically depressed or psychotic. It is important to recognize the symptoms of postpartum depression:

- Letdown feeling
- Irritability
- Loss of appetite
- Insomnia
- Anxiety

The mother cries easily and may complain of discomfort and an inability to concentrate. It is important to differentiate the symptoms of postpartum blues and postpartum depression in terms of the number of episodes, intensity, and persistence of symptoms.

Mild depression occurs in a large proportion of postpartum women. It usually begins two or three days after the delivery and disappears within a week or two. Approximately 40 percent of women with mild depression have symptoms that persist for a year.

This mother needs to know that her depression is normal and that the symptoms will disappear. She must be able to verbalize her feelings. Rest and nutrition should be encouraged and it is essential that any new mother have help in the home at least for the first few days. The cause of **postpartum depression** is not known, but it is thought to be due to hormonal changes and perhaps, partly, to the mother's reaction to her changing role. It is important to recognize the symptoms of a depressed mood throughout pregnancy as it is a significant factor when considering postpartum depression. Educating clients and their significant others (husband, partner, and/or grandparents) about postpartum depression and postpartum blues is beneficial.

About 1 to 2 percent of new mothers have severe depression that requires intervention. Severe depression affects the relationship between the mother and her infant. She may be overprotective or reject the child. She may have delusions and endanger the child's life. Severe depression has many times gone undetected until the infant has been harmed. Early detection is essential, so that appropriate care can be provided. Treatment includes medications, behavioral management, or, at times, electroconvulsive therapy.

MOTHERS WITH MENTAL DISORDERS

When a woman with a serious mental disorder is pregnant, a major consideration is the risk versus the benefit of continued use of psychotropic medication. Antipsychotics, atypical antipsychotics, mood stabilizers, antidepressants, and anxiolytic medications can have teratogenic effects on the fetus/neonate. **Teratogenic** effects that may arise from medication use are miscarriage, premature delivery, malformed neonate, and neonate adaptation problems postdelivery.

Some of the literature indicates that pregnancy and lactation in a mother with mental illness can be managed in a safe manner, especially when there is increased collaboration between the multiple providers (obstetrics, primary care, and mental health). If the mother's psychotropic medication is discontinued and an acute episode of mental illness occurs, the fetus/neonate is also at grave risk. Women with serious mental illnesses need more comprehensive education/information about day-to-day parenting skills, family planning, (birth control), mother/infant bonding, and child custody issues. Consider the fact that some mothers with mental illness are not the custodial parent, as their child/children may reside with their grandparent(s), reside in a foster home, or the parental rights of the parent have been terminated. Due to the complexity of these issues, women's mental health is a major issue of the millennium. Continued research is needed in the areas of pregnancy and lactation and their relationship to a woman's mental health and women's rights.

THE HOSPITALIZED CHILD

The child's response to hospitalization depends in part on his or her developmental stage. Very young children do not understand why they must be hospitalized and often see it as punishment. If the child has any concept of illness, it is thought to be due to disobedience. Although **regression** is a defense mechanism observed in all age groups, it is most common in the very young child. One who has been drinking from a cup may seek comfort in a bottle during hospitalization.

When the hospitalized child is removed from all that is familiar, he or she looks to the bonded person for support. If that person is missing, anxiety increases. This is known as separation anxiety, which is normally seen in children between seven months and three years of age. In the hospital, separation anxiety may be seen in children up to four or five years of age and occasionally in older children. When the parent leaves, the child exhibiting separation anxiety responds with temper tantrums, crying, and attempts at clinging to the parent. It is important to the child that at least one parent remain and participate in his or her care if at all possible. If both parents must leave, they need to understand that separation anxiety is a normal reaction. The child who is old enough to understand should be told that the parent is leaving but will return. It is best that the parent not sneak away. The nurse should be sure that the child has his or her security blanket or a favorite toy nearby.

Although preschoolers still see hospitalization as punishment, there is an increased awareness of the hospital experience. Fantasies are common; intrusive procedures can be made very frightening through fantasy. The preschooler knows the missing parent will return. However, he or she worries that the parent will not be able to find him or her, particularly if the child is moved. Bleeding is extremely frightening as children think all their blood may come out. A small bandage often lessens anxiety as effectively as a kiss.

The school-age child's hospitalization causes anxiety mainly because of immobility, a possibility of bodily harm, and a loss of friends and parents. This child may be embarrassed when forced to surrender privacy. Though he or she is not expected to have separation anxiety, the child sees the loss of parents as a stress and is relieved when the parent is around. This child's concept of illness is dependent in part on the parent's concept of illness. It is generally a simple concept: most children fear mutilation of the body.

If the school-age child is not in pain, he or she may actually enjoy staying in the hospital. It may mean a recess from schoolwork and added attention. It may represent a change in routine, and the child may enjoy experimenting with the many push buttons in the unit.

The adolescent who is attempting to gain independence is thwarted by illness and hospitalization. He or she must submit to sometimes strict rules and regulations. The adolescent may be told what he or she can and cannot eat, when and how to move, and activities in which he or she may and may not engage. Illness that affects the body image is more frightening to the young adolescent, but the increased attention of the medical and nursing staff may be welcome. The young teen often accepts the diagnosis but is optimistic about the prognosis.

The middle adolescent finds his or her independence threatened. Hospitalization limits association with friends, intrudes on privacy, and makes the teen less attractive. The more visible the condition, the more distressing it is to the middle teen.

The older adolescent is more stable. He or she can understand illness and the effects it may have on future life. The teen sees serious illness as being the most threatening. Friends primarily comprise his or her support system.

Coping Methods of the Hospitalized Child

Other factors that affect the child's response to hospitalization are past experiences, the child's support system , the child's coping methods, and parental separation anxiety. If the previous hospital experience has been good and the child has learned to trust the nursing staff, readmission is less traumatic. Almost all children benefit by the presence of the parent. Children seem to adapt to hospitalization better if they have close relationships with their parents. Nurses may find some parents difficult, but they are important to the child. Therefore, the nurse needs to make the parents feel welcome. He or she should keep the parents informed about what is happening to their child and why.

Play is a major source of support. It relieves boredom and tension. Also, the children learn through play. The child can learn about hospital procedures and better ways of handling stress. Play helps the young child communicate. All children need age-related toys (Table 8-2). Infants like bright mobiles, busy boxes, and rattles. The adolescent wants a radio or telephone.

The very young child copes by crying and clinging to the parent. The child who is able to use language may ask questions to relieve

TABLE 8-2 Examples of Age-related Toys.

INFANT	TODDLER	PRESCHOOL	SCHOOL	ADOLESCENT
Mobiles	Push toys	Blocks	Action dolls	Radio
Busy boxes	Stuffed animals	Cars	Models	Telephone
Rattles	Dolls	Trucks	Books	Puzzles
		Dolls	Puzzles	Books
		Stuffed animals	Video games	Video games

stress. *How* and *why* are common words in the preschool group. At other times, children display dependence by saying "Will you stay with me?" or hostility with "I will hit you." Regression to a more secure stage of development is most common in this age group.

Denial is the most common mechanism seen in children and adolescents, but the denial is usually temporary. Children who use denial do not accept the extent of their illness. They may be uncooperative, overcomplaisant, or even stoic about painful procedures. Another mechanism is intellectualization. Children who use this method disassociate themselves from the illness and view it objectively. They display an interest in factual aspects; it is as if they were discussing someone else.

Some children cope by acting out. Children who act out exhibit aggression and uncooperativeness. These children may disconnect IV from their arms, hide their medications, or refuse to stay in bed. Children who are depressed often act out. Almost all children use manipulation, which effectively lessens anxiety.

Children need to know what procedures will be done and forewarned about discomfort. The information needs to be presented in a way the child understands. Puppets, storytelling, games, and handling equipment are ways of preparing children for procedures. Preschool children need to follow their usual routine. School-age children need to know that their things at home will not be disturbed while they are away. All children need to have their life routines changed as little as possible for a sense of security.

SUMMARY

Pregnancy is a developmental stressor for every woman, but for the pregnant teenager stress is increased. She must cope with the stressors of adolescence as well as those of pregnancy. Her basic needs may be threatened, and she may be missing the support of her sexual partner.

Teenagers are categorized into young, middle, and late adolescence. The young adolescent often becomes pregnant following the first sexual experience. Denial is the mechanism commonly used. Blame is usually placed on the sexual partner. The baby is generally turned over to the grandmother to be raised as the mother's sibling.

The middle adolescent may choose pregnancy for various reasons. It may mean maturity and independence or it may be an act of rebellion against her parents. In some groups it is simply the "in" thing to do. Denial of responsibility is often seen is this age group. The middle adolescent needs the support of her sexual partner. She often has unrealistic and ambivalent feelings toward motherhood. The middle teen is usually an anxious and frightened child. She may be rebellious, angry, disinterested, or bored. She may offer numerous somatic complaints in exhibiting her anxiety.

The late adolescent often intends to marry her sexual partner, whose support is important to her. Although many older adolescent boys accept paternity, the vast majority still reject the girl. The older adolescent is able to recognize the many problems of being a single parent. Abortion and adoption are alternatives.

Teenagers cannot be stereotyped; it is important for the nurse to get to know the adolescent parent. Trust is an essential component of the helping relationship. Developing trust may require several visits. The nurse needs to listen, assist with meeting the needs identified by the teenager, and offer support. Education for labor and parenthood is the most common need expressed.

Communicating with a teenager may be difficult because the adolescent uses language differently and responds literally to questions. Teenagers may not be aware of their feelings or they may not have the words to express their feelings.

Nursing care should be based on an assessment of the mother's strengths and weaknesses. Since the young mother is in the hospital for such a short time, referral to a home health service is usually indicated.

Bonding is the process of establishing an intimate attachment among the infant, mother, and father. Bonding is very important to the child's future interpersonal relationships and ability to handle stress. The immediate postnatal period seems to be a critical time for bonding. Skin-to-skin contact, touching, and eye contact are essential to the bonding process. The nurse can help to enhance the bonding process by encouraging these activities.

When a malformed or deceased infant is born, the parents must grieve for the dream child before they can begin to accept the real child. Denial is a mechanism often used. It is often fostered by the health care professionals, who provide tranquilizers and may offer to move the mother off the maternity floor. The mother should be the one to make the choice of moving to a private room or to another department. If the mother decides to move, she should be visited by the nursing staff so she does not feel forgotten.

Parents need to have truthful information about their child's condition and be encouraged to talk together regarding their feelings. The nurse can best help by letting the parent know it is all right to talk about the event and by following the parent's cues. The nurse can point out the baby's healthy aspects. The child's name and sex should be used. The nurse needs to be alert to signs of anxiety in the parent.

Mild depression occurs in a large percentage of postpartum clients. It lasts only one to two weeks and requires no treatment. The mother, however, needs support, understanding, rest, and nutrition. Severe depression occurs in 1 to 2 percent of postpartum clients and requires immediate detection and treatment. When a woman with a serious mental disorder becomes pregnant, the risk versus benefit of continuing medication must be considered. Collaboration between all providers (obstetrics, primary care, and mental health) must occur as a protection to both mother and child.

The child's response to hospitalization depends on the developmental level of the child and the parents' concept of illness. Other factors are previous hospitalizations, the child's support system, and the child's coping methods.

The hospitalized child has been removed from all that is familiar. He or she is sometimes subjected to embarrassing procedures and strict rules. There is often an interruption in his or her developmental needs.

The hospitalized child should have a parent near and be told what is going to happen and why. His or her routine should be changed as little as possible. Children cope with stress in different ways. The very young child cries, has tantrums, and clings to the parent. Older children may use denial, intellectualization, acting out, and manipulation.

SUGGESTED ACTIVITIES

- Attend a prenatal class in which preparation for labor and delivery is discussed.
- Volunteer time in a home for unwed mothers, if one is available in your area.

■ Spend a day with a play therapist. Observe the therapist's responses to and effects on children.

■ Plan an age-appropriate activity for a pediatric client.

■ Make a list of bonding behaviors observed while visiting or caring for a mother and her newborn.

■ With a small group of classmates, discuss feelings towards the birth of a malformed child.

REVIEW

KNOW AND COMPREHEND
A. Multiple choice. Select the one best answer.

1. Which factor contributes to emotional manifestations of pregnancy?
   - ❑ A. psychotic disorders
   - ❑ B. somatic disorders
   - ❑ C. neurotic disorders
   - ❑ D. normal physiological changes

2. Which developmental tasks must the pregnant teen accomplish?
   - ❑ A. autonomy and generativity
   - ❑ B. trust and initiative
   - ❑ C. identity and intimacy
   - ❑ D. autonomy and identity

3. Select the factor commonly present when a middle adolescent becomes pregnant.
   - ❑ A. ignorance
   - ❑ B. failure of birth-control methods
   - ❑ C. overwhelming passion
   - ❑ D. rebellion against her parents

4. Bonding should be encouraged because it
   - ❑ A. assures that the child will not be abused.
   - ❑ B. prevents postnatal complications and depression.
   - ❑ C. aids in involution and hormonal stability.
   - ❑ D. is important in the child's future interpersonal relationships.

5. When teaching parents to hold their infants, which instruction would the nurse include to promote bonding? "Hold the infant:
   - ❏ A. no more than 17 inches from the face."
   - ❏ B. only when the child is wrapped securely."
   - ❏ C. in the football hold for safety and ease in handling."
   - ❏ D. away from the face to avoid disease transmission."

6. Which defense mechanism would the nurse expect from parents of a malformed child?
   - ❏ A. rationalization
   - ❏ B. intellectualization
   - ❏ C. denial
   - ❏ D. reaction formation

7. The mother of a malformed child can best be helped by
   - ❏ A. giving a tranquilizer to alleviate anxiety.
   - ❏ B. being transferred from the stressful maternity department.
   - ❏ C. making her face reality and forcing her to touch the infant.
   - ❏ D. allowing her to talk about her feelings if she desires.

8. Which defense mechanism is most commonly seen in the very young hospitalized child?
   - ❏ A. denial
   - ❏ B. regression
   - ❏ C. fantasy
   - ❏ D. identification

9. Select the most common defense mechanism seen in the young, pregnant adolescent.
   - ❏ A. denial
   - ❏ B. regression
   - ❏ C. fantasy
   - ❏ D. identification

10. Which stressor is most likely to cause anxiety in a hospitalized, school-age child?
    - ❏ A. immobility
    - ❏ B. lack of opportunity for creativity
    - ❏ C. missing school
    - ❏ D. loss of independence

APPLY YOUR LEARNING

B. Multiple choice. Select the one best answer.

1. Which of the following women would be best prepared to cope adaptively with the emotional stressors of pregnancy? A woman who
    - ❏ A. is actively pursuing her nursing education, with a goal to work in critical care.
    - ❏ B. was recently diagnosed with multiple sclerosis and is learning about the disease.
    - ❏ C. is resolving feelings about her abusive childhood through intensive psychotherapy.
    - ❏ D. planned the pregnancy, is excited about being a mother, and lives with a loving family.

2. The nurse meets a pregnant adolescent during her first visit to a prenatal clinic. Which comment by the nurse would be most effective to begin the relationship?
    - ❏ A. "What birth control method were you using when you got pregnant?"
    - ❏ B. "I'm a nurse. Before we talk, I'd like to show you around the clinic."
    - ❏ C. "How do you plan to continue your education during your pregnancy?"
    - ❏ D. "Are you feeling happy or sad about your pregnancy?"

3. A woman in her second trimester of pregnancy lightly massages her abdomen and smiles. The nurse would interpret that which event is occurring?
    - ❏ A. bonding
    - ❏ B. contractions
    - ❏ C. pain
    - ❏ D. spasms

4. These statements are made by women in their third trimester of pregnancy. Which woman needs nursing support for bonding?
    - ❏ A. "I like to sing to my baby, even though I'm still pregnant."
    - ❏ B. "I want to listen to my baby's heartbeat with your stethoscope."
    - ❏ C. "The fetus interrupts my sleep by moving so much."
    - ❏ D. "I think my baby has grown a lot in the last week."

5. An infant is born with a cleft palate. Which nursing strategy would be most important to the parents' successful coping?
  ❏ A. Give support and encourage the parents to hold and cuddle the infant.
  ❏ B. Explain to the parents how cleft palates develop during pregnancy.
  ❏ C. Tell the parents not to look directly at the infant's mouth.
  ❏ D. Show the parents a video about corrective surgeries for cleft palate.

C. Briefly answer the following.

1. Name four stressors of pregnancy that the teenager must face.

2. Name three actions essential to the bonding process.

3. Discuss two areas of education/information a woman with a serious mental disorder needs postdelivery of her child.

Maladaptive Behaviors

OUTLINE

KEY TERMS

maladaptive behavior

normal

abnormal

anxiety

panic

agoraphobia

phobia

obsession

compulsion

conversion disorder

hypochondriasis

anhedonia

anorexia nervosa

bulimia

associative looseness

autism

ambivalence

affect

word salad

neologism

echolalia

delusion

hallucination

tardive dyskinesia (TD)

neuroleptic malignant
  syndrome (NMS)

waxy flexibility

paranoid

schizoid

schizotypal

histrionic

narcissistic

antisocial

borderline

milieu

OBJECTIVES

After studying this chapter, the student should be able to:

- State three aspects of adaptive and maladaptive behaviors.
- Describe two psychological disorders.
- List cautions to be taken when a client is prescribed anti-anxiety medication.
- List the signs and symptoms of major depressive disorder (MDD).
- List the signs and symptoms of bipolar disorder (BPD).
- Differentiate between dysthymia and cyclothymia.
- Identify medications prescribed, benefits of use, and side effects of antidepressants and antimanic medications.
- List four types of dissociative disorders.
- List four symptoms of an eating disorder.
- Describe three positive and three negative symptoms observed in schizophrenic disorders.

- Identify three antipsychotic medications as well as the benefits of use and side effects.
- Describe the Abnormal Involuntary Movements (AIMS) test.
- Describe characteristics of three personality disorders.
- Describe characteristics of attention-deficit hyperactive disorder (ADHD).
- List five behavioral changes noted in a sleep protocol.
- Discuss milieu therapy.

Maladaptive behavior is the inability to act or react to a particular condition or situation in an appropriate manner. Maladaptive behaviors are very complex. The person with a mental illness is unable to adjust to the world in which he or she lives. During childhood, the person may have learned methods of coping that are costly in terms of adaptive energy and that may be considered abnormal by society. These coping methods may be ineffective but also may be the only way the individual knows to manage his or her problems. Maladaptive behaviors can develop at any time from infancy through old age. Three critical stages are adolescence, menopause, and old age. Stress is experienced during every developmental stage, and coping activity is required throughout the entire life cycle. Problems in any area can contribute to maladaptive behavior.

When studying mental disorders, remember the brain is a complex center with many neurotransmitters, chemicals, and critical pathways. An abnormality of structure, an imbalance of neurotransmitters, a traumatic brain injury (TBI), infectious diseases (encephalitis, meningitis), and cerebral abscesses can impair brain functioning.

THE MEANING OF NORMAL AND ABNORMAL

The word **normal** has a social, clinical, moral, and statistical aspect. It includes a wide range of acceptable behaviors. In the social sense, normal is concerned with actions that fit the social rules. The person who follows the rules of a particular society is considered normal if he or she adapts to society norms. For example, self-sacrifice is considered normal in some cultures but abnormal in other cultures. Social rules are important in any culture. People become disturbed if rules change too quickly.

Clinical normal is subjective. It is concerned with whether the individual sees himself or herself as being normal; therefore, it is a personal consideration. The question is how well the person is satisfied with self. Is he or she in control of personal behavior? Is the person happy?

Moralistic normal is an ideal. It concerns setting and attaining goals that may be expected by society or by the person. Individuals may become conditioned to a specific ideal. For example, they may continually tell themselves they are not allowed to become irritable and must remain calm at all times. Setting unrealistic or impossible goals creates unnecessary stress.

The statistical concept of normal is based on the number of people engaging in specific behaviors. Statistics deal with numbers. If a behavior is practiced by the majority of people, it is statistically normal.

There are many misconceptions concerning the word **abnormal**. To many people, the word means weird or bizarre. Some people expect to see a sharp difference between normal and abnormal, but there are many variations between the two. The disturbed person often exhibits normal behaviors. Behaviors found in persons with mental illness also may be found in the normal individual under certain circumstances. *Maladaptive behaviors* are the reaction of an individual to stress, so there is no clear-cut line between normal and abnormal.

Psychiatry categorizes patterns of behavior. The nurse must realize that clients do not fit neatly into these categories because their patterns of behavior are individual reactions to stress. A diagnosis in psychiatry is not as clearly defined as a physical diagnosis. The nurse should be fully aware that the client does not necessarily conform to a set standard of diagnosed behavior.

PSYCHOLOGICAL DISORDERS

Psychological disorders are emotional disturbances characterized by maladaptive behavior aimed at avoiding anxiety. These disorders were formerly classified as psychoneuroses or neuroses. Since the psychological disorder represents a poor adaptation to stress, there is a crippling of personality growth. Suffering from a psychological disorder keeps a person from attaining full potential. A psychological disorder may occur at any time during the life cycle. Bed-wetting, temper tantrums, extreme shyness, nail biting, excessive fear, and a poor school record may be early symptoms of a psychological disorder.

Individuals with psychological disorders maintain contact with their environments. However, people with psychological disorders lack awareness and so lack control over their behavior.

Common psychological disorders are:

- Panic disorder
- Anxiety disorder
- Phobic disorder
- Social phobia/anxiety disorder
- Obsessive-compulsive disorder

Anxiety Disorder

Every individual experiences **anxiety** at some time during the life cycle (see Chapter 4). A situation such as a final exam can produce symptoms of anxiety. These symptoms include nausea, anorexia, dry mouth, diarrhea, tachycardia, difficulty in swallowing, and a nervous stomach. Anxiety may be classified as mild, moderate, or severe. During mild or moderate anxiety, there are usually manifestations of rapid speech patterns and irregular voice tones. There are attempts made to block communication, such as changing the subject of the conversation. When anxiety is so widespread that it is not associated with a specific object or situation, it is called free-floating anxiety. Severe, overwhelming anxiety is called panic. Panic causes the individual to feel helpless and immobilized.

An anxiety disorder is characterized by anxiety that is disproportionate to stressors. The anxiety may occur periodically or it may be constant. Anxiety attacks may be brought on by even mild stress, or they may occur for no apparent reason.

The person with an anxiety disorder cannot relax. He or she becomes restless and irritable and continually overreacts to stressful situations. The person may experience loss of appetite, heart palpitations, and increased respirations. If the anxiety is severe or prolonged, these symptoms intensify and the person may need to be hospitalized. Antianxiety medication may be given (Table 9-1).

Panic Disorder

Panic attacks can be spontaneous or situational and characterized as major or minor attacks with anticipatory anxiety or situational **panic**. Sudden anxiety attacks occur with little or no provocation. Some anxiety episodes occur when a person anticipates facing a fearful situation. Repeated spontaneous panic attacks cause anticipatory anxiety that results in avoidance behaviors. An example is **agoraphobia**, the irrational fear of being in open spaces (e.g., shopping malls and sports arenas). Symptoms of panic include difficulty breathing, rapid and/or irregular heart rate, chest pain, choking or smothering sensation, dizziness, fear of dying, sweating, trembling or shaking, and fear of going crazy. A panic attack diary is important and should include: type of attack, length, intensity, time of day, number of symptoms and precipitating events.

Anxiety attacks may be caused by repressed feelings of anger and frustration. They may also be caused by trying to achieve unrealistically high goals and standards. Anxiety disorders include several subtypes: social phobia, phobic, and obsessive-compulsive disorders.

TABLE 9-1 Antianxiety Medications

TRADE	GENERIC
BuSpar/buspirone HCl	Klonopin/clonazepam
Xanax	Alprazolam
Ativan	Lorazepam
Valium	Diazepam
Librium	Chlordiazepoxide HCl
Benefit gained:	Short-term relief from intolerable anxiety
Side effects:	Increased appetite
	Headache
	Muscular weakness
	Poor coordination
	Impaired judgment
	Menstrual irregularities
Caution:	*Never* drink alcohol while on this medication
	Watch for drowsiness—do not drive a car
	or operate heavy equipment
	Dependence and tolerance may occur
	Abrupt discontinuance may result in
	insomnia
	agitation
	nervousness with trembling
	seizures

Social Phobia/Anxiety

A person with social phobia has anxiety or fear of particular situations (for example, public speaking, eating in public, using public restrooms, making a telephone call from a public phone). This anxiety is based on humiliation or embarrassment, and the coping pattern is avoidance or escape from the situation. Serious consequences resulting in impaired relationships, failure to achieve educational or vocational goals, and financial difficulties can lead to the comorbidity of depression and/or alcohol or substance abuse.

Phobia Disorder

A **phobia** is an abnormal, excessive fear of a specific situation or object. The person with a phobia realizes that the fear is unreasonable, but he or she is not able to control it. Phobias usually begin with repressed conflicts that produce anxiety. In an effort to control the anxiety, the person converts the anxiety into fear of a specific object. The person can then avoid the object and thus control the anxiety.

When a phobia is limited, the person can live a reasonably comfortable life simply by avoiding the object of fear. However, phobias often spread to include associated objects. When this happens, it may be difficult or impossible to keep the phobia from interfering with daily living. One treatment often used to help people overcome phobias is desensitization.

Phobias include exaggerated fears of death, snakes, dogs, open spaces, confinement, or heights. Table 9-2 lists some common phobias.

Obsessive-Compulsive Disorder

Although different in meaning, obsession and compulsion often occur together. An **obsession** is a persistent, recurring thought or feeling that is overpowering. A **compulsion** is an irresistible urge to engage in a behavior. Compulsion may be in the form of frequent handwashing or shoplifting. Whatever the compulsion may be, it has a symbolic meaning. The behavior is engaged in because it lowers anxiety. When the anxiety level builds up, the obsessive-compulsive act is performed again. This process is cyclic and may occupy the person's entire life.

It is not unusual for a person to experience recurrent thoughts periodically or to engage in ritualistic behaviors (handwashing, counting and recounting, checking and rechecking). However, in the person with an obsessive-compulsive disorder, these thoughts and ritualistic actions interfere with daily living. The person is unable to control his

TABLE 9-2 Some Common Phobias

PHOBIA	FEAR OF	PHOBIA	FEAR OF
Acrophobia	Heights	Laliophobia	Speaking
Agoraphobia	Open spaces	Necrophobia	Death
Algophobia	Pain	Olfactophobia	Odor
Androphobia	Man	Ophidophobia	Snakes
Claustrophobia	Being closed in	Pharmacophobia	Medicine
Cynophobia	Dogs	Phasmophobia	Ghosts
Demophobia	Crowds	Ponophobia	Work
Gamophobia	Marriage	Pyrophobia	Fire
Hodophobia	Travel	Traumatophobia	Injury
Kainophobia	Change	Triskardekaphobia	Number 13
Kakorrhaphiophobia	Failure	Vaccinophobia	Vaccination

or her thoughts and actions even though the person knows they are irrational; however irrational, they release pent-up anxiety and tension.

Obsessive-compulsive behavior is often caused by repressed thoughts and feelings. It is an attempt to relieve anxiety and is another example of converting anxiety into other symptoms.

Somatoform Disorder

Somatoform disorders are characterized by a loss or an alteration of physical functioning that has no physical basis. It is thought the physical impairment is caused by a psychological conflict or need of the person. However, it must be remembered that the symptoms are very real—the person does not have conscious control over them. Somatoform disorders are divided into several subtypes. Two common subtypes are *conversion disorder* and *hypochondriasis*.

Conversion Disorder

Conversion disorder was formerly known as hysterical neurosis. In **conversion disorder**, the person converts his or her overwhelming anxiety into physical symptoms. This is an unconscious response. The person may experience paralysis of an extremity, blindness, deafness, or numbness. The disability has no physical basis. Individuals usually complain about their pain and discomfort but are calm and indifferent about their symptoms. The physical symptom is symbolic of the unresolved anxiety producing the conflict. The symptoms enable people to avoid actions that are unacceptable to them. They also enable people to get attention and support from others that they might not get otherwise.

Hypochondriasis

Hypochondriasis is an abnormal anxiety about one's health. This disorder was formerly known as hypochondriacal neurosis. People with hypochondriasis are preoccupied with their bodies and their imaginary illnesses. They have unrealistic fears or beliefs that they are ill despite medical assurance that this is not so. Such people have difficulty establishing meaningful relationships with others since much of their time and energy is spent worrying about themselves. Hypochondriasis can affect both social and occupational functioning.

Adjustment Disorder

Maladaptive coping to a life event that is stressful is an adjustment disorder. The DSM IV-TR lists several subtypes; the most commonly seen are adjustment disorder with anxiety and/or depression and adjustment disorder of mixed disturbance of mood and conduct. The client appears worried and upset about an event that occurred in the past three months and describes trouble handling the stressors. Usually, there is no personal or family history of mood disorders, although a personality disorder needs to be ruled out.

MOOD/AFFECTIVE DISORDERS

As the name may suggest, affective disorders deal with emotions and mood. Included in this category are:
- Major Depressive Disorder (MDD)

  dysthymia
- Bipolar Disorder

  cyclothymia

The National Institute of Mental Health (NIMH) estimates that 36 million Americans are depressed at some time in their lives. Depression is a major public health problem. Research is indicating a corollary between depression and brain biochemicals (i.e., norepinephrine and serotonin deficiency). There is a problem with the transmissions of neurotransmitters across a brain synapse. Literature points to depression being biologically determined and influenced by multiple situational factors.

Researchers are gathering data on seasonal affective disorder (SAD), whereby an individual is depressed in winter when there is less light available.

Major Depressive Disorder (MDD)

With major depression, the symptoms have been present for a two-week period and represent a change from previous functioning. Depressed mood and **anhedonia** (a loss of interest or pleasure) are present most of the day. Subjectively, the client reports feeling sad or empty or is observed by others to be sad or tearful. Other symptoms include significant weight loss, insomnia, hypersomnia, psychomotor agitation, or retardation. Clients endorse feelings of worthlessness, excessive guilt, and diminished ability to think; they often have recurrent thoughts of death or suicide. Depression over time that is chronic and recurrent can manifest as psychosis, which is an inability to recognize reality and communicate or relate to others.

Elderly persons often experience depression. The elderly person's self-perception may become distorted and he or she may feel worthless and ashamed. A decrease in self-confidence and loss of self-esteem may occur. A negative self-concept results in irritability, apathy, and a lack of humor. Activities of daily living become a problem, and hair and clothing may appear disheveled. Movements are slow, posture is stooped, the brow is furrowed, and crying spells may be frequent. In the depressed elderly person, there is an intense preoccupation with health. Complaints of vague aches and pains, constipation, and anorexia are common. The severely depressed can become extremely agitated and appear totally miserable.

Dysthymic Disorder. The person experiencing a dysthymic disorder has a prolonged feeling of extreme sadness that is accompanied by guilt feelings, self-deprecation, and social withdrawal. The disorder is usually associated with a loss, such as loss of a loved one, possession, or self-esteem. The person feels rejected, helpless, and worthless. He or she is indecisive and disinterested in the surroundings and unable to experience pleasure in life. He or she has a low energy level and is always tired. The person may either be unable to sleep or may sleep excessively. The depressed person dwells on the negative aspects of life, which only add to his or her feelings of displeasure and guilt. He or she may cry often and easily and may have serious thoughts of suicide.

A dysthymic or depressive disorder often results from people feeling (1) that they have no control over their lives, (2) that they are failures because they have been unable to attain desired goals, or (3) internal anger. Critical periods in the life cycle when a dysthymic disorder is more likely to occur are adolescence, menopause, and old age.

During adolescence, depression must be differentiated from temporary states of sadness. Adolescents are subject to emotional ups and downs. However, when a lack of feelings or a sense of emptiness becomes a dominant mood, this is considered a dysthymic or depressive disorder. The adolescent with a dysthymic disorder is unable to deal with or express his or her feelings. Boredom and restlessness can result. Drug use and unwarranted risk-taking can be symptoms of hidden depression.

During menopause, women must cope with physical changes as the aging process occurs. Menopause may have physical symptoms such as hot and cold flashes, pressure headaches, heart palpitations, insomnia, and persistent fatigue. Some of these symptoms are caused by the changed hormonal balance between estrogen and progesterone. Depression can be caused by a perceived loss of womanhood and childbearing abilities.

Women are not the only people who must contend with the effects of menopause. Men may also experience menopausal changes, which accompany the normal diminution of sexual activity that occurs with advancing age. They may reduce their social interaction at this time and become preoccupied with feelings of guilt. They may communicate depression via facial expressions of sadness or negative verbal remarks. Daily stressors encountered on the job may have an increasingly negative impact on their outlooks. The effects of the aging process on men may also become cause for heightened concern.

Social isolation and boredom may be symptoms of a dysthymic disorder. The individual has a facial expression of sadness, a blunted or flat affect, and decreased verbal communication. With lessened energy levels and migratory aches and pains, they frequently withdraw from activity. With social interactions reduced, feelings of guilt and sadness prevail. Some people experience agitation and restlessness that result in pacing the floor and wringing the hands. The menopausal person who feels useless and less attractive turns feelings of rejection inward. These feelings of self-anger and destruction can make a person with a serious dysthymic disorder a real suicide risk. Any indications of suicidal thoughts should be dealt with. (See Chapter 10 Violence and Disturbed Behavior.)

Some antidepressant medications are listed in Table 9-3. The selective serotonin reuptake inhibitors (SSRI) subdue hyperarousal symptoms, decrease avoidance symptoms, and decrease emotional dyscontrol symptoms: anger, hostility, and irritability. Examples of SSRIs include fluoxetine (Prozac), sertraline (Zoloft), and paroxetine (Paxil). The side effects to be monitored are irritability, insomnia, and seizures.

TABLE 9-3 Antidepressant Medications

TRADE	GENERIC
SSRIs	
Tofranil	imipramine HCl
Norpramin	desipramine HCl
Elavil	amitriptyline HCl
Aventyl	nortriptyline HCl
Sinequan	doxepin HCl
Desyrel	trazodone HCl
Prozac	fluoxetine HCl
Zoloft	sertraline
Paxil	paroxetine
Celexa	citalopram
Luvox	fluvoxamine

(Continues)

TABLE 9-3 (Continued)

TRADE	GENERIC
Major side effects of SSRIs	Headache; lightheadedness; nausea; jitteriness; insomnia; sexual dysfunction including loss of libido, erectile problems, and delayed ejaculation; weight changes; apathy, fatigue

Miscellaneous

TRADE	GENERIC
Wellbutrin-SR	bupropion
Effexor	venlafaxine
Serzone	nefazadone
Remeron	mirtazapine
Benefit gained:	Improved outlook on life, better concentration, improved sleep, appetite, increased energy level
Side effects:	Blurred vision, dry mouth, drowsiness, nausea, dizziness, light headedness
Caution:	Medication is **highly lethal**, nonaddicting
	Be alert to suicidal clients stockpiling medication for a lethal overdose.
	Advise client to get up from a lying-down position slowly because he or she may experience dizziness; with client or inclient, monitor B/P in sitting and standing positions; may have orthostatic hypotension.
	Keep all medication out of reach of children. Watch for drowsiness—do not drive a car or operate heavy machinery.

Monitoring laboratory results is important. There may be impaired hepatic metabolism (lab: LFT—liver function test), thyroid dysfunction (lab: T3, T4, TSH), elevated prolactin levels (lab: prolactin level), excessive weight gain (lab: FBS—fasting blood sugar, to rule out Type II diabetes), and anorexia. Yearly labs include but are not limited to complete blood count (CBC) and urinanalysis (UA).

When the client's medication is being discontinued, it is important to have the dosage gradually reduced with no abrupt discontinuance. The client should be educated about the importance of daily medication compliance as intermittent noncompliance and the resulting stop-start syndrome does not contribute to medication bioavailability and, therefore, good medication effects. Research is reflecting that medications need to be taken a minimum of ninety days for efficacy and perhaps even six months before they are beneficial.

Bipolar Disorders (BPD)

Bipolar mood disorders are complex. Researchers are looking at biochemicals (i.e., melatonin, phenylethlymine) that influence brain function. A deficiency of dopamine and serotonin transmitters has been discovered in mania. Internal biological rhythms (circadian) are being carefully observed. Other studies are focused on the effect of light on mood patterns. It has been found that people with mood disorders may have abnormal thyroid studies including, T3, T4, and TSH. Electroencephalograms (EEGs) may indicate a picture of a complete or partial seizure. In England (1988), DNA markers for bipolar disorder were located on chromosome 2, thus increasing our knowledge of the role of genetics. Bipolar disorders deal with moods of elation and depression. They are subtyped as bipolar disorder, manic; bipolar disorder, depressed; and bipolar disorder, mixed. Lithium and anticonvulsants are mood-stabilizing medications frequently given for bipolar disorder (Table 9-4).

In the manic phase, individuals' appearances and behaviors are hyperactive. They speed up physically, mentally, and emotionally. They generally feel they are too busy to waste time on eating and sleeping. These thought processes may be so rapid that they are difficult to follow. This is called a *flight of ideas*. Manic people are happy and witty. Their moods may shift from euphoria to exaltation to frenzy. They have an overoptimistic, perhaps delusionary, view of their own powers. They often meddle in the affairs of others and are aggressive in their social behavior. Their angry outbursts, loudness, and manipulative ploys only increase their sensory overload.

The depressed phase is characterized by moderate to severe depression. The level of depression may fluctuate spontaneously throughout the day. These clients are high suicide risks even though depression appears to be only moderate. During the depression stage, the individual's appearance and behavior are hypoactive. Feelings, thoughts, and actions are abnormally decreased. He or she complains of being tired. Body functions slow, so anorexia and constipation are common. The person is negative and hostile, and actions are characterized by agitation, restlessness, pacing, and wringing of the hands. He or she has the appearance of being sad, remorseful, and dejected. After each episode of misery, the depression slowly lifts.

TABLE 9-4 Antimanic Medications

TRADE	GENERIC
Lithium	lithium carbonate
Benefit gained:	Controls episodes of mania
	Long-term use prevents recurrences of manic and depressive episodes
	Continue to experience emotions
Side effects:	Diarrhea, dizziness, dry mouth, increased thirst, increased urination
	CNS symptoms and toxicity:
	tremors, lethargy, confusion, nausea, diarrhea, slurring of speech, muscle weakness, blurred vision
Caution:	Take this medication immediately after meals or with food or milk to lessen stomach problems
	Contraindicated in pregnancy, breast-feeding
	Laboratory tests are necessary to determine that the proper amount of medication is in the client's system; the blood drawn for a lithium level should be secured 8–12 hours after the last lithium dosage
	Therapeutic blood level: 0.6-1 mcg/L.
	Monitor client and laboratory reports
	Dietary: drink 8–12 full (8 oz) glasses of water or other fluids each day; use normal amounts of table salt on your food
	Lithium toxicity: mild to moderate can be reversed by discontinuing or decreasing the dosage. Acute toxicity can lead to coma and death.

Newer Medications

Depakote	divalproex
Lamictal	lamotrigine
Neurontin	gabapentin
Tegretol	carbamazepine
Topamax	topiramate

Cyclothymic Disorder. The person with a cyclothymic disorder experiences alternating moods of depression and elation. During the elation stage, the person is warm and friendly. During the depression stage, the person isolates himself or herself and withdraws from social activity. The person may experience normal moods between or intermixed with the elation and depression. The person is oriented to reality and has no delusions or hallucinations.

A cyclothymic disorder is a mild form of bipolar disorder. If the person is not treated, the disorder can become more serious.

Dissociative Disorders

Dissociative disorders were formerly classified as hysterical neuroses. This disorder is characterized by changes in consciousness and identity. Psychogenic amnesia, psychogenic fugue, multiple personality, and depersonalization disorder are included in this category.

Psychogenic Amnesia. The person with psychogenic amnesia has a sudden loss of memory regarding important personal information that is too extensive to be considered ordinary forgetfulness. There is no damage to the nervous system. Psychogenic amnesia usually follows a stressful event and is thought to be a way of escaping conflicts and relieving overwhelming tension.

Psychogenic Fugue. Psychogenic fugue involves sudden and unexpected travel away from home or work with the inability to remember the past. The person experiencing psychogenic fugue assumes a new identity. Fugue often occurs following severe stress. Usually it lasts for several hours to several days and involves only limited travel. In some rare cases, however, it may last for many months and involve extensive travel. The recovery is rapid, and recurrences do not usually occur. This disorder is more common after a natural disaster or during wartime. No damage to the nervous system is involved.

Dissociative Identity Disorder. Dissociative identity disorder (formerly called multiple personality disorder) refers to the existence of two or more distinct personalities within the same individual. Each of these personalities is dominant at a particular time. The personality that is dominant determines the behavior of the individual. Each personality is complex and has its own behavior patterns. The secondary personalities are usually quite opposite to the original personality. The original personality is not aware of the other personalities, although the secondary personalities are often fully aware of the thoughts and actions of the original personality. Transition from one personality to another is sudden and usually follows stress. This disorder is extremely rare.

Depersonalization Disorder. Depersonalization disorder involves a change in the person's perception of himself or herself. A sense of the person's own reality is lost. People are cut off from their own awareness. They feel disassociated from their minds and bodies and may view themselves from a distance. They function in a dream state or mechanical fashion. Their senses are dulled, and they have a feeling of not being in complete control of their speech and actions.

This disorder often occurs after severe stress, depression, recovery from intoxication, fatigue, toxic illness, or physical pain. Onset is rapid but recovery is gradual. People with a depersonalization disorder may experience dizziness, anxiety, hypochondriasis, and a disturbed sense of time. They may even feel that they are going insane or will die.

Nursing Care

Coping with the individual with a psychological disorder may be very difficult for the nurse. Nurses may feel that this person is a malingerer or fake. It must be recognized, however, that this individual needs help. The nurse should never deny the client's illness. All complaints should be recognized as legitimate. The client is always the best source of information. A medical examination should be done to rule out the possibility of physical illness.

Nursing care of the psychological client focuses on reducing anxiety. The person with a psychological disorder is often treated with minor tranquilizers and/or psychotherapy. Clients often feel that medication will help them. On the unit, psychological clients need to be involved in making their own decisions. This decreases their fears and anxieties. The nurse can increase clients' ability to socialize by encouraging participation in unit activities. Keeping the client busy and giving verbal praise for achievements increases the client's self-esteem. Verbalization is very important for these clients. Clients should be encouraged to talk freely concerning themselves and their experiences.

The nurse should not ridicule the client's ritualistic behaviors. It would be better to set limits that the client can tolerate or attempt to distract the client with diversional activities geared to his or her particular interests. If the nurse can gain insight into what motivates the client's behavior, he or she can be observant of precipitating factors and plan appropriate nursing interventions.

Clients suffering from a bipolar disorder need acceptance and approval to diminish their fears of inferiority and rejection. While in the manic state, they can be very dramatic and exhibit overwhelming enthusiasm and talkativeness. In contrast, they can also be very critical, sarcastic, and dominating. The nurse should reinforce positive behavior.

The nursing care plan for bipolar clients must be consistently carried out by all nursing personnel. The ability to recognize manipulative behavior and set firm limits is essential. Manipulation is any action/behavior the individuals purposefully direct toward others in order to meet a need of their own. Remember, manipulation can be viewed as a positive or negative action. Individuals who engage in manipulation frequently evoke anger in others, yet their behavior is a form of guarding a very fragile self by attempting to control others. Therefore our goal is to strengthen individuals' inner, personal control. All staff must approach clients with a firm, consistent manner. Avoid acting in a judgmental way toward clients; rather, recognize your own feelings of resentment. Our goal is directed toward maintaining the self-esteem of our clients.

Begin by stating clearly your own expectations of the client at an interdisciplinary meeting where everyone should agree on one planned approach. Clarify with the client if there is a reason for this behavior and then state clearly why the behavior is unacceptable. Clearly state the team's expectation. Offer alternatives by stating choices or options (either/or statements). By having choices, the client will begin to feel more in control and will learn how to choose alternatives that work positively for him or her. The staff must practice attentive listening (what is this client really trying to say?). Help the client verbalize his or her feelings in a more appropriate way. Be alert for increased anxiety and refocus clients when they become distracted. Remember that you are working together to achieve a change in behavior.

Frequently a written contract works best. A contract clearly states the mutually agreed upon expectations and the way to arrive at this goal. Look at the client's strengths, resources, and energy for change. Maybe the client is currently in just a survival pattern that will need to be addressed. We want to make reasonable requests so that the client can be held accountable, and we want small success experiences so that we can give the client positive feedback. Areas to consider when writing a contract are personal safety, amount of sleep and rest, food intake, structured time, activities of daily living, problem-solving techniques, and the client's level of social interaction.

The bipolar client's concentration is lessened, and he or she is easily distracted and provoked. Social activities must be planned with this in mind. Exercise can be advantageous, but competitive activities may increase anxiety and frustration levels. Many clients enjoy writing down their thoughts, although they are usually fragmented.

During the depressed stage, clients become weary and despondent. Their feelings of hostility are directed inward. Safety of the client is one of the major responsibilities of the nurse. Whenever there is a suspicion that clients may be suicidal, they must be observed carefully. Showing a genuine caring attitude may help prevent a suicide attempt.

Bipolar clients need sufficient rest to avoid fatigue and irritability. They may become so absorbed in their overenthusiasm or pessimism that basic hygiene is not remembered.

The psychological client usually has poor eating and sleeping habits. The nurse can encourage proper eating habits, provide adequate nutrition, and provide the environment for restful sleep.

In dealing with the psychological client, nurses need to frequently reevaluate nursing goals and their effectiveness. They also need to be aware of their own feelings of frustration and helplessness.

EATING DISORDERS

In our culture, much emphasis is placed on the ideal female figure. The modern female is believed to be influenced by multiple cultural and social pressures to be physically attractive or slim. To attain this ideal figure, females very often engage in reduced food intake. At times, dieting can go too far, and a clinical syndrome characterized by a voluntary refusal to eat occurs. This is called **anorexia nervosa**. The incidence of anorexia nervosa has been estimated at between 0.24 and 1.6 annually per 100,000 population. Mortality rates range from 3 to 5 percent. This disease is most prevalent (95 percent) in females—adolescent girls and young women. Hilde Bruch described anorexia nervosa as "relentless pursuit of thinness." Characteristics of anorexia nervosa include

- Excessive weight loss with refusal to maintain weight
- Body image distortion with intense fear of becoming fat (25 percent of ideal body weight)
- Obsessional thoughts
- Hyperactivity (excessive exercising)
- Shy and introverted
- Sense of inadequacy
- Conscientious and perfectionist behavior
- Inability to trust the reliability of own emotions
- Amenorrhea

People with anorexia nervosa will rigidly and severely restrict their food intake and genuinely feel this is a positive achievement. The starvation syndrome simplifies their living. The anorexic's excessively thin body, which looks like a prepuberty figure, can help her avoid the conflicts of autonomous growth, competition, sexual identity, and social independence. Many anorexia nervosa clients have experienced family life with overprotectiveness, conflict avoidance, and rigidity. This family experience has been described as *enmeshment*. The family input fails to verify the developing child as a competent person who can function in an independent way.

Bulimia is an eating disorder characterized by the consumption of a large amount of food in a short period of time (one to two hours, 50,000 calories) followed by self-induced vomiting. This cycle is called binging and purging. Other characteristics of bulimia include

- Extreme dieting
- Laxative abuse
- Diuretic (water pill) abuse
- Preoccupation with food and eating
- Extreme sensitivity to body, shape, and weight
- Self-deprecating thoughts
- Impulsivity
- Depression
- Proneness to addiction
- Possible suicide risk

There are serious physical complications to eating disorders. Complications include the following:

- Electrolyte imbalance (potassium, chloride, sodium)
- Cardiac irregularities
- Kidney dysfunction or failure
- Neurological disturbances
- Edema and dehydration
- Gastrointestinal disturbances

With bulimia, the person can experience painless swelling of his or her salivary glands. It is speculated that the swelling is caused by a combination of nutritional deficiencies, electrolyte imbalances, and trauma caused by excessive vomiting. Also, the gastric acid from self-induced vomiting in bulimia can cause gum and teeth deterioration.

Many of the deaths in anorexia nervosa and bulimia result from compromised cardiac functioning. With the profound depletion of the electrolytes—potassium, chloride, and sodium—abnormalities can result in serious heartbeat irregularities (arrhythmias) and sudden death.

Some researchers believe that anorexia and bulimia are compulsive-obsessive disorders. Clients with these disorders appear to have difficulty separating and individuating from their families. One sees much ambivalence and unexpressed anger. When taking a family history, the professional may note that the family has continuously used food to express its love or to gain control. Many eating disordered clients have been well-behaved, perfectionist youths who restricted their personal feelings and did not verbally communicate. A self-sacrificing attitude prevails. Initially, eating disordered clients must be closely evaluated. Do they need a hospital admission to stabilize them metabolically? Will close observation with a behavioral approach be beneficial? Couple or family therapy can be indicated. Bulimics appear to progress with group therapy. Community education programs are a necessity in a time when eating disorders are of epidemic proportion.

SCHIZOPHRENIC DISORDER

The National Institute of Mental Health (NIMH) describes schizophrenia as the most prevalent, malignant, and baffling of all mental illnesses. It can be severe, persistent, and disabling. An estimated 2 million Americans will be stricken with schizophrenia each year. Current research into the contributing factors to the disease of schizophrenia include molecular pathology, cerebral atrophy, ventricular enlargement, and evidence of neurological disease. A dysfunction of the dopamine system may be involved in schizophrenic symptoms. A link is being sought between genetic factors and biological vulnerability. In 1989, NIMH's National Plan for Schizophrenia Research Data derived that schizophrenia occurs at an equal rate among various ethnic and racial groups; however, limited information is available on blacks, Hispanics, and Native Americans. Important data pointed to the fact that schizophrenia is found among the poor in disproportionate numbers (eight times higher). Poverty destroys the chance of earning a living and therefore, some sense of job satisfaction or the maintenance of a decent standard of living. Unemployed, uninsured, indigent people have increased environmental stressors, greater biological risk, and a diminished quality of life.

Kraeplin's (1919) studies described dementia praecox (a premature brain deterioration). Bleuler (1950) stated that schizophrenia describes the splitting of the mind's functions and introduced the four "A"s of schizophrenia: associative looseness, autism, ambivalence, and change of affect. **Associative looseness** is defined as the personalized interpretation of reality that is usually disorganized and fragmented. **Autism** is characteristic of a person who is focusing exclusively on his or her own feelings. When positive and negative feelings toward a person or object occur simultaneously it is called **ambivalence**. **Affect** describes a feeling state, usually flat with no expression or inappropriate giggling and laughing. A fifth "A" cited by some authorities is auditory hallucinations. Basically, schizophrenia is a thought disorder with disorganized thinking and faulty communication and social interaction.

One of the most important factors in a schizophrenic disorder is loss of self-esteem. This may be manifested in sudden and violent outbursts. It may result in dissociation or an exaggerated concern over body functions and appearance. Disturbances in thinking may range from a lack of clarity in the person's ideas to total incoherence. His or her thoughts are illogically connected, so they are difficult to understand. The person may jumble words so they make no sense; this is called **word salad**. He or she may make up words to express confused thoughts; these are called **neologisms**. **Echolalia** is the purposeless repetition of a word or phrase.

Characteristics of schizophrenia include delusions, hallucinations, disturbed thought processes, and peculiar behavior. **Delusions** are false ideas that cannot be changed by logical argument. Delusions are often associated with hallucinations. They may occur in any type of psychotic reaction.

Delusional ideas may be in the form of guilt or persecution. Clients may feel that they have committed grave sins or they may exaggerate a slight misdeed. People with delusions of persecution believe that an organized group intends to harm them. They may perceive all happenings in relation to their delusion, using even unrelated events as proof of the delusion. Persons with schizophrenia may also have delusions of grandeur, believing that they have great power. They may see themselves as Napoleon or Jesus Christ.

Hallucinations are perceptions that occur in the absence of stimuli and have no basis in reality. They include hearing nonexistent voices (auditory), having visions (visual), smelling (olfactory) or tasting things (gustatory), or having a sensation of being touched (tactile). Command hallucinations can be very frightening for the client and may command the client to do something dangerous to self or others.

An important part of behavior disturbance of clients with schizophrenia is their progressive withdrawal. They substitute fantasy for real life. Their actions may seem inappropriate to the situation because they become increasingly indifferent to their outside environment and feel alienated and isolated.

In an acute onset of schizophrenia, there is usually normal IQ, a normal brain functioning, the absence of negative symptoms (Table 9-5), and a good response to antipsychotic medications. With a slow onset, there are enlarged central ventricles, prominent negative symptoms, and a poor response to antipsychotics.

Antipsychotic medications possess many side effects that need to be carefully assessed by the nursing staff and reported to the psychiatrist (Table 9-6). A serious, irreversible side effect is **tardive dyskinesia (TD)**. To detect TD at its earliest stages, an abnormal involuntary movement scale (AIMS) needs to be done at a minimum of every six months (Table 9-7).

TABLE 9-5 Positive and Negative Symptoms of Schizophrenia

POSITIVE:		NEGATIVE:
outward, more visible, increased or grossly distorted behaviors or experience	**Behavior**	a lessening or loss of normal functioning
Hostility	**Affect**	Flattened, restricted
Excitement	**Emotions**	Blunted—diminished range Anhedonia—inability to express joy or pleasure
Delusions, disorganized thinking, hallucinations	**Thought**	Content—poverty of content, disorganized Profess—hallucinations, delusions, ideas of reference
Feelings of persecution	**Personal**	Social withdrawal Psychomotor retardation Lack of sense of purpose, direction Impaired self-care Bizarre behaviors
Poor	**Judgment**	Poor
Poor	**Insight**	Poor

All clients on antipsychotic medication need to be observed for **neuroleptic malignant syndrome (NMS).** It is a serious, life-threatening syndrome of sudden onset with the following symptoms: increased temperature and blood pressure, diaphoresis, tachycardia, disorientation, and confusion. Immediate intervention must be made to prevent death. Blocking dopamine receptors improves the positive symptoms but frequently causes extrapyramidal symptoms (EPS). Studies have shown that negative symptoms may result from excess serotonin. Research is looking at control of negative symptoms by blocking serotonin.

There are several types of schizophrenia: disorganized, catatonic, paranoid, and undifferentiated. Again, the nurse must be cautioned that clients with schizophrenia do not exhibit clear-cut patterns. Each client responds with his or her own characteristics. As his or her anxiety increases, the person turns from the real world and withdraws into a personal world.

TABLE 9-6 Antipsychotic Medications

TRADE	GENERIC
Haldol	haloperidol
Prolixin	fluphenazine HCl
Mellaril	thioridazine HCl
Thorazine	chlorpromazine
Stelazine	trifluoperazine HCl
Navane	thiothixene
Loxitant	loxapine
Trilafon	perphenazine

DEPOT NEUROLEPTICS

Haldol decanoate	haloperidol decanoate
Prolixin decanoate	fluphenazine decanoate

Depot neuroleptics are designed for individuals who need antipsychotic medication yet have difficulty remembering to take it or have paranoid ideation. Medication is injection form and usually given every two weeks for Prolixin decanoate and every four weeks for Haldol decanoate. Administer intramuscularly (IM) into gluteus maximus muscle with an 18g, 1/2" needle.

Benefit gained:	Think more clearly
	Elimination or significant reduction of hallucinations, delusions, anxiety, and troublesome thoughts, feelings, and behaviors
Side effects:	Blurred vision, dry mouth, constipation, urinary retention
Neurological:	**Akinesia**—changes in posture, shuffling gait, muscular rigidity, drooling, slowed movements
	Akathesia—squirming, restlessness, fidgeting, agitation
Tardive dyskinesia:	Sucking movements, involuntary chewing, tongue protrusion; this is often irreversible
Caution:	Do not use alcohol
	Avoid prolonged exposure to sun; if outside, use a sunscreen with PABA—the higher the number, the greater the protection.

ATYPICAL ANTIPSYCHOTICS

Clozaril (clozapine)	Atypical antipsychotics that are both
Risperdal (risperidone)	dopamine- and serotonin-type antagonists
Zyprexa (olanzapine)	

*Mellaril (thioridazine) requires periodic ECGs and tests for potassium levels to monitor for a potentially fatal arrhythmia, torsades de pointes.

TABLE 9-7 Aims-Abnormal Involuntary Movements

CLIENT ACTION	STAFF OBSERVATION
Open mouth Protrude tongue	Tongue at resting Tongue movements
Tap thumb with each finger as rapidly as possible (approx. 10–15 seconds)	Facial and leg movements
Extend both arms in front, palms down	Trunk, leg, mouth movements
Walk a few paces, turn and walk back	Hand and gait
Sit in chair with hands positioned on knees, legs slightly apart	Entire body for movements
Record abnormalities on scale of minimal,mild, moderate, severe Check mouth for candy, gum, dentures	

Adapted from The Abnormal Involuntary Movements Scale (AIMS)

Disorganized Type. This category was formerly classified as hebephrenic schizophrenia. The disorganized schizophrenic exhibits inappropriate behavior, smiling and giggling frequently at everything or nothing at all. There are gross thought disturbances, including the use of word salad and neologisms. Delusions and hallucinations are common, as is extreme social withdrawal.

Catatonic Type. The catatonic person's behavior varies, but there is usually an acute onset. Behavior may take the form of stupor or excitement. In catatonic stupor, the client is immobile, mute, and negative. There is no interest in the environment; this apathy completely cuts the client off from outside stimuli. He or she may remain in one position with very rigid muscles or possess **waxy flexibility** (a condition in which a limb remains in one position, even a very uncomfortable one, for a period of time).

Catatonic people exhibit unpredictable behavior because their behavior is controlled by their delusions and hallucinations. Stupor may change rapidly and unexpectedly to excitement. At these times, they are extremely restless and may become violent. The client with catatonic schizophrenia exhibits two peculiar mannerisms—*echolalia* and *echopraxia*. Echolalia is an involuntary repetition of words spoken by others. This is often accompanied by muscle twitching. Echopraxia involves imitating the motions of others.

Paranoid Type. Clients with **paranoid** schizophrenia are suspicious, aggressive, and hostile. They suffer from suspicion and jealousy, and delusions of grandeur and persecution. Hallucinations are common. Clients often hear voices commanding them. They may become combative. For example, they may break the television set because they believe it is sending them bad messages or perhaps reading their mind. At the beginning, other symptoms may be difficult to detect. As the condition progresses, behavior becomes more inappropriate and unpredictable. Since their delusions are often bizarre, they can be dangerous.

Undifferentiated Type. Undifferentiated schizophrenia is diagnosed when the symptoms do not fit in other categories for schizophrenia. Symptoms may include delusions, hallucinations, incoherence, and grossly disorganized behavior.

Psychosis, NOS (Not Otherwise Specified)

A deterioration in functioning and a lack of recognition of reality is termed *psychosis*. Usually, psychosis, NOS is a brief psychotic disorder of no longer than one month. A serious stressor may or may not be present. Note whether delusions or hallucinations (specify auditory, visual, olfactory, or tactile) are present and specify a general medical condition that may be present. If the psychosis is substance-induced, specify the substance that was used and whether the client is intoxicated or in withdrawal.

PARANOID DISORDER

Clients with a paranoid disorder, like the client with schizophrenia, suffer from persistent delusions. These delusions are generally delusions of jealousy, persecution, or sometimes grandeur. The paranoid client does not have hallucinations but possesses a heightened suspiciousness that may progress to psychosis. The client is fearful and guarded and uses the defense mechanism of projection.

Clients with paranoid disorder usually do not show disorganization of their personalities, other than the delusions. Their actions seem to be appropriate to their delusionary experiences. There is seldom further deterioration in their personality. They speak and act rationally and are well oriented to time and place. They may be able to carry on a productive occupation even when their condition is well developed. However, social and marital functioning are usually adversely affected.

Feelings of anger and resentment are common with a paranoid disorder. These clients can be dangerous as they may strike out in self-defense. Bizarre deterioration or incoherence is not seen in these clients.

Nursing Care

Nursing care for the client suffering from a schizophrenic or paranoid disorder must be based on an assessment of behavior and problems because these clients have an individualized array of symptoms. Clients with schizophrenia have a pattern of isolation motivated by a fear of rejection. His or her behavior reflects a lack of self-confidence. The nurse needs to demonstrate a hopeful attitude consisting of acceptance, security, and confidence. Avoiding the client only reinforces his or her feelings of low self-esteem. The nurse should observe the client with schizophrenia for any special interests. Involving him or her in a variety of activities such as checkers, card games, crafts, or hobbies can be a method of stimulating the senses. Genuine praise can reinforce confidence. It may be therapeutic to change the environment by walking outdoors or taking a ride in the country.

For a client with a paranoid disorder, a flexible but consistent approach should be maintained at all times. This client's trust in others must be strengthened. It is important for the nurse to be aware of his or her own behavior. Whispering or pointing when in the client's environment must be avoided. Probing questions may provoke paranoid behavior. The paranoid client requires calm, soothing voice tones at all times.

The nurse's goal is to provide support and structure for the client in order to decrease his or her anxiety and decompensation. A firm, consistent environment will facilitate the client's recovery from a state of inner disorganization.

In preparation for a return to the family and their community, clients with schizophrenia need to be educated about the warning symptoms of a relapse of the disease. A sign-of-relapse checklist would be beneficial for clients and their families and would be an excellent method of education as part of discharge planning. Warning signs of relapse include a loss of interest in doing things, eating, and attending to activities of daily living; trouble concentrating or thinking straight; fast thoughts; increased trouble with decision making; preoccupation with religion; fear of others hurting them or that others are playing with their minds; increased irritability over little things; thoughts of hurting or killing self; and an increased use of alcohol or drugs. These warning signs indicate that a relapse may be coming and the client needs to seek professional help. In extreme presentation of symptoms, the client needs to go to the emergency room of their hospital. Each client needs an emergency plan for severe relapse.

Hildegarde Peplau (1962) stated that to help clients is to remember and understand fully what is happening to them in the present situation. You want to assist clients in integrating this with other experiences in their lives. Avoid isolating the experience because that will only increase thought fragmentation. Assist clients to recognize maladaptive behavior and its causes, motives, and consequences. Assist clients to look for alternate choices for their behavior and increase their constructive, productive lifestyle. The nurse is building trust and nurturing the client, which is called a corrective emotional experience.

PERSONALITY DISORDER

Personality can be defined as an individual's character traits, attitudes, thoughts, behaviors, and habits. It encompasses the individual's behavioral and emotional tendencies. It also involves the individual's adaptation to internal and external problems.

Personality disorders are maladaptive patterns of seeing, relating to, and thinking about the environment and relationships with others. Since the patterns are inflexible and deeply ingrained, there is impairment in adaptive functioning. Disturbances in emotional development and equilibrium are seen. There is a maladjustment to the social environment. Some personality disorders are associated with changes in the normal levels of neurotransmitters

The *American Psychiatric Association's Diagnostic and Statistical Manual* (Text Revision) (DSM-IV-TR) lists several subdivisions under the category of Personality Disorders. These subdivisions and characteristics are shown in Table 9-8. Personality disorders can begin in childhood but usually are manifested at adolescence, and interfere with social or role functioning. Often, persons with personality disorders do not seek mental health care.

Nursing Care

People with personality disorders are very difficult to deal with, and treatment may be ineffective. In caring for these clients, the nurse should be able to handle the frustrations caused by their behavior. He or she also should be aware that some clients may be very manipulative. Manipulative clients want all needs to be met immediately and may become aggressive or hostile when they are not met. Respond to manipulation with consistent reinforcement of limits.

The nurse might directly tell clients with a personality disorder that their blaming, accusing, and intimidating manner alienates people.

TABLE 9-8 Personality Disorders

DISORDER	SPECIFIC CHARACTERISTICS	GENERAL CHARACTERISTICS
Paranoid	Unwarranted suspicions and mistrust; hypersensitivity; exaggeration of difficulties; inability to relax; cold and unemotional	Odd
Schizoid	Lack of warm tender feelings for others; indifferent; few close friends; "loner"	Difficulty in maintaining satisfactory relationships
Schizotypal	Social isolation; oddities of thinking and speech; illusions; suspicious; hypersensitivity	Eccentric
Histrionic	Overly dramatic expressions of emotion; overreaction to events; self-indulgent; constant drawing of attention to self; irrational outbursts; inconsideration of others; vain and demanding; constant seeking of reassurance; lack of genuineness; craving of excitement	Dramatic and emotional
Narcissistic	Exaggerated sense of self-importance; need for constant attention and admiration; preoccupied with fantasies; vacillates between emotional extremes; lacks ability to recognize how others feel	Self-centered
Antisocial	Seeks immediate pleasure; selfish; poor occupational performance; unable to maintain lasting relationships; poor sexual adjustment; failure to accept social norms; irritability and aggressiveness; failure to plan ahead (impulsive); disregard for the truth; reckless violation of the rights of others	Defective judgment At risk of substance abuse and harm to others
Borderline	Impulsive and unpredictable; unstable interpersonal relationships; frequent displays of anger; identity problems, shifts in moods; intense discomfort when alone; physically self-damaging acts; recurring feelings of boredom and emptiness	Erratic
Avoidant	Hypersensitivity to rejection; social withdrawal; low self-esteem	Anxious
Dependent	Lacks self-confidence; avoids relying on self; allows others to assume responsibility	Fearful
Compulsive	Preoccupation with trivial details; overly conventional and serious, insists on own way; indecisive	Perfectionist
Passive-aggressive	Indirectly resists demands for adequate performance; intentional inefficiency; forgetful; stubbornness; procrastination; dawdling; resentful	Incompetent Overly dependent

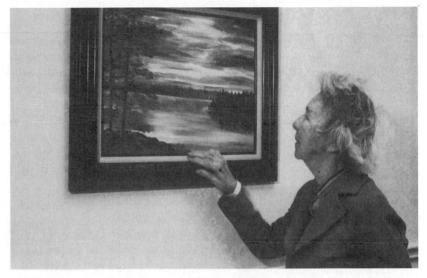

FIGURE 9-1 A small success experience for clients may be seeing their artwork displayed; this builds self-esteem.

Peer pressure can frequently be used to modify behavior. Guidance in assertiveness is helpful for some clients. These clients need positive feedback for open, direct communication. The nurse should encourage relaxed rather than hostile exchanges. He or she should set appropriate limits and be sure the client knows the limitations. Diversional activities are important. The nurse might help by presenting growth opportunities, chances to assume responsibility, and small success experiences (Figure 9-1). There is now a move toward special residential homes for some clients with personality disorders.

Impulse Control Disorder

Clients with an impulse disorder have uncontrollable impulses that result in harmful behaviors to self or others. Their poor insight and inability to reflect and think of an alternative behavior results in exciting, dangerous behaviors that reduce their sense of tension and pleasure. As a result, they experience relief. Impulsive behaviors include kleptomania, pyromania, pathological gambling, trichotillomania, and compulsive skin picking (sometimes to the point of excoriation). Some of the literature also includes compulsive buying as an impulse disorder. Comorbidity with other disorders, such as bipolar disorder, psychoactive substance use, attention deficit/hyperactive disorder (ADHD), and/or borderline and antisocial personality disorders need to be assessed.

Attention Deficit/Hyperactive Disorder (ADHD)

Symptoms of ADHD include a persistent pattern of inattention, hyperactivity, and impulsivity with the following observable behaviors: fidgeting, distractability, interrupting, inattention, and difficulty with waiting, following instructions, sustaining attention, and remaining task-focused.

A neuropsychological assessment for a differential diagnosis is important as the complexity of a multiple diagnosis or dual diagnosis will influence the use of medications and treatment interventions. Comorbidities include learning disorders, mood disorders, and substance abuse or use. Many youths with ADHD have concurrent social and behavioral problems that place them at risk for committing crimes and becoming involved in the criminal justice system.

Medications prescribed are Ritalin (methylphenidate) and Cylert (pemoline). However, the subject of medication usage for treatment of ADHD is controversial, and the reliance on drugs for children and adolescents is being questioned. Continuing research in genetics, brain injury, and psychopharmacology is likely to contribute to a better understanding of this disorder and effective treatment approaches.

SLEEP DISORDERS

More than 30 million Americans will be affected by insomnia at some point in their lives. Hauri (1988) defined three types of insomnia: transient insomnia caused by a brief period of stress or when one travels from different time zones, insomnia caused by poor sleeping habits or drug and alcohol dependence, and chronic insomnia. If excessive, loud snoring is present, the client needs to be evaluated by the pulmonary department, which assesses breathing functions and then consults with a sleep disorders clinic. Many people experience shallow, fragmented sleep and never feel rested or refreshed. Studies suggest sleep protocols that involve no naps; arising from bed when you cannot sleep and doing some quiet activity for approximately ninety minutes, then retiring to the bed; learning and practicing relaxation techniques.

MILIEU THERAPY

Milieu includes all surroundings in the physical environment and those interpersonal interactions that contribute to the individual's personal growth and adaption. The environment is structured to provide security and safety. On admission to the unit, the stimuli may be decreased while trust is built, but gradually increased responsibility and involvement is encouraged. The environment is flexible, yet limit setting is consistent. Personal respect and cooperation modeled by the staff increases the self-confidence and sense of autonomy of the client. The eventual goal for the client is increased motivation and socialization. The milieu aids in the recognition of maladaptive behaviors and allows for confrontation of the client when these behaviors are observed.

The physical environment needs to be clean and safe. Harmonious colors and comfortable and safe furnishings contribute to the overall sense of well-being. Milieu includes many therapy modalities: group therapy, art and music therapy (a means to socialize and structure free time and increase self-confidence), pet therapy (comfort with the expression of caring through touching), horticulture (gardening and its responsibilities), nutrition counseling, occupational therapy (maximizing strengths and one's response to the environment), vocational work (counselor explores work and job options), and educational groups (communication skills, self-esteem, social interaction, financial planning). An interdisciplinary team coordinates these treatment activities and evaluates the client's participation and progress at weekly team meetings. An individualized care plan facilitates the client's participation through the client's review of the plan and consent (either verbal or written) that he or she accepts the treatment plan.

Another aspect of the milieu is the community meeting. A community meeting is a scheduled meeting with a set time and predetermined decision that there will be no interruptions by staff or clients. On admission to the unit the client is an observer at the meeting but then becomes a participant. The community meeting gives everyone a voice in decision making. It provides a time to review problems and tensions on the ward and decreases conflict through discussion. Unit rules and roles are clarified and enforced in a consistent manner. At times, unit upkeep may be the meeting focus, with assignments of chores or tasks. The main concept is to increase client responsibility and accountability and thereby increase self-awareness and self-esteem.

Frequently requests for a therapeutic pass are generated at the community meeting. A therapeutic pass is a leave of absence (LOA) from the hospital for two or more hours. It is authorized by the physician. Before the pass is issued, a member of the team meets with the client, and they decide on the purpose of the leave. Papers are filled out and handed in on return that reflect the positive and negative aspects of the LOA. The client may visit with family, run errands, or seek aftercare placement. This is an important part of the discharge plan because it promotes the client's resocialization and assists him or her to identify and cope with stressors and begin to utilize community support. Many third-party reimbursement agencies do not allow therapeutic passes.

SUMMARY

Maladaptive behaviors can develop anytime from infancy through old age. Three critical times are adolescence, menopause, and old age. Coping activity is required throughout the life cycle.

The word *normal* can be viewed in a social, clinical, moral, or statistical way. There is no sharp distinction between normal and abnormal. Psychiatry categorizes patterns of behavior, but it must be remembered that clients do not fit neatly into these categories. Each client has an individual reaction to stress and therefore an individual pattern of behavior.

Psychological disorders are disturbances characterized by maladaptive behavior aimed at dealing with high levels of anxiety. Anxiety disorders, somatoform disorders, affective disorders, and dissociative disorders are some common psychological disorders. Nursing care focuses on reducing anxiety.

Affective disorders deal with mood and emotions. This category includes dysthymic, depressive major, cyclothymic, and bipolar disorders. Bipolar disorders are subtyped as manic, depressed, or mixed. Dissociative disorders are characterized by changes in consciousness and identity. This category includes psychogenic amnesia, psychogenic fugue, multiple personality, and depersonalization disorder. Schizophrenia is characterized by delusions, hallucinations, disturbed thought processes, and peculiar behavior. Persons with schizophrenia experience conflicting feelings and demonstrate inappropriate affect, word salad, neologism, delusions, and hallucinations. The types of schizophrenia are disorganized, catatonic, paranoid, and undifferentiated. The client with a paranoid disorder suffers from persistent delusions, generally of jealousy, persecution, or grandeur. Personality disorders involve an individual's adaptation to internal and external problems. The disorder interferes with social or role functioning.

Many psychiatric clients are high risk for suicide. The depressed client is the client most likely to commit suicide. The nurse should be able to recognize indirect cues that the client may be considering suicide. Talking about suicide is a plea for help and must be recognized as such. (See Chapter 10, Violence and Disruptive Behaviors.)

SUGGESTED ACTIVITIES

■ Visit a mental health center. Observe nurses as they relate to clients.

■ In a class discussion, correlate the developmental stage of adolescence with the development of an eating disorder.

■ Investigate the admission procedure to a day-treatment center or mental health unit in your community. Report your findings to the class.

■ Obtain and review pamphlets from:

American Psychiatric Assn., Division of Public Affairs
1400 K Street, NW
Washington, D.C. 20005
1-202-682-6220

Anxiety Disorders Association of America (ADAA)
11900 Parlawn Drive, Suite 100
Rockville, MD 20852-2624
1-301-231-9350
www.adaa.org

Children and Adults with Attention Deficit Disorders (C.H.A.D.D.)
499 N.W. 70th Avenue, Suite 101
Plantation, FL 33317
1-800-233-4050
www.chadd.org

Food and Drug Administration (FDA)
5800 Fishers Lane
Rockville, MD 20857
1-800-332-0178
Med Watch: 1-800-332-1088
www.vm.cfsan.fda.gov

National Alliance for the Mentally Ill (NAMI)
200 North Glebe Road, Ste. 1015
Arlington, VA 22203-3754
1-800-950-NAMI

National Depressive and Manic Depressive Disorders Association.
730 N. Franklin Street, Suite 501
Chicago, 60610
1-800-826-3632
www.ndmda.org

National Foundation for Depressive Illness, Inc.
PO Box 2257
New York, NY 10116
1-800-239-1265
www.depression.org

National Institute of Mental Health
6001 Executive Boulevard
Room 8184 MSC 9663
Bethesda, MD 20892
1-301-443-4513
www.nimh.nih.gov

National Mental Health Association
1021 Prince Street
Alexandria, VA 22314
1-800-969-6642
www.nmha.org

Obsessive-Compulsive Foundation
337 Notch Hill Road
North Branford, CT 06471
1-203-315-2190
www.ocfoundation.org

■ Group discussion on following:
Mosby, Communication Series Communicating with Clients from Different Cultures, 1996.

REVIEW

KNOW AND COMPREHEND
A. Multiple choice. Select the one best answer.

1. An abnormal, excessive fear of a specific situation or object is called a/an
   ❑ A. obsession.
   ❑ B. compulsion.
   ❑ C. phobia.
   ❑ D. psychosis.

2. A recurring overpowering thought or feeling is called a/an
   ❑ A. obsession.
   ❑ B. compulsion.
   ❑ C. phobia.
   ❑ D. psychosis.

3. An irresistible urge to engage in a behavior is called a/an
   - ❏ A. obsession.
   - ❏ B. compulsion.
   - ❏ C. phobia.
   - ❏ D. psychosis.

4. The type of schizophrenic disorder characterized by stupor and waxy flexibility is called
   - ❏ A. disorganized.
   - ❏ B. catatonic.
   - ❏ C. undifferentiated.
   - ❏ D. paranoid.

5. The affective disorder that deals with alternate moods of depression and elation is the
   - ❏ A. dysthymic disorder.
   - ❏ B. depersonalization disorder.
   - ❏ C. psychogenic fugue.
   - ❏ D. bipolar disorder.

6. For most individuals, use of compulsive behavior results in which of the following?
   - ❏ A. occupying the mind
   - ❏ B. manipulating the environment
   - ❏ C. lowering anxicty
   - ❏ D. preventing mistakes

7. Psychogenic amnesia is classified as a/an
   - ❏ A. affective disorder.
   - ❏ B. personality disorder.
   - ❏ C. dissociative disorder.
   - ❏ D. conversion disorder.

8. The person with a conversion disorder
   - ❏ A. converts anxiety to bodily symptoms.
   - ❏ B. experiences severe mood swings.
   - ❏ C. is cut off from his or her awareness.
   - ❏ D. worries about self obsessively.

9. Behavior that the person with an antisocial personality is likely to display is
   - ❏ A. withdrawing from group activity.
   - ❏ B. mechanical obedience.
   - ❏ C. manipulation of others.
   - ❏ D. ritualistic behavior.

10. Which of the following clients would have the highest risk for suicide? A client diagnosed with a/an
    ❑ A. psychogenic amnesia.
    ❑ B. antisocial personality disorder.
    ❑ C. major depression.
    ❑ D. cyclothymic disorder.

APPLY YOUR LEARNING

B. Multiple choice. Select the one best answer.

1. A client diagnosed with paranoid schizophrenia tells the nurse, "I'm Jesus Christ, your Lord and Savior. Confess your sins to me." Which response by the nurse would be most appropriate?
   ❑ A. "I am of the Jewish faith and do not accept Jesus as Lord and Savior."
   ❑ B. "Your admission papers do not list your name as Jesus."
   ❑ C. "You are out of touch with reality. Your belief is a symptom of your illness."
   ❑ D. "I respect your belief but I do not share the belief."

2. A client with catatonic schizophrenia is mute and sits for hours in a rigid posture. Which communication strategy would be most appropriate for the nurse to use?
   ❑ A. Frequently pat the client's shoulder to demonstrate caring.
   ❑ B. Avoid verbal interaction until the antipsychotic medication takes effect.
   ❑ C. Ask the client's significant other to obtain information from the client.
   ❑ D. Offer short, caring phrases to communicate concern for the client.

3. A client has a medical diagnosis of bipolar disorder, manic phase and a nursing diagnosis of imbalanced nutrition, less than body requirements. Which nursing intervention would be most important?
   ❑ A. Record how much the client eats at each meal.
   ❑ B. Ask the client to keep a journal about eating habits.
   ❑ C. Record the client's intake and output.
   ❑ D. Frequently offer the client snacks and beverages.

4. The nurse prepares to administer fluphenzine decanoate (Prolixin decanoate) 37.5 mg IM to a client diagnosed with paranoid schizophrenia. Which needle should the nurse select?
   - ❏ A. 18 g, 1/2"
   - ❏ B. 20 g, 1 1/2"
   - ❏ C. 22 g, 3/4"
   - ❏ D. 25 g, 2"

5. The nurse prepared to administer haloperidol decanoate (Haldol decanoate) IM to a client diagnosed with paranoid schizophrenia. The nurse could use any of the following sites *except*:
   - ❏ A. the abdomen.
   - ❏ B. deltoid.
   - ❏ C. gluteus maximus.
   - ❏ D. vastus lateralis.

6. The nurse gathers information for a newly admitted client diagnosed with an eating disorder. What information would have the highest priority to obtain?
   - ❏ A. age
   - ❏ B. heart rate and rhythm
   - ❏ C. menstrual pattern
   - ❏ D. body image

7. A client with bipolar disorder takes lithium. Which finding would prompt the nurse to withhold the next dose and promptly notify the physician?
   - ❏ A. constipation
   - ❏ B. infrequent urination
   - ❏ C. lethargy and confusion
   - ❏ D. increased thirst

8. The nurse finds a client, who is diagnosed with major depression, alone and crying. Which response by the nurse would be most therapeutic?
   - ❏ A. Administer the client's antidepressant medication.
   - ❏ B. Offer to sit quietly with the client.
   - ❏ C. Ask the client, "What's the matter?".
   - ❏ D. Offer the client a recreational activity.

C. Match each item in column II with the statement describing it in column I.

<table>
<tr><th>Column I</th><th>Column II</th></tr>
<tr><td>1. Inability to act or react in an appropriate manner</td><td>a. Delusion</td></tr>
<tr><td></td><td>b. Dysthymic disorder</td></tr>
<tr><td>2. Having positive and negative feelings simultaneously</td><td>c. Maladaptive behavior</td></tr>
<tr><td></td><td>d. Echolalia</td></tr>
<tr><td>3. Prolonged feeling of extreme sadness accompanied by guilt feelings and social withdrawal</td><td>e. Echopraxia</td></tr>
<tr><td></td><td>f. Hallucinations</td></tr>
<tr><td></td><td>g. Ambivalence</td></tr>
<tr><td>4. False ideas that cannot be changed by logical argument</td><td>h. Anxiety disorder</td></tr>
<tr><td></td><td>i. Neologism</td></tr>
<tr><td>5. Perceptions that occur in the absence of stimuli</td><td></td></tr>
<tr><td>6. Imitating motions of others</td><td></td></tr>
<tr><td>7. Involuntary repetition of words spoken by others</td><td></td></tr>
<tr><td>8. Made-up words to express confused thoughts</td><td></td></tr>
<tr><td>9. Characterized by anxiety that is disproportionate to the stresses of daily living</td><td></td></tr>
</table>

D. Briefly answer the following.

1. Differentiate between moderate and severe anxiety and panic.

2. List four types of schizophrenic disorders.

3. Describe day-treatment centers.

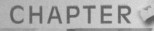

Violence and Disturbed Behaviors

OUTLINE

KEY TERMS

violence	victimization
aggression	seclusion
anger	restraint
conflict resolution	least-restrictive mode
direct message	behavioral flagging
active listening	contraband
explore alternatives	teen suicide
contract	homicide
talking down	Duty to Warn
therapeutic neutrality	perpetrator
impulse control	rape
macho image	shaken-baby syndrome
suicidal ideation	incest

OBJECTIVES

After studying this chapter, the student should be able to:

- Identify predisposing signs, sociocultural variables, and precipitating factors to violence.
- Recognize the importance of understanding anger and alienation.
- Identify verbal intervention techniques.
- Identify important criteria for placing clients in seclusion and/or restraints and discontinuing seclusion/restraints.
- Describe techniques needed to restrain an assaultive client.
- Identify important areas of nursing documentation.
- Gather data about the suicidal/homicidal client and identify intervention techniques.
- Describe nursing interventions in the planning of the care of the rape victim.
- List five behaviors of the abused child.
- List six characteristics of the abusing parent.
- Describe conditions in which child abuse should be suspected.
- Describe nursing interventions in the planning of the care of the victim of incest.

Violence is an urgent public health concern, with homicide being the second leading cause of death in our society for people between the ages of fifteen and thirty. In New York, homicide is the leading cause of death among youths fifteen to nineteen years old. Many people are witnesses of homicide and subsequently experience posttraumatic stress disorder, depression, and anxiety disorders. Enough violence has occurred in the workplace that a Violence Workplace Awareness Week was designated for the month of October. Our society also has seen an increase in the number of people exposed to violence who survived terrorism, deprivation, losses, assaults, rape, and murder attempts. Part of the broad spectrum of violence is current murder-suicide pacts.

The Centers for Disease Control and Prevention (May 1995) define *violence* as the threatened or actual use of physical force or power against another person, against oneself, or against a group or community that results in injury, death, or deprivation. It includes societal violence and deprivation of equality and justice.

The management of violence, both physical and psychological, is a neglected problem in America. Violence is seldom addressed in textbooks; you may see suicide listed but not other topics such as homicide, violence, assault, aggression, or agitation. When violence is the behavior, the *DSM IV-TR* assists the clinician with a differential diagnosis: substance intoxication, bipolar disorder (manic episode), dissociative identity disorder, antisocial personality disorder, impulse control disorder, and/or intermittent explosive disorder. When a person loses control and the aggression is directed toward property or people, gather information from the client for a diagnosis of intermittent explosive disorder.

There are also rampant acts of victimization (e.g., spouse, child, and elder abuse, rape, and incest) that are forms of perpetrated violence. Violent behavior among hospitalized medical and surgical clients has been on the increase, and the incidence of clients approaching facilities with concealed weapons is now a known fact.

We may expect the sick, suffering client to become suicidal or depressed but are taken aback when the client rejects our help or makes unreasonable demands and becomes caustic, unruly, and angry. Additionally, many psychiatric clients have a dual diagnosis (e.g., paranoid schizophrenia and substance abuse), which increases the risk of violent behaviors.

The management of disruptive, assaultive, or out-of-control behavior requires the development of a sound knowledge base and practical intervention skills, as well as training in and the practice of techniques for the client with disturbed behavior. Prevention of violent episodes before they escalate is the best way to intervene.

AGGRESSION

There are many points of view concerning **aggression**. Freud viewed aggression as an inborn drive or an impulse, with the aim of destruction, which requires discharge either directly or indirectly. Horney rejected this theory and stated that aggression and hostility are a response to basic anxiety. Horney believed that aggression is hostility turned inward and is self-destructive behavior, whereas hostility turned outward is an aggressive act toward others.

Lorenza correlates genetics with the environment and believes that aggressive behavior is innate (inborn), demands expression, and stems from the internal excitation that increases aggression, impulsivity, and criminal violence. However, this evidence is fragmentary, and Lorenza's XYY genotype has never been proved. Lorenza states that aggression can be beneficial if slowly siphoned off or subliminated. However, if it is stored up it can be explosive and destructive.

The frustration-aggression view states that aggression is the result of frustration. When the achievement of a goal is blocked and frustration builds, it is released as aggression because the tension is too much for the individual to endure. Environmental, behavioral, and learning theories are addressed in the frustration-aggression view.

Social learning theory states that aggression is acquired through direct experience or by imitating the behaviors of others. Social learning theorists believe that positive and negative reinforcers are more responsible for aggressive behavior than internal, inborn processes.

ANGER AND ALIENATION

Anger is an emotion/feeling that usually follows people's realizations that they do not like what is happening and it must stop.

It is often our own anxiety and anger that makes rebellious people look so threatening to us and compels us to take flight or fight. We need to reflect about the nature of our anger, anxiety, and fears. They tend to reinforce these same feelings in our clients and possibly will lead to violent behaviors. Remember that none of us are strangers to anger and its destructive power. Self-righteousness and self-deception arising from anger can give us an excuse to carry out a decision that has been made in anger.

Anger can be destructive; it can, however, also be constructive (which we rarely recognize) (Table 10-1). A key to use in reducing anger is to give the angry person something he or she can accept. Since anger is usually based on an unrealistic expectation of oneself, someone, or something else; courtesy, tolerance, and a willingness to help make deescalation work.

TABLE 10-1 Anger: Constructive and Destructive Uses

CONSTRUCTIVE USE	DESTRUCTIVE USE
1. View as normal, natural, healthy	1. Makes you distrustful
2. Take responsibility for your own feelings	2. Weakens self-esteem
3. Remember you have control over your anger and how you handle it	3. Masks "real" feelings
4. Recognize what triggers your anger	4. Stops communication
5. Defuse self	5. Destroys relationships
6. Increase assertiveness skills	6. Leads to physiologic problems
7. Deal with issues as they arise	7. Increases feelings of isolation
8. Increase personal self-esteem	8. Accumulates and leads to hostility and rage
9. Develop mutual understanding and forgiveness	

Conflict resolution is a method of resolving these feelings of alienation and anger. Conflict resolution contains the following: a *direct message, active listening, exploring alternatives,* and a *contract.* Each of these areas can be defined as follows:

- **direct message**: clear message of what you want, do not want, or feel; "I want you to stop yelling obscenities."

- **active listening**: being attentive, verifying by stating: "I heard you say."

- **exploring alternatives**: consider alternatives and look at possible options.

- **contract**: either a verbal or written contract. The objective is that both people clearly understand and agree upon alternatives and are committed to following through on them.

TALK DOWN

The prevention and management of disturbed behavior is based on early, safe, effective interventions accompanied with careful consideration of the client, self, and environment. **Talking down** is verbal deescalation.

It is very important to be aware of sudden changes (escalation) in the normal behavior patterns of the client. These can include pacing, restlessness, wringing of the hands, kicking, throwing things, grimacing and withdrawal, fault-finding, shouting, unwarranted joking at another's expense, refusing medications, arguing, refusing to obey unit rules and schedules, cursing, sarcasm, and constant demands on the staff.

Physical changes caused by a chronic illness and the prolonged use of therapeutic drugs increase the incidence of assaultive behaviors. Organic brain syndrome, brain lesions, and metabolic or endocrine disorders can also cause disruptive behaviors. One needs to carefully observe the client's condition and drug regimen, because an agitated client may be manifesting symptoms of toxic drug levels or interactions and a delirium syndrome (Table 10-2).

Research reveals that causes of disruptive behaviors include fear, frustration, reality testing, rejection, feelings of inferiority, intrusion of personal space/lack of privacy, and grief. Common behavioral disorders can occur as either defensive or offensive actions. A client's feelings of fear and helplessness are motivated by a sense of self-preservation. Offensive actions are actually meant to destroy or punish one's self. It is possible that this can result in suicide. Sarcasm, arguing, and physical aggression to self or others is seen. On the other hand, clients with passive behaviors are unable to accept and acknowledge their feelings of anger. These clients will usually withdraw.

Disturbed behavior moves along a continuum from verbal to physical violence to destruction of self or others. There is usually a

TABLE 10-2 Therapeutic Drugs Associated with Delirium

ACTH	lithium
alprazolam	meperidine
amantadine	naproxen
aminophylline	prednisone
amphetamines	propanalol
amphotericin B	theophylline
cimetidine	clonidine
digitalis	ephedrine
isoniazid	lidocaine

Anticholinergics produce delirium

CNS stimulants produce paranoid psychosis

Corticosteroids produce affective (mood) changes

Beta blockers produce depression

hierarchy of violent behaviors (Figure 10-1). An important aspect of the control of the anger and alienation is personal self-awareness. This self-awareness can prevent escalating anger and alienation. Learn to trust your own feelings and judgments.

From your own viewpoint, when you have a gut feeling of uneasiness, look at the following feelings: fear, anger, anxiety, need to act out, frustration, helplessness, guilt, denial, withdrawal. Observe the environment and factors that influence that environment.

With regard to clients, watch for periods of increased activity followed by periods of inactivity on your units (i.e., during shift report or the idle time before bedtime where limits can be tested). Observe the unit organization of males and females and the age variable. On the psychiatric unit, there will develop a client hierarchy of social status and power influence. This can be assessed at unit community meetings.

We, as health professionals, can inadvertently reenact destructive patterns in the client's history and increase the insecurity that duplicates relationships outside the hospital. So one concept important to understand is **therapeutic neutrality**. Therapeutic neutrality is not a blank screen, not a deprivation, not unresponsiveness; it is a response that is neutral and devoid of needs, values, and morality. It is predicated on what is helpful to that particular client rather than the professional.

As staff on a psychiatric unit, we need to review our behavior regularly and process our feelings. We need to assess whether the need is ours or theirs. We need to ask: Are my feelings of powerlessness related to my interaction with a client? Do I fear loss of control? Finally, we need to remember that powerlessness is difficult to deal with in our culture because we do not value weakness and vulnerability.

An important characteristic of the unit milieu is the allowance of open dialogue. Communication needs to be undistorted and unconstrained. In open dialogue, no topics are off-limits. There are always four directions of communication: client-staff, staff-client, staff-staff, and client-client.

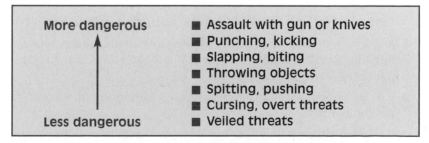

More dangerous	■ Assault with gun or knives
	■ Punching, kicking
	■ Slapping, biting
	■ Throwing objects
	■ Spitting, pushing
	■ Cursing, overt threats
Less dangerous	■ Veiled threats

FIGURE 10-1 Hierarchy of dangerous behaviors.

- Not setting enough limits or limits with unclear expectations
- Staff approaches that are inconsistent
- Offensive attitudes
- Arguing, joking, ridiculing
- Veiled hostility . . . Mask of kindness
- Seductive behavior
- Labeling a client
- Inappropriate touching
- Pushing for disclosure
- Attention given only when inappropriate or out-of-control

FIGURE 10-2 Staff behavior increasing possibility of violence.

Sometimes we model our client's communication patterns rather than offering a new communicative style. In our self-assessment we need to find out what pushed our button. Is one pushed by hostility, profanity, out-of-control people, or seductiveness? Do I respond to the client in a competitive manner?

Staff also need mutual support so that they can individually and together work on issues and begin to deal with them. Increasing your knowledge base of psychopathology is very helpful, as is the development of treatment interventions. Remember that inappropriate or negative staff behaviors can lead to violence (Figure 10-2).

Working with a violent client is less anxiety-provoking when a systematized approach to assessment is followed. Even a thumbnail assessment of violence can be most helpful. Collect data on

- *previous history of violence:* Do you tend to be a fighting person? What is the most violent act that you have engaged in? (ask nonjudgmentally)

- *methods of violence available:* knives, guns, black belt in karate?

- *problems with* **impulse control**: a history of substance abuse, difficulty keeping a job, multiple AMA (against medical advice the client leaves the hospital)

- *a recent or threatened loss:* illness, death, abandonment, divorce, unemployment

- *a* **macho image**: tough, brave, fearless, volatile, abandonment, unpredictable (can be male or female)

■ **suicidal ideation**: suicide often is the acting out of rage felt toward someone else and directed toward the self; remember that suicide and homicide are the opposite sides of a coin

■ *tension in a relationship:* teasing in a hostile way, caustic humor, provocative and unpredictable behaviors

■ *psychosis:* assess history of hallucinations, delusions, and thought processes. Are the client thoughts logical, sequential, and relevant?

■ *cognitive impairment:* assess confusion, disorientation, impaired judgment, and concentration

■ *history of* **victimization**: assess for child/adult abuse, neglect, incest, or witnessing victimization

SECLUSION AND RESTRAINT

Seclusion is the placement of a client, alone, in a specifically designated, lockable room with direct observation available through a window. Seclusion should be considered a treatment intervention before progressing to the ultimate act of **restraint** of the client. Remember that we are always looking for the **least-restrictive mode** that provides verbal/chemical intervention before initiating seclusion.

Seclusion is influenced by unit philosophy, staff attitude, staff availability, staff/client ratios (increased census, decreased staff), general milieu (anxiety, hostility), and the staff's regular, routine training in the prevention and management of disturbed behavior. The goal of seclusion is to get the client to settle down, be cooperative, and usually sleep. Serious consideration must be given to the outcomes—the calming effect of the room versus the sensory deprivation that may lead to increased mental deterioration.

Two factors should be kept in mind when considering seclusion: the client's potential for harm to self or others and the unit environment that accelerated the client's agitation. Each unit also needs a clinical indicator checklist to initiate seclusion and a readiness-to-release-from-restraints guideline (Figure 10-3).

Each facility has a policy and procedure that directly addresses seclusion and restraint policies. Seclusion/restraint laws are state mandated. (See your individual state laws.) The procedure might involve calling a nursing alert for a violent client and a number to dial (e.g., 511) or announcing a code. This information needs to be posted where all staff have ready access to it.

At times, the facility security officers need to be called; however, the officers will only take part in the action when specifically request-

- Orientation—Responds to name, direct eye contact
- Hallucinations/delusions—No longer active
- Medication—Effective response
- Threats—No longer making physical/verbal threats
- Self-control—
  1. Able to state what self-control means for him or her
  2. Cooperate with simple instructions
  3. Noted decreased impulsivity
- Readiness—
  1. Client able to state he or she is ready to be released from restraints
  2. Confer with staff for assessment of readiness

FIGURE 10-3 Readiness to release client from seclusion or restraints guidelines.

ed to do so by the clinical staff member directing the action or take-down. Remember that the takedown and placing of the client in restraints is equivalent to the code 99 cardio-pulmonary resuscitation procedure on medical-surgical units. A takedown is based on speed, surprise, and the break and escape methods. Be certain to have sufficient help for physical restraining and always be keenly aware of client safety issues. Team work is important; however, one leader will direct the situation as the charge person. Be ready.

Have the team ready and the restraints keys and a complete set of restraints ready. The staff must have confidence with their personal safety techniques; that is, providing personal space and lunge room, punch blocking, and handling grabs and hair pulls.

A new technique utilized by some facilities is the hang technique. Three persons are needed for this technique: Two grab one arm each and hang with their dead weight; the third person steers the client by holding the disruptive client's belt. The hang technique is used until the client drops to one knee, is then in a controlled position, and can be carried to the seclusion room where the restraints are applied. A clinical record of visual client checks made every fifteen minutes (q15m) are initiated. Remember that these checks are mandatory (Table 10-3).

A registered nurse (RN) who initiates the seclusion or restraint procedure is legally accountable, but all staff are responsible for their own behavior. An order for restraint then must be obtained from the physician and must be rewritten every twenty-four hours. The time of initiating restraints and the time of the notification of the physician must be carefully noted. Clear, concise charting is especially important.

TABLE 10-3 Clinical Record: Seclusion and Restraints, Visual Checks Made on Client Every 15 Minutes

DATE _____

CODE # AND ACTIVITY	NIGHTS	DAYS	EVENINGS
1. Yelling or screaming	12:00 _____	8:00 _____	4:00 _____
2. Cursing	12:15 _____	8:15 _____	4:15 _____
3. Standing still	12:30 _____	8:30 _____	4:30 _____
4. Lying down on cot	12:45 _____	8:45 _____	4:45 _____
5. Sleeping	1:00 _____	9:00 _____	5:00 _____
6. Fluids given	1:15 _____	9:15 _____	5:15 _____
7. Restraints released	1:30 _____	9:30 _____	5:30 _____
a. right wrist	1:45 _____	9:45 _____	5:45 _____
b. left wrist	2:00 _____	10:00 _____	6:00 _____
c. right leg	2:15 _____	10:15 _____	6:15 _____
d. left leg	2:30 _____	10:30 _____	6:30 _____
8. Range of motion	2:45 _____	10:45 _____	6:45 _____
a. right arm	3:00 _____	11:00 _____	7:00 _____
b. left arm	3:15 _____	11:15 _____	7:15 _____
c. right leg	3:30 _____	11:30 _____	7:30 _____
d. left leg	3:45 _____	11:45 _____	7:45 _____
9. Medication	4:00 _____	12:00 _____	8:00 _____
	4:15 _____	12:15 _____	8:15 _____
	4:30 _____	12:30 _____	8:30 _____
	4:45 _____	12:45 _____	8:45 _____
	5:00 _____	1:00 _____	9:00 _____
	5:15 _____	1:15 _____	9:15 _____
	5:30 _____	1:30 _____	9:30 _____
	5:45 _____	1:45 _____	9:45 _____
	6:00 _____	2:00 _____	10:00 _____
	6:15 _____	2:15 _____	10:15 _____
	6:30 _____	2:30 _____	10:30 _____
	6:45 _____	2:45 _____	10:45 _____
	7:00 _____	3:00 _____	11:00 _____
	7:15 _____	3:15 _____	11:15 _____
	7:30 _____	3:30 _____	11:30 _____
	7:45 _____	3:45 _____	11:45 _____

STAFF SIGNATURES AND INITIALS

_____   _____   _____

_____   _____   _____

_____   _____   _____

- Seclusion or restraint used only as last resort, and only after FAILURE OF LESS-RESTRICTIVE MEASURES
- Use facility's policy/procedure standards as guidelines
- Alternatives and/or interventions and results
- Client's behavior necessitating seclusion/restraints
- Time placed in restraints
- Medications effectiveness, any changes in meds, any side effects
- Time physician notified
- Fifteen-minute checks and interventions
- Progress note every two hours
- Assessment note at the beginning and end of each shift
- Nursing conference
- Nursing conference recommendations

FIGURE 10-4 Seclusion/restraint documentation.

There are many critical documentation areas in the seclusion/restraint procedure (Figure 10-4). For documentation purposes, many facilities require an *RN progress note* in the chart every two hours.

Remember that the client in restraints is a critically ill client. Tell the client in a calm manner that he or she is now safe and protected and that close supervision will be provided.

Immediately following a seclusion or restraint action, the nurse in charge needs to conduct a conference with all staff members involved to evaluate the manner in which the action was carried out. The conference notes will be used as a guide to assess the restraint action and any need for improvement. Continual monitoring and assessing of the use of seclusion and restraining will ensure that this treatment alternative is utilized judiciously, safely, and therapeutically.

If a client remains in seclusion/restraints for a period of twenty-four hours, a nursing care conference should be held. The conference includes the nursing staff, the clinical nurse administrator, and the clinical nurse specialist assigned to that unit. An evaluation would consist of indicators similar to the following:

- What is the need for continued seclusion/restraint?
- Does an objective assessment verify this decision?
- Is the documentation clear; can it meet review criteria?
- Is the medication regime effective?

- Does the documentation state that the seclusion/restraint action occurred *after* least-restrictive measures were utilized?
- Are the facility's policy/procedure standards met?
- Have attempts been made to remove the client from restraints or reduce the level of restraints?

Results of this nursing care conference will be posted in a staff-only area for all staff to read and initial. This conference provides objectivity and peer support as well as an opportunity to vent feelings. Many facilities have a monthly report of restraint and seclusion that must also be completed and submitted to a Risk Management or Quality Improvement committee. Lately facilities have been marking charts or designating on computer entries when a client has a history of assaultive behavior. This is called **behavioral flagging** and remains a controversial issue.

SUICIDAL CLIENTS

Many clients under psychiatric care pose some risk for suicide. Suicidal clients have feelings of depression and guilt and frequently relate feelings of hopelessness and helplessness. Self-esteem is also very low. Suicidal clients turn their hostility inward until it becomes self-destructive.

Genuine caring and helping the client feel worthwhile may help prevent an attempt at suicide. Letting the client know that there are alternatives and that others are willing to help find solutions may be beneficial.

However, clients may seem determined to destroy themselves. They secretly collect razors (or any other sharp items), ropes, pills, or belts and attempt suicide the first chance they get. These items are contraindicated on the psychiatric unit and are called **contraband**. Contraband checks are very important when clients are initially admitted to a unit or if a client is returning from a pass. Contraband may be sent in the mail or included in a present to the client.

The majority of suicidal clients are not so intent on ending their lives as they are giving a cry for help. The nurse must watch for the direct or indirect pleas for help. Suicidal clients may give some indications of intention, perhaps by saying, "Life isn't worth living," or "Here, take my camera, I won't be needing it anymore." Others may openly or jokingly mention suicide. The old notion that a person who talks about suicide will never do it is simply not true. In fact, once a person has attempted suicide, they are likely to attempt it again. Other significant behavioral clues include the following:

■ Despairing mood

■ Prolonged depression

■ Change in eating or sleeping patterns

■ Problems with school grades for the adolescent

■ Loss of previous interest in social situations

■ Uncharacteristic behavior such as reckless driving or serious drug abuse

■ A vacant stare

As previously stated, adolescence, menopause, and aging are critical events in the life cycle. During these stages there are many stressors that may culminate in suicidal tendencies. Immediately precipitating factors may include loss of a loved one, rejection, divorce, or fear of a physical or mental breakdown. These factors plus a sense of social isolation and nothingness can provoke a suicide response.

Teen Suicide

Teen suicide is an ever-increasing problem. The depressed adolescent is of growing concern to the community. It is important that the client be identified as quickly as possible so that proper treatment can be started. Usually teens thinking of individual suicide or teen suicide pacts give one or more of the following clues. They express their intentions or feelings to someone. They withdraw to an abnormal degree. Grades usually drop drastically, and they pay less attention to appearances. Teens sometimes overindulge in alcohol or drugs, and their driving becomes more reckless. It is suspected that many deaths attributed to accidents are in reality suicides.

Why this problem exists is not readily known, but there are several possible factors that contribute to the adolescent's decision to end his or her life. The many stressors teens must face in their transition to adulthood are often overwhelming. They may be unable to cope with a loss such as rejection by a girlfriend or boyfriend or the actual death of a friend. They may fear that they cannot meet the life expectations that have been set by self or parents, or they may simply be lonely and bored.

There seems to be an increase in teen suicide when there is little or no adult guidance or support, where drugs and alcohol are abused, in teens who are pregnant, or where a friend or classmate has committed suicide. Adolescents most apt to take their own lives feel that they have no purpose. They feel they are of little value because they contribute nothing worthwhile to society. Their self-esteems are low. Because they have no control over their lives, they cannot change things.

If the nurse suspects that a teen may be thinking of suicide, he or she should verify the suspicions. Not only is it proper to ask the clients about their intentions, but it is a responsibility. Teens are usually very willing to talk about their intentions. The nurse can say, "Have you had any thoughts of suicide?" or "Are you planning to hurt yourself?" Direct questioning should be done for all suicidal clients, not just teenagers.

The teenager contemplating suicide needs to be placed in a protective environment. Certainly, if the causative stressor is one that can be changed, it should be taken care of immediately. If it cannot be changed, the client needs to be watched very carefully. Sometimes a written no-suicide contract is used to prevent teens from making suicide attempts while treatment is in progress. Adolescents are asked to promise in writing that they will not try to harm themselves for a specific period of time. At the end of each period, the contract is renewed. Even though teens may use the threat of suicide to gain attention, it is more often a cry for help. A threat, whether expressed or intimated, should never be ignored. If clients have the opportunity, they will probably attempt suicide and may be successful.

Nurses can help suicidal teens by encouraging activities that will improve self-image and by showing the clients that the nurse cares about them personally. Teens need adult guidance in developing goals and support in adjusting to their changing status. They need to develop better coping mechanisms and to learn problem-solving methods. Most basically, they need to know that someone is listening and really hearing them. For more information on depression and suicide, see Chapters 11 and 12. Assess the client for a suicidal plan of action, as a plan increases the risk of suicide and need for closer observation. The nurse must connect with the suicidal client and attempt to build a relationship. To prevent self-destructive actions, the nurse first observes the client closely.

Suicidal Assessment

Intent or plan: fleeting thoughts of suicide versus a specific plan (low, medium, or high lethality)

History: Assessment of previous attempts (how many, types, lethality) and impulsivity

Recent losses

Drinking/drug abuse

Depression

History of mental illness

Another high-risk time for suicide is when a person is coming out of depression and now has the energy to conceptualize and carry out a suicide plan. The staff of a medical-surgical area in which suicidal clients are being cared for until they are medically stable for transfer to a psychiatric setting needs to recognize ways to safely alter a common environment.

Staff and client safety is important when clients who have a potential for violence are being treated outside of a psychiatric unit. If the client is housed on a nonpsychiatric unit and is experiencing any degree of suicidal ideation, high-risk suicide precautions will immediately be initiated and a nursing staff member will be assigned to monitor the client on a one-to-one basis (within arm's length) at all times. The client is to remain in his or her pajamas, restricted to the unit, and not allowed the use of any metal or sharp objects. Imposed restrictions are a restriction of the client's rights; however, the restriction is justified because of the client's risk to self. The rationale for these actions should be clearly explained to the client. The nursing staff member assigned to the client will document the client's clinical status every two hours in the medical record. Assessment is frequently made for the lethality of the client's thoughts or plans. Time is then planned to sit with the client and encourage verbalization. This will acknowledge the person's feelings of helplessness and provide an opportunity to discuss alternatives to suicide. Listening and reflecting back feelings expressed demonstrates to the suicidal person that you are aware of his or her pain and willing to stay and provide a safe environment.

Suicide assessment includes the level of lethality (low, moderate, high), a distinct plan (client states, "I will take this ballpoint pen and stab myself in the chest"), and gathering family history of suicide attempts and client's history of previous attempts.

Look at the history of impulsive acting out by this client and his or her current life stressors. Are thought problems, such as hallucinations, delusions, or thought broadcasting present? Has the client been finalizing his or her life by giving things away? What are this particular client's personal strengths, resources, and support systems?

If the client appears to have no energy to act, do not decrease vigilance because the client remains at serious risk. Place the client on Suicide Precautions to ensure protection and safety. A client placed on high-risk precautions needs a staff member on a one-to-one basis. This places the client under constant observation, and the staff member stays directly with the client. Previous attempts, that is, suicidal gesturing or manipulative or serious suicidal attempts, are the best predictors of a client at risk. Research indicates that suicide occurs at a far greater rate among alcoholics and other substance abusers than it does among the general population.

When the client is being discharged from the hospital to the community, check the client's resources for: family, relatives, close friends, physicians, clergy, professional therapists, and agencies. Does this client have other people to communicate with? Is there a support system? Are there positive thoughts about the future or an attitude that there is no point in living?

Suicide research is currently needed in certain areas. These include genetic factors inlcuding the part that they play in suicide, and differences in suicide in a variety of cultures—men, women, young, old, white, Hispanic, Asian, and African-American.

▧ Nursing Care Plan: ▧
The Client with Suicidal Tendencies

Tim James, a fifteen-year-old, is a lanky, six-foot-tall high-school basketball player. He studies hard and tries to get good grades because his father expects him to excel and his aunt is a teacher at the local high school. His peer group teases him because he is so tall and has bright red hair. The courses he is taking this semester are challenging, and his grades are beginning to slip. His father is putting pressure on him to study harder. In the last month his girlfriend, whom he had been dating for a year, decided she wanted to date other guys. Tim has become very quiet and started spending more time alone listening to music in his room. At the last basketball game, the score was tied with thirty seconds to go and he was at the foul line. He missed both shots. The other team got the ball and made a three-point basket right before the buzzer sounded the end of the game. Tim blames himself for the team not winning the game. His mother talked to his aunt about his recent behavior, and his aunt told the school counselor. When Tim and the counselor talked, he said, "I am so tall and ugly. No girl will ever want to date me. I can never please my dad. I can't even play basketball good any more. Last night I started to take a whole bottle of aspirin but my mom knocked on the door and wanted to talk to me, so I didn't take them." The counselor recommended Tim see the nurse practitioner on the psychiatric unit to do a suicide-risk screening. After the initial interview and testing, the nurse practitioner recommended that Tim be admitted to the adolescent psychiatric unit. Tim and his parents consented and Tim is admitted.

NURSING DIAGNOSIS 1

Risk for self-directed violence, related to recent increased pressures in life.

Nursing Outcomes

Tim will verbalize a desire to live by _____.

Nursing Interventions / Rationales

Nursing Interventions	Rationales
Examine Tim's personal belongings for contraband.	Inspecting Tim's belongings for contraband protects him from harming himself and conveys concern.
Acknowledge Tim's thoughts of suicide.	Discussing Tim's suicidal ideas encourages him to process his feelings and thoughts.
Establish a trusting, supportive relationship.	By establishing trust and support, Tim will be comfortable to share his thoughts and feelings.
Reinforce Tim's self-evaluation and attempts at looking forward to future events.	Reinforcing Tim's self-evaluation encourages him to grow and make plans for the future.

Evaluation

After three days on the psychiatric unit, Tim is expressing a desire to live and has contracted with the clinical specialist to share any returning thoughts and feelings of suicide.

NURSING DIAGNOSIS 2

Ineffective coping related to insufficient psychological resources to cope with increased pressures as evidenced by the lack of self-esteem, self-derogatory statements, self-doubts, and desire to commit suicide.

Nursing Outcomes

1. Tim will identify three activities that he does well by _____.
2. Tim will state needs and feelings assertively _____.
3. Tim will list coping mechanisms he can use to manage stressful situations at discharge.

Nursing Interventions	Rationales
1a. Encourage Tim to identify activities he does well.	1a. By identifying activities he does well, Tim can take pride in these and build his self-esteem.
1b. Acknowledge Tim's positive aspects.	1b. Reinforcing Tim's assets will build his self-esteem.
2a. Encourage Tim to keep a journal of his feelings and thoughts.	2a. Writing feelings and thoughts in a journal gives Tim a nonthreatening way to vent.
2b. Develop a relationship of trust with Tim so he feels free to share his needs and feelings.	2b. An open, trusting relationship will help Tim feel more free to share his feelings.
2c. Share ways Tim can express himself assertively.	2c. By expressing himself more assertively, Tim will be able to verbalize his needs and feelings.
2d. Refer Tim to an assertiveness class.	2d. An assertiveness class will teach Tim new ways to communicate effectively.
2e. Discuss healthy ways Tim can communicate and interact with his friends.	2e. Discussing healthy communication and interactive skills with Tim exposes him to new ways to interact with his peers.
3a. Encourage Tim to list positive and negative methods he has previously used to handle stress.	3a. Listing past coping methods assists Tim in identifying positive and negative coping mechanisms.
3b. Discuss healthy methods Tim can use to handle stress.	3b. Discussing healthy methods to handle stress gives Tim more options to handle stress effectively.

Evaluation

Tim acknowledges that he is a good basketball player and has received high marks on creative writing assignments. He begins keeping a journal to catalog his feelings. Although nervous, he agrees to enroll in a teen assertiveness class.

NURSING DIAGNOSIS 3

Compromised family coping related to unrealistic expectations of father and Tim as evidenced by father's pressure on son to achieve and Tim's feelings that he lost the ball game.

Nursing Outcomes

1. Family will participate in family therapy sessions (3x week) until treatment is ended.
2. Family will learn effective communication skills and provide a supportive environment for each other.

Nursing Interventions	Rationales
1a. Establish a trusting relationship with the family.	1a. Family will feel free to share feelings and thoughts.
1b. Discuss need for family to attend therapy sessions.	1b. Involvement in therapy sessions will show Tim that the family is concerned about him and willing to change.
2a. Model supportive, therapeutic communication skills.	2a. Role-modeling communication techniques provides an example to the family.
2b. Encourage family to attend sessions on effective family communication.	2b. Family will learn effective, supportive communication.

Evaluation

Tim's family is attending therapy and communication sessions. Tim is sharing his thoughts and feelings with the family. Tim's father is examining reasons he is expecting so much of Tim.

HOMICIDE

Homicide is an act of violence directed toward another with an intent to kill. It is our responsibility to focus attention on the client's mental status and look for increased agitation, specific threats, and their view of this violent act as their only recourse. Assessment must be made of the availability of both a weapon and a victim. An open-ended approach where clients are asked directly about their desperate thoughts is an effective and safe way to handle client care.

A landmark case, *Tarasoff vs. Regents of the University of California*, California Appellate Court, 141 Ca. 92 (1977) brought to focus the rights of the client versus the rights of the public. A client communicated to the provider (a psychiatrist) an actual threat of violence or the means of harm to a reasonably identifiable victim. Statements were made to the psychiatrist indicating imminent danger to that person and that physical violence would be used to cause serious personal injury. In this particular case, the victim was murdered, and the family brought suit against the psychiatrist. This court decision brought about (in most states) the health provider's **Duty to Warn**.

In September 1987, the state of Indiana stated that providers of mental health services have a duty to warn of a client's violent behavior. Providers include hospitals, private institutions, physicians, psychologists, social workers, nurses, and college counseling centers. Reasonable efforts must be made to notify a police department or other law enforcement agency having jurisdiction in the client's or victim's place of residence. A civil commitment to take custody of the client may need to be sought. The mental health professional who provides information that must be disclosed to comply with this act is immune from civil and criminal liability under state statutes that protect the client's privacy and confidentiality. If the victim is a minor, the parents must be notified. Current hospital policies and procedures need to reflect the provisions of this act, and mental health providers must research the laws of their particular state.

RISE IN CHILD AND ADOLESCENT VIOLENCE

In 1990, more than 4,000 teenagers were killed by firearms. Many attribute the rise in violence in this age category to low socioeconomic status, high population density, availability of guns, substance abuse, poor academic performance, child abuse, or a culture of violence. A priority for youth by the year 2000 by the public health service is reduction in assault injuries (age twenty-three and older), reduction in physical fighting (age fourteen to seventeen), reduction in weapon-carrying adolescents (age fourteen to seventeen), and coordination of a comprehensive violence-prevention program. Since violence is an interpersonal conflict, a range of nonviolent options and responses must be available. School education strategies may include conflict resolution and mediation, crime prevention, law-related education, handgun violence education, life skills training, self-esteem development, public education, and media education.

A creatively designed program to resolve conflict may focus around less physical violence in the classroom, less name calling, fewer verbal put-downs, more caring behaviors, and increasing willingness to cooperate, understand, and look at the other points of view. Peer education with straight talk about risk and firearm safety courses have been implemented in some school programs.

ABUSE

With increased media coverage, there is awareness and emphasis on family and social violence. It is a complex social problem. A violent act has a victim, a **perpetrator**, and frequently witnesses. There are female and male perpetrators. Multiple stressors contribute to violence (Table 10-4).

Adult Abuse

Family violence is an important public health problem in the United States. Reports indicate that more than 12 million women are abused by partners during their lives, with 25 percent of women seen in the emergency rooms having injuries from abusive relationships. Battery of pregnant women is a critical problem, with 21 percent of prenatal clients having a history of abuse and subsequent referrals to a shelter. Victims are traumatized physically, emotionally, psychologically, and spiritually. They are pursued and terrorized by their partners. The perpetrator is the one attempting to gain power and authority through abusive threats and controlling behaviors that lead to the use of violence. Victims of domestic violence need to be given power and control with resources and alternatives. For example, having critical phone numbers close at hand may help victims of domestic violence in the advent of a crisis (Figure 10-5). Emergency room personnel are being

TABLE 10-4 Stressors

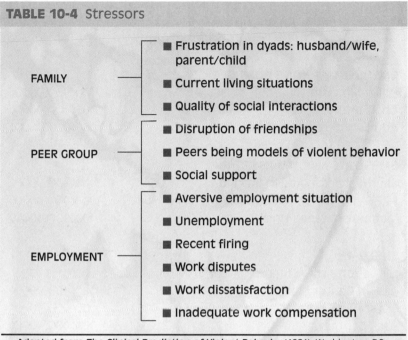

FAMILY	■ Frustration in dyads: husband/wife, parent/child ■ Current living situations ■ Quality of social interactions
PEER GROUP	■ Disruption of friendships ■ Peers being models of violent behavior ■ Social support
EMPLOYMENT	■ Aversive employment situation ■ Unemployment ■ Recent firing ■ Work disputes ■ Work dissatisfaction ■ Inadequate work compensation

Adapted from *The Clinical Prediction of Violent Behavior* (1981). Washington, DC: Government Printing Office DHHS Pub. No. ADM 81 921

educated to identify the abused person and utilize the Adult Abuse Protocol (Figure 10-6). Previously, personnel may have distanced themselves to avoid feeling vulnerable or overwhelmed with the severity of the injuries or wounds (e.g., enucleation of an eye). The battered person/victim may describe his or her injuries as accidental, self-inflicted, or undefined. Victim's behaviors frequently are evasive, fearful, depressed with numbness, rationalization, self-blame, and denial. If learned helplessness has been part of his or her lifestyle, there is a belief that the victim has no control over life's events. Usually he or she has participated in a victim/perpetrator (abuser) relationship in which tension builds. The perpetrator has an explosion of rage and batters the victim. A honeymoon period filled with apologies and possibly gifts follows. All too soon, an altercation occurs and the cycle of violence begins over and over again.

**DOMESTIC VIOLENCE RESOURCE
AND REFERRAL CARD**

EMERGENCY PHONE NUMBERS	911
Police Emergency	XXX-XXX-XXXX
Crisis Intervention	XXX-XXX-XXXX
Adult Protective Services	XXX-XXX-XXXX

EMERGENCY VICTIM ASSISTANCE	
Sheriff's Victim Assist. Program	XXX-XXX-XXXX
PREVAIL	XXX-XXX-XXXX
Victim Assistance Unit	XXX-XXX-XXXX

SHELTERS	
*Salvation Army Emergency Lodge	XXX-XXX-XXXX
*Julian Center Shelter	XXX-XXX-XXXX
Dayspring Center (after-hours shelter)	XXX-XXX-XXXX
Care Center	XXX-XXX-XXXX
Holy Family Shelter (emergency)	XXX-XXX-XXXX
Mount Olive Care Crisis Center	XXX-XXX-XXXX

*Priority to battered women

SUPPORT GROUPS/COUNSELING FOR DOMESTIC VIOLENCE	
Breaking Free	XXX-XXX-XXXX
Family Service Association	XXX-XXX-XXXX
Julian Center	XXX-XXX-XXXX
PREVAIL	XXX-XXX-XXXX
Salvation Army Social Service Center	XXX-XXX-XXXX

OTHER IMPORTANT NUMBERS	
To check jail status	XXX-XXX-XXXX
Prosecutor's Office	XXX-XXX-XXXX
Family Helpline 7:30-5PM (TTY/TDD)	XXX-XXX-XXXX
Helpline (TTY: 9:25-7104)	XXX-XXX-XXXX
Legal Serv. Org. IN. Inc (low income civil cases)	XXX-XXX-XXXX

FIGURE 10-5 Sample Domestic Violence Resource and Referral Card and Safety Plan. (Adapted from Domestic Violence Network Cards, Indianapolis, Indiana, 1996.) (English and Spanish.)

**VIOLENCIA FAMILIAR Y TARJETA
DE INFORMACION**

TELEFONOS DE EMERGENCIA

Policia Emergencia .... XXX-XXX-XXXX
Ayuda Emocional de Emergencia .... XXX-XXX-XXXX
Servicios de Proteccion para adultos .... XXX-XXX-XXXX

ASISTENCIA PARA VICTIMAS EN EMERGENCIA

Sheriff's Victim Assist. Program .... XXX-XXX-XXXX
PREVAIL .... XXX-XXX-XXXX
Victim Assistance Unit .... XXX-XXX-XXXX

REFUGIO

*Salvation Army Emergency Lodge .... XXX-XXX-XXXX
*Sojourner .... XXX-XXX-XXXX
Dayspring Center (Alojamiento a cualquier hora
   o despues de horas regulares .... XXX-XXX-XXXX
Care Center .... XXX-XXX-XXXX
Holy Family Shelter (Alojamiento de Emergencia XXX-XXX-XXXX
Mount Olive Care Crisis Center .... XXX-XXX-XXXX
                * Priondad para mujeres que han
               sido friscamente maltradas

**GRUPOS DE AYUDA Y CONSEJO PARA VICTIMAS
DE VIOLENCIA FAMILIAR**

Breaking Free .... XXX-XXX-XXXX
Servicio Para la Familla .... XXX-XXX-XXXX
Julian Center .... XXX-XXX-XXXX
PREVAIL .... XXX-XXX-XXXX
Salvation Army Social Service Center .... XXX-XXX-XXXX

OTROS NUMEROS IMPORTANTES

Bail Commissioner (para chequear is condicion o estado de
   personas que han sido arrestadas) .... XXX-XXX-XXXX
Prosecutor's Office .... XXX-XXX-XXXX
Indiana Family-lines
   de ayuda 8am-4pm (TTY/TDD) .... XXX-XXX-XXXX

FIGURE 10-5 (Continued)

SAFETY PLAN

Safety signal (to alert neighbor to call police)

Have bag packed (include the following if possible)

- Change of clothes for yourself and children
- Address book—include phone numbers of friends, relatives, doctors, lawyers
- Money—include change for pay phone
- Extra keys—to house and car
- Emergency medicines
- Important papers—include checking and savings account numbers; copy of lease; copy of No Violent Contact Order/Protective Order; birth certificates; social security numbers for yourself, children and partner; ADC/SSI/Medicaid cards; etc.

REMEMBER: Avoid long distance calls if possible (long distance numbers can be traced). Advise school system, court, welfare not to give out any information.

NOTE: To be notified when your batterer is released from jail, call: XXX-XXX-XXXX

This second printing Funded by: The Indianapolis Foundation, Indiana University Community Child Abuse Projects, Domestic Violence Network of Indianapolis, St. Francis Hospital, and numerous other interested professionals and agencies. To obtain cards or donate to this cause, call XXX-XXX-XXXX

FIGURE 10-5 (Continued)

PLAN DE SEGURIDAD

PLAN DE SEGURIDAD (para alertar a sus vecinos en casos del emergencia)

Advierto a sue vacinos o planee con dilos una senal para que en caso de emergencia ramen a la Policia

- Ponga en una maleta pequena, o boisa suficiente ropa para Ud. sus ninos y acompanante
- Un directorio (libreta) contelefonos y direcciones de famillares y amigos, medicos de la familia y elde sus abogados
- Incluya dinero con suficiente cambio o sencilo para el telefono publico
- Liaves Extra para su casa y carro
- Medicinas de emergencia

- Papeles Importante: partidas de nacimiento de Ud sus hjos y personas que la commpanen, tarjetas de social security, medicaid, ADC/SSI, copoias dela ordende proteccion en contra de su esposo para Ud y su famila, documentos de propiedad, o contato de su case o vivienda, numeros de cuertas bancaries bien seen de ahorros o cheques. Y cualquier otro tipo de documentacion que sea de importancia para su familla.

RECUERDE DE NOTIFICAR: Sile es posible irate de no hacer byebadis de karge dustabcua (ye que estas pueden ser facilmente localzades). Advierta o comuniquese con les escueles de sus hjos, a la Corte, y a el Departmenento de Ayuda Social de no der ningun tipo de informecion acarca de Ud o de su familla sin su autortzacion.

Funded by:

IU Community Child Abuse Projects, Domestic Violence Network, Methodist Hospital, Inc. and others

FIGURE 10-5 (Continued)

ADULT ABUSE PROTOCOL

- Consent for photos of injuries

- Detailed description of the battered (victim)

- Detailed description of the incident

- Involve family, friends, clergy, police, prosecutor's office

- Legal interventions: restraining order, no-contact order for one year, prosecution of assault/battery charges, which may be a misdemeanor or felony. A safety plan needs to be given to the battered person, including a safe environment and assessment of the level of violence, availability of weapons, previous experiences with the court system, and police interventions. Long-term goals would be to increase services to battered pregnant women, education to healthcare providers, and social community support systems. Public-service announcements would increase awareness. It is interesting to note that there has been an increase in physical assault of men by women. Female-only violence is often denied because many assume that such violence is reciprocal. The female uses minor or severe violence and the abuse occurs among couples dating, cohabiting, or married.

FIGURE 10-6 Adult abuse protocol.

Client Abuse

Client abuse includes mental, physical, sexual, and verbal abuse. This act is forbidden: no client is to be mistreated or abused in any way. Client abuse is not allowed even if the employee feels provoked by the actions of the client. Abuse considered to be of a minor nature (teasing a client, speaking harshly, rudely) can result in reprimand, suspension or demotion. The penalty of serious abuse is removal from the facility. Further, any employee who witnesses any unkindness, rudeness, or violence of any kind toward the client and does not promptly report it is also subject to disciplinary action and there is a risk to the nurse's licensure. Employees need to be closely advised of the client's rights. Remember that intentional omission of care is also abuse, and disciplinary action is warranted.

Sexual Abuse

Rape is a sexual assault: a forcible, degrading, and humiliating act. It is sexual intercourse by force, without consent of the partner. It is an act of aggression and a violent sexual crime.

The nurse in the emergency room may be confronted with a client who has experienced a sexual assault or rape. Rape occurs to both men and women. The emergency care for the rape victim needs a multifaceted approach (Figure 10-7). The need for sedative medication must be carefully evaluated. The client's psychological needs are also great. She feels frightened and vulnerable. Her self-esteem is damaged and she often feels embarrassed. Often, she feels guilty ("What has happened to me is my own fault").

Frequently, her thought processes are disorganized. When talking to the client, the nurse should speak slowly and allow time for comprehension.

The police must be notified at once. They will also question her in the emergency room. She needs emotional support during this questioning because it is often a traumatic experience.

As part of the medical process, any wounds must be dressed and medication must be given to prevent pregnancy and sexually transmitted disease (STD), even though pregnancy seldom results from rape.

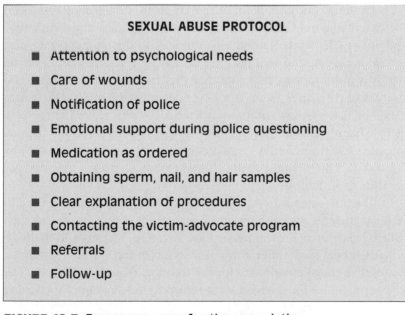

SEXUAL ABUSE PROTOCOL

- Attention to psychological needs
- Care of wounds
- Notification of police
- Emotional support during police questioning
- Medication as ordered
- Obtaining sperm, nail, and hair samples
- Clear explanation of procedures
- Contacting the victim-advocate program
- Referrals
- Follow-up

FIGURE 10-7 Emergency care for the rape victim.

(Scientists suspect that the hormonal balance of the victim is upset by the rape, thus preventing conception.)

Rape kits are available in emergency rooms. These kits contain materials for collecting proof of the occurrence of a rape (such as sperm). The emergency room staff must be careful about collecting and handling evidence. This proof, such as clippings of fingernails and combings of pubic hair, might be compared by the police to the skin and hair samples of a possible suspect. A rape victim will want to take a shower or bathe, but the nurse should not permit this until all evidence has been collected.

It is extremely important that the victim understand each procedure and the reason for it. No one other than the doctor, nurse, and police is allowed access to the evidence. All slides and smears must be protected. If there is a victim advocate program in the area, the staff should be contacted. Someone from the program will usually come to the emergency room to provide support for the victim. Later, someone from the program will visit her for counseling and referral.

The nurse should be aware of the sociological aspects of rape. The attacker is usually a person with a strong hostility toward women. He has the need to control by sexually dominating women. Rape may give the man a sense of power, and he feels that power will ensure potency, since many rapists have difficulty with erection or ejaculation.

From the woman's point of view, rape inflicts a feeling of loss on the victim. She may develop a wide range of feelings—anger, mistrust, and anxiety. This internalized rage can lead to depression. The nurse should anticipate the victim's grief caused by the degradation of the self. It is important to also note that she may not receive loving and supportive responses from significant persons in her life. Some husbands or fiancés may withdraw from her. Others reject the woman, using a blaming statement such as, "Things like this just don't happen to good girls." Even family members may ask questions such as, "Why did you walk alone in the dark?" "Couldn't you have screamed louder?" or "Didn't you fight back?"

The nurse needs to recognize that significant others may need to ventilate their feelings as they search for a rational explanation for such violent behavior against someone they love. Rape victims and their significant others can suffer a traumatic disruption of their lifestyles. Counseling may be necessary for the woman, spouse, and family. The long-term goal is for the woman to return to independent functioning in all phases of her life.

CHILD ABUSE

Child abuse is defined as maltreatment of a child by the child's caretaker. It is not a new phenomenon. Children from birth through adolescence have been victims of physical and sexual mistreatment and neglect throughout history. Recently, national attention has focused on the **shaken-baby syndrome**, which occurs when a caretaker violently shakes an infant or young baby. The severe head trauma causes retinal hemorrhage, subdural hematomas, and cerebral edema with intracranial pressure leading to serious impairment or death. If nurses work with children, they will at some time become involved with a child who has been abused. In most states, nurses are part of the group required to report suspected cases of child abuse.

Abuse can be suspected when the parent's story does not explain the injury or when the parents frequently change doctors or clinics. Abuse also may be suspected when there are many unexplained old injuries or when there are multiple scars in various stages of healing. An abused child may be aggressive or apathetic and unresponsive (Figure 10-8). There may be an unrealistic fear of adults or an overattachment to the parents. In some instances, the child may become the caretaker of the parent. Most abused children protect their parents because of fear of abandonment or reprisal. It is a nurse's obligation to report suspicions to social service agencies.

COMMON BEHAVIORS OF AN ABUSED/NEGLECTED CHILD

- Shows little or no distress at being separated from parents (frightened of parents)
- Acts unpleasant, demanding
- Causes trouble or interferes with others
- Unusually shy or fearful
- Often does not obey
- Wears long sleeves or other concealing clothing to hide injuries
- Clothes dirty or wrong for weather
- Tired, no energy
- Hungry
- Frequently breaks or damages objects
- Evidence of bruises, burns, bite marks

Adapted from Frisch & Frisch. (2002). *Psychiatric mental health nursing* (2nd ed.). Albany, NY: Delmar.

FIGURE 10-8 Common behaviors of an abused/neglected child

The majority of abusing parents are not psychotic. They care about their children and have no desire to seriously hurt them. The abusing parent comes from all economic and educational levels. The average abusing parent has a low self-concept and poor coping ability (Figure 10-9). He or she lacks parenting skills and often was abused as a child. This parent has unrealistic expectations of the child due to a knowledge deficit and employs physical means of discipline almost exclusively. He or she is usually dependent and has a spouse that is too passive to meet dependency needs. The average abusing parent relates poorly to others and has marriage difficulties. As a result, he or she is often lonely.

There is apt to be a lack of bonding. The child who is abused is often seen as different from others in appearance and/or behavior. Most severe damage is done to small children. Two-year-olds and those between thirteen and fifteen years of age are often abused because they are difficult to care for and place added stress on the parent.

It is not easy, but if the nurse is going to help prevent child abuse, he or she must look beyond the injured child. If abuse is to stop, the parent must be helped.

The abusive parent may use abuse as a disciplinary technique. The twelve-month-old may be beaten because he is not yet able to walk. The toddler may be burned because she wouldn't stay away from the stove. A school-age child may be whipped with a belt because that's the way the child's father was disciplined. The school-age child may be

- Comes from all economic and educational levels
- Has low self-concept
- Has poor coping ability
- Lacks parenting skills
- Was abused as a child
- Has unrealistic expectations of the child
- Primarily uses physical means of discipline
- Has a dependent personality
- Has a passive spouse
- Has poor interpersonal relationships
- Is lonely
- Has marriage difficulties
- Has not bonded to the child
- Cannot handle criticism well

FIGURE 10-9 Characteristics of the abusing parent

shoved or thrown against a wall because he disturbs a parent. The thirteen-year-old may be beaten and confined to home indefinitely because of a rule infraction. The parent may expect complete obedience, which is impossible for the thirteen-year-old.

Abusing parents, like all dependent people, cannot handle criticism well. The person who is trying to help must be nonjudgmental and nonauthoritarian. The helper must develop a trusting relationship with the parent, which may take weeks or months, and must also supply the nurturing support the parent is lacking. The helper needs to allow the parent to be dependent while guiding the parent toward growth and independence.

Since stress is a factor, the nurse needs to determine where the parent is on Maslow's hierarchy of needs (see Chapter 3 Understanding Self and Others). If physical needs such as food, shelter, and employment are not being met, the parent should be referred for help in these areas. Marital or personal counseling by a psychologist or professional nurse counselor may be needed. The parent may also benefit from assistance in budgeting, marketing, and child care. Growth and development of the normal child are often unclear to the abusing parent. The self-concept can be improved by providing success experiences for the parent and offering realistic compliments.

Parents Anonymous is a self-help group of abusing parents who have joined together to help each other learn to handle stress and do problem solving. Homemaker home health aides and nonprofessionals trained to help abusing parents in their homes provide assistance and support.

Child abuse is a widespread and complex problem that requires a multidisciplinary approach. Nurses can play an important role because they can represent a knowledgeable but nonauthoritarian figure to the parent.

ELDER ABUSE

It is estimated that approximately one million elderly persons are mistreated. Most abuse occurs in the home by family members, but abuse also happens in institutions. Elderly persons may be psychologically, physically, and financially mistreated. They may be abandoned, exploited, or neglected. Abuse does not have to result in fractures, malnutrition, or bruises. Not giving the elderly person glasses, hearing aides, or dentures could be considered abuse. Failure to bathe or shave a resident can be considered neglect. Speaking in a loud voice or disrespectfully is verbal abuse. Holding a resident too firmly and causing bruising is physical abuse. These acts are abusive whether or not they are intentional.

Just as in child abuse, elders are more likely to be abused by someone who is frustrated, fatigued or overstressed. Abusers are often elderly themselves. They tend to have unrealistic expectations of the older person's abilities. For instance, a caregiver may be unable to accept incontinence in the elderly parent. The frustration the caregiver feels is translated into humiliation for the elderly person and rough handling each time the elder person is found wet.

Abused elders are withdrawn, frightened, or aggressive and may be unresponsive, particularly with strangers. They may complain of abuse, but usually they do not. They remain quiet because of a fear of retaliation. The abused is most often female and dependent. The abuser is very similar in personality to the child abuser—he or she has a low self-concept, poor coping skills, and unrealistic expectations; lacks interpersonal skills; and has a poor support system (see Chapter 8).

INCEST

Incest is defined as a sexual relationship between blood relatives. It can be either a forced or a consensual relationship. These relationships may involve father and daughter, mother and son, or brother and sister. This section will deal only with forced incest. The sexual relationship may include foreplay, caressing, kissing, mutual masturbation, or intercourse.

This experience can be a very traumatic one for young children and adolescents. It may predispose them to sexual maladjustment or psychological problems such as phobias and depressive reactions. According to Briere (1989), postincestuous relationships have three phases: reaction, adaptation, and survival. During these phases the victim is going to deal with intrusive (flashbacks, nightmares, reliving of the incest) and avoidant symptoms (withdrawal and dissociation). Anxiety, depression, and anger are the emotional effects. Impulsive behaviors, that is, self-mutilation, drug/alcohol abuse, hypersexual activity or suicide, may occur.

In therapy, the victims need to be reminded how far they have come and how much they have accomplished. It must be realized that there is much numbing, emotionally and sexually. Briere (1989) discusses an impaired self-reference (Where do I start? Where does he or she stop?). The victim, who is now the survivor, will have difficulty with the consolation of self; therefore, the therapist must align with the survivor's strong, healthy parts.

Understand two things when approaching the client: stay with reality and provide concrete information. Many of the survivor's symptoms have served a purpose and provided him or her with a more adaptive way of dealing with their abuse. The basic philosophy of their treatment is respect, positive regard, and the assumption of the victim's own personal growth.

SUMMARY

Violence in our society is rampant. We must learn to understand our roles in the prevention and management of our clients' violent behaviors and also our roles in the nursing care of the victims. The care provider's own fear and anger must be dealt with appropriately and personal safety issues explored.

Violent, assaultive behavior is a true emergency. A safe, systematized approach and learned and practiced management techniques will provide therapeutic interventions for the violent clients. If necessary, this will involve restraint. Postconferences after a violent episode allow time for the staff to discuss their personal safety needs and feelings. During the seclusion/restraint time period, careful and thorough documentation must be followed.

Child abuse is defined as maltreatment of a child and most often occurs by the child's caretaker. Children of all ages are abused, though the very young are usually the most seriously injured. Nurses are required to report suspected cases of child abuse. Abuse can be suspected when the parent's story does not explain the injury or when parents frequently change doctors or clinics. It may also be suspected when there are many unexplained old injuries and when there are multiple scars in various stages of healing. The behavior of an abused child may range from aggression to apathy. The abused child usually protects the parent.

Abusing parents come from all economic and educational levels. Stress seems to be an important factor. The child that is abused is often seen as different in appearance or behavior.

If the nurse is to help prevent child abuse, he or she must look beyond the injured child and assist the parent. Abusing parents need help in handling stress; learning new ways to discipline; getting information on normal growth and development; and providing child care. They may need professional counseling to aid in personality growth. Child abuse is a widespread problem that requires a multidisciplinary approach. Health care professionals are mandated to report suspected child (and elder) abuse. (See individual state laws.)

Family and social violence are complex issues in our culture. As health professionals we need to deal with our own beliefs and biases. Rape and incest are difficult areas for care providers, and knowledgeable, supportive care must be given.

SUGGESTED ACTIVITIES

- Collect newspaper articles in your community over the period of a week and look at the most-reported areas of violence.
- Look at your anger in the present and in the past and allow yourself to view the differences. List constructive-destructive elements of your own personal anger.
- Write a script and role-play a specific aggressive, acting-out behavior and way of deescalating the behavior.
- Role play a postconference on a psychiatric unit after a vigorous takedown and placement of the client in restraints. A team member has been injured and is currently in the emergency room.
- Discuss current issues of consensual sex and rape. Look at the myths versus reality.
- Invite a guest speaker to discuss child abuse and the problems in your own community. Recognize available community resources.
- Discuss gun rights versus gun control and societal implications.
- Discuss appropriateness and effectiveness of metal detectors to curtail the growing problem of weapon-carrying students.
- Address underlying social and psychological causes of aggressive behavior.

REVIEW

KNOW AND COMPREHEND

A. Multiple Choice. Select the one best answer.

1. The second-leading cause of death in our society for people between the age of fifteen and thirty is
   - ❏ A. suicide.
   - ❏ B. homicide.
   - ❏ C. cardiac arrests.
   - ❏ D. cancer.

2. Conflict resolution with an angry client would include all of the following *except*:
   - ❏ A. giving a directive.
   - ❏ B. direct message.
   - ❏ C. active listening.
   - ❏ D. negotiation and contract.

3. Which staff behavior may increase the possibility of violence?
   - ❑ A. negotiating with a client.
   - ❑ B. contracting with a client.
   - ❑ C. labeling a client.
   - ❑ D. actively listening to a client.

4. Constructive uses of anger include all of the following except
   - ❑ A. increasing assertiveness skills.
   - ❑ B. increasing feelings of isolation.
   - ❑ C. developing mutual understanding.
   - ❑ D. increasing personal self-esteem.

5. A suicide attempt on the part of a teenager is usually a
   - ❑ A. means of getting attention.
   - ❑ B. psychotic behavior.
   - ❑ C. result of a dare.
   - ❑ D. call for help.

6. The parent who abuses a child should be
   - ❑ A. understood and counseled.
   - ❑ B. locked away in jail.
   - ❑ C. admitted to a psychiatric hospital.
   - ❑ D. encouraged to give up custody of his or her child.

7. Which of the following is a major factor in child abuse?
   - ❑ A. the parent's economic level.
   - ❑ B. the parent's age
   - ❑ C. stress coupled with poor coping skills.
   - ❑ D. the number of children in the home.

APPLY YOUR LEARNING

B. Multiple choice. Select the one best answer.

1. A depressed, suicidal client is admitted to the psychiatric unit. Which personal possession should the nurse remove from the client?
   - ❑ A. The client's wedding band
   - ❑ B. A cardboard nail file
   - ❑ C. A battery-operated CD player
   - ❑ D. A leather belt

2. The nurse administers PO medication to a client on suicide observation. Which action should occur afterward?
   - ❑ A. Perform a mouth check to confirm the medication was swallowed.
   - ❑ B. Tell the client the name and purpose of the medication.
   - ❑ C. Ask the client if he/she swallowed the medication.
   - ❑ D. Check the client's identification bracelet.

3. An eighty-two-year-old widow is admitted with major depression. Since her husband died two years ago, she has not resumed her normal social activities, lost 23 pounds, and stopped taking medication prescribed for her cardiac problems. Which action by the nurse would be most important?

❏ A. Weigh the client every morning after breakfast.

❏ B. Record vital signs q2h, including the apical heart rate.

❏ C. Ask the client if she is having suicidal thoughts.

❏ D. Initiate a moderate exercise program for the client.

4. A hospitalized client diagnosed with an antisocial personality disorder throws a chair against the wall. The registered nurse says to the practical nurse, "I'm going to call a code and assemble the team to place this client in seclusion." Which response by the practical nurse would be most appropriate?

❏ A. Move other clients on the unit to safety and prepare to assist the team with placing the client in seclusion.

❏ B. Tell the registered nurse, "I have an excellent relationship with this client. I'd like to try to talk him down first."

❏ C. Recommend to the registered nurse that the client should be restrained rather than secluded.

❏ D. Call the physician and get a telephone order for seclusion or restraint.

5. The nursing team discusses a recent increase in violent behaviors on the acute psychiatric unit. Which circumstance has most likely contributed to this situation?

❏ A. A new series of recreational therapy activities is being offered.

❏ B. The unit was recently recarpeted and repainted in bright colors.

❏ C. All staff members regularly attend the community meeting.

❏ D. Three new staff members have joined the team in the past month.

6. A twenty-five-year-old victim of date rape is brought to the emergency department. During the evaluation, the client says, "This is all my fault. I was mean to my boyfriend." Which is the nurse's best response?

❏ A. Ask the client what methods she used to try to escape from her boyfriend.

❏ B. Immediately locate a physician who can talk to the client.

❑ C. Reassure the client that the rapist will be prosecuted.

❑ D. Allow the client to express her feelings and notify victim assistance.

C. Briefly answer the following.

1. List the three chief life stressors that contribute to violent behavior.

2. List the hierarchy of dangerous behaviors.

3. List the three components of a suicide assessment.

4. List and briefly describe the three phases of postsexual abuse.

5. Describe the role of the mental health care provider in complying with the Tarasoff Duty to Warn of a Client's Violent Behavior.

6. List five behaviors that might be exhibited by an abused child.

7. List six characteristics of the abusing parent.

Geriatric Mental Health

OUTLINE

KEY TERMS

confusion

reversible confusion (delirium)

hypoxia

hypothermia

electrolytes

data collection

psychosocial history

mental status

amnesia

agnosia

aphasia

reality orientation

irreversible confusion

Alzheimer's disease

depression, endogenous

depression, reactive

pseudodementia

electroconvulsive therapy
  (ECT)

OBJECTIVES

After studying this chapter, the student should be able to:

- List categories of confusion.
- List possible causes of reversible confusion.
- List five ways to prevent reversible confusion in the elderly.
- Distinguish normal forgetfulness from dementia.
- Name three techniques to assess confusion in a client.
- Describe techniques to communicate with distressed or confused clients.
- List four nursing interventions to help confusion in the elderly.
- Define MDS and its purpose.
- Explain how prevalent attitudes affect the care of clients with irreversible confusion.
- Review physical assessment.
- List the theories explaining the causes of Alzheimer's disease.
- Describe causes of disease progression and nursing care of a client with Alzheimer's disease.
- Describe the different types of depression.
- Describe communication with an elderly client who is depressed.
- Differentiate between pseudodementia and true dementia.
- Briefly explain the nursing needs of the client with dementia.
- Briefly explain the nursing needs of the client with depression.
- Describe electroconvulsive therapy and the client's reaction.
- Briefly discuss two issues related to substance abuse in the elderly.

AGING

Old age is arbitrarily defined as sixty-five years and older. This group contains a very diverse population physically, mentally, and economically. Unfortunately, many people still believe the stereotyped picture of the aged as debilitated, poverty stricken, cranky, and confused.

Chronic diseases are more prevalent in the aged, but the percentage that is disabled is very small. Personality does not radically change as one becomes older. It gradually develops throughout the life cycle. If the individual is able to meet the developmental tasks of each age level and cope with the stressors encountered, the older person will not suddenly become cranky on his or her sixty-fifth birthday. Confusion is not a part of normal aging but a symptom of disease. Although there are certainly poor elderly, most have adequate incomes and assets to live comfortably. The aging person may be dealing with a current mental health problem as well as a general medical condition, such as heart disease, chronic obstructive lung disease, or diabetes.

The number of elderly has greatly increased in the past few years and is expected to continue to rise steadily. This is primarily due to the vast improvements in maternal and child health, increased technology in health care, as well as the large and aging baby boomer population.

There is a big difference between the old old and young old. Those who are turning sixty-five today are healthier, better educated, more affluent, and more outspoken than their older peers. They are speaking up and letting their needs be known. They are using political power to push through improvements in their lives and particularly in health care. As a result, there has been a surge of interest in the problems of the aged.

The care of the aged with mental health problems has unfortunately lagged behind. Deinstitutionalization had the effect of moving the mentally distressed elderly into nursing homes, where the facilities and preparation of the personnel are generally inadequate to care for them. Although the situation is improving, most of the health care disciplines find little challenge in working with the elderly. The more common mental health problems of the aged, namely confusion, dementia, and depression, are considered to be within the realm of the general practitioner.

Although the elderly who are mentally distressed are more concentrated in nursing homes, many are being taken care of by their families. In the future, it is likely that fewer elderly persons will be cared for in skilled nursing facilities. Nurses working in hospitals, in doctors' offices, and in the community are more apt to be the first to see these clients. If nurses are able to recognize the different types of problems, they may be able to save some clients great expense in terms of time, money, stress, self-esteem, and independence. More than a few elderly whose problems are reversible find themselves in institutions rather than living independently at home simply because the confusion was not treated.

CONFUSION

Confusion is not clearly defined. It means different things to different people. Clients can be termed confused if they do not know where they are or the day's date. If the answer to a question is inappropriate or behavior does not meet acceptable standards, the older person will be labeled confused. If they appear to have a blank stare or ignore simple directions, older people will most certainly be considered confused.

Confusion is one of the most common problems in old age and is extremely detrimental to the quality of life in later years. Confusion is not a normal part of aging but can result from the internal and external stressors on any of the older person's body systems. Confusion is divided into three main categories: (1) confusion referred to as delirium, results from acute illness, drugs, emotional stress, or environmental factors (this is the most common type of confusion seen in this age group and is generally reversible if treated early); (2) confusion resulting from brain damage, commonly referred to as dementia; and (3) confusion associated with affective disorders and psychosis.

REVERSIBLE CONFUSION (DELIRIUM)

Before labeling a client as confused, the nurse must be certain that the problem is not a result of factors that mimic confusion (Figure 11-1). It is assumed that everyone living in the same area shares the same culture and speaks the same language. It is hard for most young people to realize that the culture of the elderly is quite different from the culture today. The customs and manners learned in youth are carried into old age. The elderly person's own culture continues to influence his or her behavior even though the world around is changing. For example,

> Mrs. Jones, age seventy, was admitted to the hospital two days ago. Her nurses had labeled her confused. While growing up in the old country, her family ate lunch at noon and dinner at 10:00 P.M., a custom she continued to date. When her dinner tray was served at 5:00 P.M., she refused to eat because it was not her dinnertime. At 10:00 P.M., after everyone was in bed, she demanded her dinner, stating that she had had nothing to eat since noon. Although her nurses did

not understand this, Mrs. Jones was simply following accepted behavior for the only culture she knew, her family pattern.

Normal hearing loss limits the older person to the lower pitched tones, so that parts of a question can easily be missed. Rather than admit to a hearing loss, older people often answer the question they thought they heard. A misperception of the environment, particularly when the older person is not wearing glasses, may be incorrectly labeled as a visual hallucination.

Sensory losses caused by the normal aging process can result in an incorrect diagnosis of confusion in yet another way. The changes have the effect of lessening sensitivity to stimuli, resulting in sensory deprivation. Because the normal loss of hearing and sight is within a given range, there is also the possibility of sensory overload. When the individual turns on a favorite program, he or she has to turn up the volume to hear the higher pitched tones. The lower tones are also turned up. Because the person can hear these within normal range, the increased volume bombards the brain and thus results in sensory overload.

When the elderly person is admitted to the hospital, the new environment is strange. When one day is like the next, it is easy to lose track. If no large clocks or calendars are around, it is easy for everyone to forget the date or the time. Unfortunately, when the older person does this, he or she is termed confused.

When first admitted to the hospital, elderly clients may wake up in the middle of the night and wonder where they are. They may get out of bed and wander in an attempt to orient themselves. They may be trying to figure things out, resulting in a blank, lost look on their faces. Such clients will no doubt be considered confused, and in all probability, they will be put back to bed and restrained. As a result, they will remain lost, and the nursing staff will have unwittingly added to the misdiagnosis.

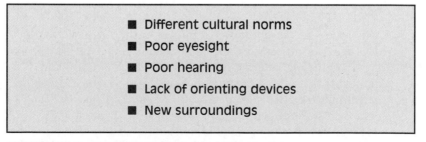

- Different cultural norms
- Poor eyesight
- Poor hearing
- Lack of orienting devices
- New surroundings

FIGURE 11-1 Conditions that mimic confusion.

Causes of Reversible Confusion

Reversible confusion is the most common type of confusion in the aged. Until definitely proved otherwise, all confusion should be considered reversible so that attempts will be made to find and eliminate the causes (Table 11-1).

Hypoxia is a lack of oxygen in the brain. Approximately 20 percent of the total oxygen consumption is used by the brain. Nerve cells cannot live for more than a few minutes without it. Because there is no storage area, the brain must get a continuous supply of oxygen. Conditions such as respiratory disease, cardiac problems, hypothyroidism, hypotension, and anemia affect the oxygen supply to the body and thus to the brain.

Hypothermia is a lowering of the body temperature. The elderly are very sensitive to this condition. They do not sense cold as easily as younger people do, and their temperatures can drop to dangerous levels very quickly. A temperature over 102° F is considered hyperthermia, and it, too, can present as confusion in the elderly.

Thirst is often ignored by older people. They may not be aware of water's importance to them, it may be too much trouble to get a drink, or water may be inaccessible to them. Dehydration is a very dangerous condition for the aged, and the only symptom may be confusion. This is especially true when electrolytes are involved. **Electrolytes** are chemicals necessary for the functioning of the nerve cell. Unless they are in balance with each other, confusion results.

TABLE 11-1 Causes of Reversible Confusion

CONDITION	EFFECT
Hypothermia	Slows brain cell functioning
Hypoxia	Diminishes cell functioning and can kill brain cells if prolonged
Dehydration	Ineffective brain cell functioning because of a lack of electrolytes
Drugs	Adversely affect brain environment
Constipation	Diminishes brain cell functioning
Sensory deprivation	Changes brain environment
Depression	Slows brain cell functioning
Malnutrition	Diminishes brain cell functioning by changing the brain's environment
Pain	Diminishes brain cell functioning as a result of stress effects

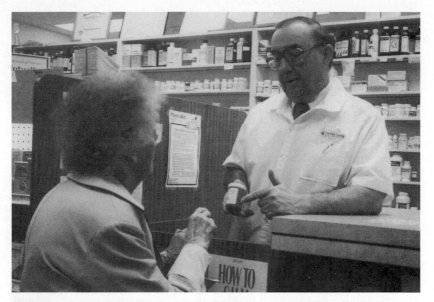

FIGURE 11-2 Elderly clients take many medications, some of which can cause confusion.

The elderly take many drugs, and some of them can lead to confusion (Figure 11-2). Tranquilizers and sedatives lessen stimuli to the brain, a condition that can be sufficient to cause deprivation. Drugs such as diuretics, hormones, and alcohol affect the fluid and electrolyte level of the brain. Medications, such as digitalis, that are used to treat hypertension and cardiac problems can cause a lessened blood supply.

Some narcotics depress the respiratory center of the brain and thus decrease oxygen supply. Besides oxygen, the brain requires a constant supply of glucose to function effectively. Hypoglycemics used to treat Type II diabetes mellitus lessen the amount available. Anticholinergics, which dry secretions, and antidepressants, which alter the chemicals in the brain, can also affect the brain's environment adversely. Antibiotics, so necessary to treating infections, have also caused confusion. Drug-induced confusion is more common than previously thought (Table 11-2).

Medications can have adverse effects in the elderly, even medications that have been taken for years. A medication or dosage change may be needed.

Sometimes the confusion can be totally due to the drug. Sometimes a person with dementia also has confusion as a result of drug therapy. In other words, a reversible confusion can be superimposed on an irreversible one. People with this problem have increased

TABLE 11-2 Drugs That Can Cause Confusion in the Elderly Client

DRUG	EFFECT
Tranquilizers and Sedatives	Lessen stimuli to the brain, resulting in sensory deprivation
Diuretics	Affect fluid and electrolyte balance
Alcohol	Affects fluid and electrolyte balance
Hormones	Affect fluid and electrolyte balance
Digitalis	Lessens oxygen to the brain by slowing heartbeat
Narcotics	Lessen oxygen to the brain by depressing respirations
Hypoglycemics	Lessen glucose available for the brain
Anticholinergics	Dry secretions, thus changing the environment of the brain
Antidepressants	Affect the brain's environment
Antibiotics	Affect the brain's environment

confusion, part of which is treatable. If drug-induced confusion is recognized, another drug can be substituted that increases clarity in the client's mind. Too often confusion is attributed to old age and is not treated at all.

Mrs. Stevens, age eighty-five, was visiting her daughter. The daughter noticed that her mother seemed confused. She set her suitcase down and the next minute could not find it. She turned the faucet on, saying she wanted a drink of water, but then quickly forgot and left the water running.

She never did get her drink. Even though she had been in the house many times, she could not seem to remember where the bathroom was. The daughter took Mrs. Stevens to see the doctor, who admitted her to the hospital.

Mrs. Stevens had been on a maintenance dose of digitalis following a heart attack several years ago. She told the nurses that she did not want her heart pill anymore. Because it was believed that she needed the drug, it was given to her by injection. As time went on, she became more confused. Finally, the doctor told Mrs. Stevens's daughter that she must consider nursing home placement for her mother. "After all, your mother is eighty-five. It is time," the doctor reasoned. The daughter reluctantly did as directed. She then sold her mother's house and disposed of most of her furniture, clothes, and household goods. After all, her mother had no use for them anymore, and she needed the money to pay the expensive nursing home bills.

In the nursing home, Mrs. Stevens told the new nurses that she did not want her "little yellow pill," the digitalis. When it was brought to her, she clenched her teeth and steadfastly refused to take it. This time, no injections were given. The drug was offered to her when it was due, but if she refused, no attempt was made to force her to take it. Mrs. Stevens's confusion, having been caused by the digitalis, began to clear up, and eventually she was discharged. Unfortunately, by that time she had no home to go to and no belongings to call her own. This happened because the confusion was wrongly assumed to be irreversible.

Mr. Roberts fared a little better. He was diagnosed as having Alzheimer's disease. He was confused, presented bizarre behavior, and was hostile toward his wife. When the diagnosis was made, his wife got him to sign a power of attorney and then admitted him to a nursing home. Because the nursing home was in another town, the client had to have another doctor. The new doctor saw no reason why phenytoin (Dilantin), an anticonvulsant, had been ordered and began to wean the client from it. As the Dilantin level fell, Mr. Roberts' confusion began to clear up.

The nursing staff noticed the change in his behavior and soon questioned his diagnosis. They asked the doctor to order a serum phenytoin (Dilantin) level, which was done. Although Mr. Roberts was improving, his Dilantin level was dangerously high. With the problem recognized and treated, however, he continued to improve.

He went to senior citizen centers and to church socials. He made many friends and one lady friend in particular. First, he got his power of attorney back and then decided to divorce his wife in order to be with his new friend. He was able to leave the nursing home and move in with his lady friend for a happier ending.

In addition, simple things like constipation, pain, immobility, and other forms of emotional and physical stress can also cause confusion in the elderly.

Data Collection

The first part of the nursing process is assessment; **data collection** contributes to the total assessment. The LPN/LVN gathers data and gives information to the RN. Before doing any assessment for confusion, the nurse must see that clients have their glasses and hearing aids, if needed. The nurse also must be certain that he or she knows the answers to the questions. For instance, to test long-term memory, the nurse can ask "What is your birth date?" Clients may be confused and have no idea, but they may know enough to realize that the nurse is asking for a date and give one. To recognize a change, the nurse must be aware of the client's history and past behaviors. This information should be contained in a good **psychosocial history**.

A psychosocial history contributes to determine the type of confusion and is the first step in assessing confusion or any of the other problems of the aged. If there is reason to believe that the client is confused, information should be obtained from family members or at least verified by them. It is best to obtain the history in an informal setting (see Chapter 7 for interviewing techniques).

The family and/or client must first be aware of the reason for the history. Time should be taken to establish some rapport. This can be done by talking about noncontroversial subjects like the weather. The basic identifying information can be collected easily after that. Client's name, address, marital status, number of children, religious preference, type of work done, and educational level are examples of basic identifying information (Figure 11-3).

Assessment tools are also available. Commonly used tools are the Brief Cognitive Rating Scale (BCRS) and the Mini-Mental Status Exam (MMSE). These tools look at changes in cognition or mental status.

The minimum data set (MDS) or another approved form containing the same information, is required to be used by all nursing homes having certified Medicare beds (see Appendix). It is a comprehensive assessment tool, but it is a minimum data set and other information may be needed. This assessment *must be started on admission* and completed within fourteen calendar days. The assessment, along with its accompanying protocols and trigger rap sheets, help the nurse determine needs and transfer these needs to the care plan. Protocols help the nurse understand the problem he or she has assessed and to think about other problems that might be related. The rap key gives the nurse guidelines in care planning. The MDS must be coordinated by a nurse, but other disciplines may complete aspects of the MDS.

Arizona Elks Major Projects, Inc.
LONG TERM CARE UNIT   DATE: _____
SOCIAL HISTORY   Hospital No: _____

The information on this form will be used solely to aid in the adjustment of your relative and you to the nursing home life. You are not obligated to answer any questions that you deem intrusive or unnecessary, but all information given will be considered confidential.

Client's name: _____   Date admitted: _____

Age: _____ Date of birth: _____   How long in Tucson: _____

Marital status: M ( ) W ( ) D ( ) S ( )   Previous area: _____

Religion: _____   Clergyman's name: _____

Responsible person: _____   and address: _____

Diagnosis: _____   Relationship: _____

  I. PRIOR TO ILLNESS

   A. Tell me about _____   _____

      before he became ill.   _____

      (What type of person was he?)   _____

      (How would you describe him?)   _____

   B. How would you describe his   Relative's Name: Relationship: _____

      relationship with his family?   _____

      (Are they able to visit?)   _____

   C. How would you describe his   _____

      relationship with friends?   _____

      (Are they able to visit?)   _____

   D. Was religion an important   Yes ( ) No ( ) Comment: _____

      factor in his life?   _____

   E. What kind of work did he do?   _____

      (Educational level?)   _____

      (How long unemployed? retired?)   _____

   F. How did he usually handle   _____

      problems or difficulties?   _____

 II. AFTER ILLNESS

   A. Date of onset.   _____

   B. Which of the changes that you   _____

      have noticed concerned you   _____

      the most?

   C. What factors did you consider   _____

      before deciding on nursing   _____

      home placement?

III. LIKES AND DISLIKES

   A. Does he have any talents?   _____

      (singing, dancing, painting,   _____

      writing, etc.)

FIGURE 11-3 Psychosocial history and assessment samples.

B. What things does he
   particularly like? (Food,
   objects, attitudes, actions,
   activities)
   _____
   _____
   _____

C. What things does he
   particularly dislike?
   (Objects, attitudes, actions,
   activities)
   _____
   _____
   _____

D. Describe his daily routine prior
   to coming to the Elks.
   _____
   _____

E. What possessions are most
   important to him?
   _____
   _____

LONG TERM CARE UNIT PSYCHOSOCIAL EVALUATION

Name: _____   Hospital No.: _____

Marital status: M ( ) W ( ) D ( ) S ( )   Age: _____

Admitted from: _____   Admitted to ward: _____

I. <u>CLIENT'S</u> <u>STRENGTHS</u> <u>AND</u> <u>WEAKNESSES</u>

A. Family support   Yes ( ) No ( )

   1. Who visits?   Comment: _____

   2. Frequency

   3. Client's reaction to visits

   4. Family reaction to client

B. Adjustment to illness

   1. Knowledge of illness   ( ) unaware   ( ) limited
                                           ( ) moderate   ( ) well aware

   2. Stage of loss   ( ) denial   ( ) anger
                                           ( ) bargain   ( ) acceptance

   3. Independent as much as   Yes ( ) No ( )
      possible?   Comment: _____

C. Adjustment to the institution

   1. Accepts therapeutic   Yes ( ) No ( )
      program   Comment: _____

   2. Accepts need to be in   Yes ( ) No ( )
      nursing home   Comment: _____

   3. Occupies time   Yes ( ) No ( )
      constructively   Comment: _____

D. Socialization

   1. Relates well to other   Yes ( ) No ( )
      clients   Comment: _____

   2. Participates in activities   Yes ( ) No ( )
                                           Comment: _____

FIGURE 11-5 Continued.

E. Mental Capacity

    1. Alert   Yes ( ) No ( )

    2. Oriented   Time ( ) Person ( ) Place ( )

    3. Appropriate reactions   Yes ( ) No ( )

                                   Comment: _____

    4. Memory   Past events ( ) Present events ( )

F. Personal Characteristics

    1. Outgoing   Yes ( ) No ( )   7. Mature   Yes ( ) No ( )

    2. Intelligent Yes ( ) No ( )   8. Sensitive   Yes ( ) No ( )

    3. Quiet   Yes ( ) No ( )   9. Happy   Yes ( ) No ( )

    4. Aggressive Yes ( ) No ( )   10. Demanding Yes ( ) No ( )

    5. Altruistic   Yes ( ) No ( )   11. Coping

    6. Selfish   Yes ( ) No ( )   Mechanism _____

II. <u>LIKES AND DISLIKES</u>

  A. Activities: _____

  B. Food: _____

  C. Objects: _____

  D. Attitudes _____

III. <u>FAMILY</u>

  A. Stage of loss   Denial ( ) Anger ( ) Bargain ( )

                       Depression ( ) Resignation ( )

  B. Relationship with client: _____

IV. <u>POTENTIAL PROBLEMS</u>

  A. Lack of stimulation   ( )

  B. Disorientation   ( )

  C. Lack of family support   ( )

  D. Adjusting to institution or illness ( )

  E. Family needs   ( )

  F. Lack of strength   ( )

  G. Poor coping mechanism   ( )

  H. Memory loss   ( )

  I. Tension   ( )

  J. Dependence on staff   ( )

  K. Other comments   ( )

<u>COMMENTS:</u>

_____

_____

_____

_____

_____

FIGURE 11-3 Continued.

The psychosocial history provides a baseline to which present behavior can be compared. It provides information on the client's strengths and support system available to him or her. The history can help determine whether the confusion is reversible and provide clues as to the cause and treatment of the condition. The history can be taken at a formal setting, but more often the information is obtained through informal conversations (Figure 11-4).

After receiving the basic identity information, the nurse can ask the family for the major problem, the behavior that led them to believe the client needed help. How the family views the confusion and how they talk about their elderly relative will give the nurse an idea of the amount and type of family support available. The number of friends with whom the client still has contact and the strength of religious beliefs are also indicators of support available to the client.

To determine whether the present behavior is a change, the nurse needs to know what the client was like previously. Was he outgoing or a loner? Was she fastidious or sloppy? Did he sleep well at night or wake often? Was she practical or a dreamer? Did he drink or abuse drugs? Did she keep busy or appear bored? Did he hold his problems in or did he talk them out? What was a typical day like?

Concerning the confusion, the nurse should ask questions such as the following: "When did the confused behavior start?" "Was the onset gradual or sudden?" "Can the family think of some stressful event that happened just before the confusion began?" "What kind of behavior does the client exhibit now?" "Has the confusion gotten worse or better?"

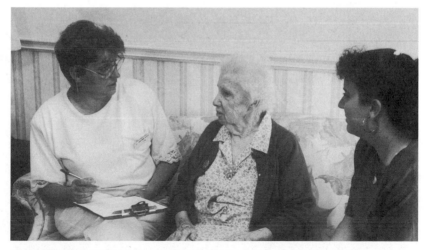

FIGURE 11-4 Taking a psychosocial history can be done in an informal setting.

Information about the client's favorite belongings, personal habits, food likes and dislikes, and perhaps long-time pet will give the nurse what he or she needs to help foster reality.

MENTAL STATUS

Following the psychosocial history, the nurse can determine the client's **mental status** through observation and questioning. First, the nurse needs to know the client's previous intellectual ability. This can be obtained, at least in part, by how far the client went in school and the occupation in which he or she engaged.

Again, before starting the mental status exam, the client should be given glasses and hearing aid, if needed. There are several areas in assessing mental status. The first three can act as a screening. If correct answers are given in these areas, the rest of the exam does not have to be given.

Memory. Memory loss can be either short or long term. Sample examples of questions to determine short-term memory, which is three to five minutes, are

1. What is your age?

2. What is your address?

3. What did you do this morning?

4. Give the client a series of numbers, an address, or a statement and ask him or her to repeat it for you in a few minutes.

For long-term memory, the nurse can ask

1. When did you get married?

2. What kind of work did you do?

3. What date were you born?

4. Where were you born?

When interviewing an elderly client, you may note an intentional effort to cover up memory losses. This filling-in of the memory gaps with their own stories is called confabulation. They may also answer questions vaguely. Many times they also answer questions with only rote memory and do not initiate conversation.

Orientation. Orientation is an awareness of time, place, person and situation. Questions that help assess orientation are

1. What is your name?

2. What is this place?

3. What state are we in?

4. What is today's date?

5. What year is this?

It is possible for a person to make a mistake with the day's date without being confused. The year is another matter. If it is 2002 and the client says it is 1945, confusion is present. Time is the most easily lost sphere of orientation; therefore it is important to determine all four spheres.

Abstract Thinking. This is the ability to generalize and categorize things. It is a higher cognitive power that is lost when confusion sets in. To test abstract thinking, the client can be asked to interpret a proverb such as "The grass is always greener on the other side." Some other proverbs are "A stitch in time saves nine" or "don't count your chickens before they are hatched." If the client is still able to think abstractly, he or she will be able to generalize the proverb. For instance, the confused person may interpret the first proverb as "The neighbor has greener grass." This is concrete. If the client is able to generalize, he or she will say that it means that people often see others as having things better than they have.

Another way to test for abstract thinking is to ask such questions as

1. How are an apple and an orange alike?

2. How are a bird and a plane alike?

It does not matter what the client answers as long as he or she uses the words *they both*. The client can say "They both eat, they both have hair, or they both make good pets." What the nurse is looking for is the ability to generalize. "The cat has hair and the bird has feathers" is a concrete answer. The client responding in this way would fail the test. However, proverbs are culturally influenced; if English is his or her second language, the client will not understand the proverb.

Judgment. The client who loses judgment is unsafe. A person who is not confused will give answers to the following questions that reflect his or her understanding of safety: "What would you do if you saw someone drop a lighted cigarette on the carpet?" "How would you get something from a high shelf?"

State of Consciousness. This area is observed. Do clients show an interest in things around them? Are they alert and aware of their environment? Do they remember personal belongings? Do they recognize themselves in the mirror?

Intellectual Functioning. The client's ability to communicate is an indication of his or her intellectual functioning. Can the client carry on a logical conversation? Does he or she use words correctly? Is the conversation consistent? Are the answers relevant? If the client is post-stroke, the client may have:

■ **amnesia**–an inability to recall past experiences (complete or partial)

■ **agnosia**–failure to recognize or identify objects. Sensory ability is intact.

■ **aphasia**–difficulty or inability to express words and phrases

A couple of other ways to assess intellectual functioning are to see if the client can follow at least a three-step instruction. "Take this paper, fold it in half, then fold it in half again, and then tear it along the folded lines" is an example of a multiple-step direction. The client can also be asked to do a mathematical problem such as serial threes or sevens.

Emotions. The nurse must observe the client's behavior. Does is seem inappropriate? If it does, the nurse must then determine whether it is a change in behavior. Regardless of how bizarre or inappropriate the client's behavior, he or she cannot be considered confused unless the behavior is a change.

> When Shirley Adams, age eighty-two, was admitted to the hospital, she was in need of a bath. Her hair was mussed and her clothes were dirty and torn. Shortly after admission, she had acquired a stack of paper cups, towels, pins, scratch pads, and pens. She had hidden them in her bedside table. This behavior does not meet acceptable standards so she would most certainly be considered confused. However, if a social history had been taken, it would have revealed that Shirley had been this way all her life. She was brought up in a very poor family. Water was a precious commodity and there was little for bathing and washing clothes. The family had very little, so they saved whatever items they could find. This was done in case there was a use found for them later. Shirley's actions were part of her life-long pattern. She was not really confused.

Has the client recently shown signs of depression, anxiety, or paranoia? These conditions, which are treatable, have been known to cause confusion.

TABLE 11-3 Physical Observations

Vital signs	Temperature, pulse, respiration, and blood pressure Quality of the pulse and respiration
Hydration	Skin turgor, intake and output Blood chemistry Urinalysis
Elimination habits	Frequency Characteristics of stool Problems with constipation or diarrhea
Nutritional status	Amount and type of food eaten Weight and height Appearance
Mobility and activity level	Range of motion Ability to ambulate Amount of assistance needed
Heart and lung functioning	Heart and lung sounds Color and condition of the skin Quality of the pulse and respiration
Vision	Need for glasses Client's ability to read a selected paragraph
Hearing	Need for hearing aid Client's ability to hear when voice comes from behind him or her
Pain	Presence of pain Type, severity, duration Any relief measures taken

Physical Changes. There are several physical factors that must be assessed to first rule out physiological causes (Table 11-3 and Figure 11-5).

Areas to be assessed include the following:

1. Vital signs. These are very sensitive indicators of change in the state of the elderly's health. They can indicate dehydration, poor circulation, and the presence of disease.

2. Hearing. The nurse must ask simple yes-and-no questions. He or she can also ask a client to repeat what was heard.

3. Vision. The client can be asked to read several sizes of print.

4. Hydration. Is the skin dry? Is there an adequate urinary output?

5. Nutritional Status. Has there been a weight change? Are there loose dentures or bad teeth? How good is the client's appetite? What kinds of food is he or she eating? Who does the cooking? How many meals per day?

6. Environment. Has there been a recent change in the client's life? Does he or she have familiar things around? Is there enough sensory stimulation without being too much? Are there orienting items around such as clocks, calendars, and newspapers? Is there a window so the client can see night and day? Is there a night-light turned on?

7. Elimination. Is there a problem with constipation or diarrhea? Is the client able to get to the bathroom? Is there embarrassment about using a bedpan? What does the client usually take for constipation?

8. Pain. Is pain present? Where is it? When did it start? How severe is it? Is it constant or intermittent? Is there anything that triggers it? Does the ordered medication help?

9. Mobility. The nurse must determine whether clients are able to walk with or without assistance. Are they likely to fall? Are they able to turn themselves in bed?

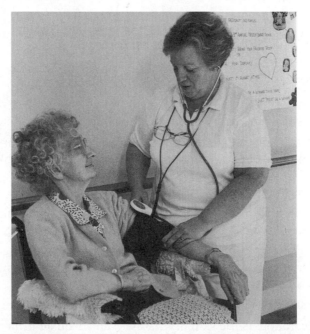

FIGURE 11-5 Physical assessment is necessary in the care of the aged.

10. Chronic Disease. Has there been a change in any of the present chronic diseases? The nurse needs information about the diseases that affect the circulation or endocrine systems in particular because these are most likely to cause confusion.

11. Medications. It is important to determine what medications the client is taking. Is the client taking any over-the-counter drugs? When it is determined that confusion results, the nurse should think about medications first. There are many medications that cause confusion in the elderly.

12. Activity. How much activity does the client have? What kind of activity does he or she enjoy?

The nurse is only one of many who assist in determining whether confusion exists. If it is determined to exist, the confusion should always be thought of as reversible. The psychosocial history and the assessment should give clues as to the cause. Treat the cause and the confusion will disappear. It is important to remember that there can be a reversible confusion superimposed on irreversible confusion.

Nursing Care of the Confused Client

Reversible confusion can be prevented. Nurses have control over many of the aspects that can cause or contribute to the confusion. That means there is much they can do to prevent it. Whenever nurses have an elderly client admitted to their care, they should see that the client has orienting items in the environment such as clocks, calendars, and reality orientation boards. They should encourage visits by family and friends who have familiar faces. It is important, too, that they make sure their elderly client has sufficient fluids. Nurses must attend to other activities of daily living as well, such as adequate nutrition, good hygiene, and physical activity. Be alert for sundowner syndrome. This client confuses day and night and wants to sleep all day and be awake all night. The client can become agitated and quite difficult to redirect.

Reality Orientation

Reality orientation is a process by which confused people are reminded of orienting cues in the environment. They are taught to use these cues to reorient themselves in time and place. Reality orientation goes on for twenty-four hours a day. *Immediacy*, simplicity, and consistency are the main factors. Immediacy means that the nurse must respond to clients quickly. If he or she asks them a question, she must allow them time to answer, but not so much time that clients lose interest. Clients' questions must be answered right away, and they should not be kept waiting to have their needs met. The attention span is short, which makes immediacy important. *Consistency* means that all personnel treat clients in the very same way. A written orientation plan is necessary to assure this.

Reality orientation is based on repetition, with everyone saying and doing the same things over and over again. This helps the confused person to relearn and lessens the extraneous stimuli with which he or she must cope. *Simplicity* demands that all responses to the client be in simple, concrete terms. Pictures are more concrete than words; therefore, they should be used often when giving directions. Instead of telling a client to go to the bathroom, the nurse can show him or her a picture or place a picture on the door of the bathroom. Only one-step directions should be given. The nurse does not tell a client to comb his or her hair. The client may not remember how. Besides breaking the task down to its simplest terms, the nurse can also put a comb in the client's hand and then move the hand through the motions. He or she can repeat this many times, but eventually the client should learn to do it alone. It is important that the nurse get the client's attention before starting to speak and that he or she maintains that attention with eye contact. This way the client is not confused about who the nurse is talking to. The conversation needs to be concrete, and the nurse needs to remain calm and relaxed. Touch is essential to keeping this client in reality (Figure 11-6).

Reality orientation is the most useful tool for helping confused clients. With this technique, clients are directed back to reality. "This is Wednesday and you are in Atlanta." The nurse should never argue with the client. If the situation tends to get out of hand, the nurse can use distraction therapy—change the subject and get the confused person's mind on something else.

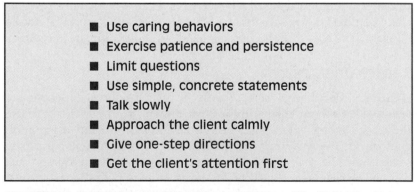

- ■ Use caring behaviors
- ■ Exercise patience and persistence
- ■ Limit questions
- ■ Use simple, concrete statements
- ■ Talk slowly
- ■ Approach the client calmly
- ■ Give one-step directions
- ■ Get the client's attention first

FIGURE 11-6 Techniques for communicating with distressed or confused clients.

As with the aggressive client, all tasks need to be broken down into simple steps. The directions for each step are given one at a time. Clients then need time to respond. Their concentration is limited and memory for recent events is poor, so it is a good idea to call confused clients by their first name. Generally, the earlier something is learned, the longer it is retained.

For some clients, reality orientation takes weeks to accomplish a simple change, and for others it takes months. Some clients do not benefit from it at all. The important thing is that the nurse not become discouraged. Without consistency, the process will definitely not work. The reasons for confusion and the stage of the illness will be factors that will affect the appropriateness of reality orientation. If used at inappropriate times, it can frustrate the client.

Reality orientation goes on twenty-four hours a day. The client is told where he or she is, the day, the date, and the nurse's name first thing in the morning and several times throughout the day. Other information that can be included is the time of the next meal, the weather, or upcoming events.

A reality orientation board is often posted in a prominent place (Figure 11-7). It serves to provide the same orienting information. The board should have a colorful background. It must be at eye level. It may be necessary to have two boards, one for ambulant clients and one for those in wheelchairs. Needless to say, all reality orientation boards should be current.

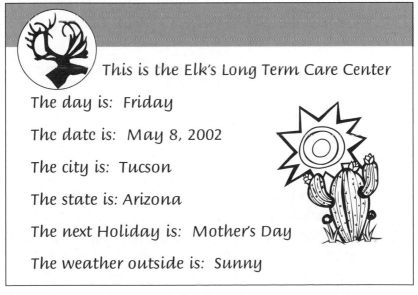

This is the Elk's Long Term Care Center

The day is: Friday

The date is: May 8, 2002

The city is: Tucson

The state is: Arizona

The next Holiday is: Mother's Day

The weather outside is: Sunny

FIGURE 11-7 Reality orientation board.

Many institutions also have a formal orientation class to supplement the twenty-four-hour program. The classes are held in a well-lighted, quiet place for fifteen to thirty minutes each day. Each class should be limited to five or six people. Besides encouraging reality, these sessions are used to help clients relearn a task such as telling time, tying a shoe, or writing with a pencil. Audiovisuals such as pictures, word and picture cards, large blocks and puzzles, felt boards, mirrors, and a tape recorder as well as mock-ups of clocks and calendars, are necessary to making the lesson concrete. Anyone wishing to start a formal program must begin by collecting all the audio and visual material available.

The class must be well planned. The leader should have a set goal and objectives in mind and should go slowly to allow each client to progress according to his or her abilities. The leader should try to keep the class lively and avoid putting any client on the spot. If he or she asks a client a question and gets no response, the nurse can reply with "I would like to help you identify this or read this or answer this," whatever the case may be. The idea is to prevent a loss of self-esteem. All correct answers or even attempts at answering should be praised. The importance of touch should never be forgotten.

A typical session may go like this:

Nurse: "Good morning, John Stevens." She would then proceed to greet each client by name. Remembering the importance of touch, she would shake their hands. "This is our reality orientation class. It is planned to help improve memory and exercise the mind. It is eleven o'clock in the morning. The sun is shining and the temperature is eighty-five degrees.

"Sam, can you tell me what season this is?" If there is no answer, she would wait a minute and then say "I would like to help you answer that question, Sam. It is summer now. Do you like summer Sam?" If Sam answers *yes* or *no*, his effort would be praised. "Of course summer is a great time, isn't it? George, can you think of some good things to do in the summertime?" If George says "Go outside," the nurse might respond with "That's right. That's a great idea. We could sit in the sun or take a walk. Andrew, do you enjoy going outside?"

Names are always mentioned first when a question is to be asked. This alerts the client to the coming question. The confused clients should never be given a nickname by the caregiver, including "Pop," "Hon," or "Dear."

Not all clients will succeed to the same degree, and some will not succeed at all. It is essential that the personnel dealing with them do not become discouraged. Reality orientation takes time.

Reminiscing is an integral part of orientation and involves the discussion of life experiences within a group. Because the person with dementia will remember past events longer than current ones, the past events provide a topic for communication. Communication is the means by which people validate their self worth. If a person feels accepted by a group, self-esteem will be improved. Most often the group becomes supportive. Their acceptance acts as a buffer against the many losses felt by the elderly.

Verbalizing about life experiences gives clients an opportunity to rethink and reorganize their lives. They can then see the meanings of some past events and find new meanings for others. These meanings help to validate the worth of the clients' lives.

Reminiscing provides a means of effective interaction with the mentally impaired elderly. It also provides a tie to present-day reality. The nurse or therapist takes people from where they are in memory and guides them to the present.

IRREVERSIBLE CONFUSION

There is no sure way to tell whether a client has reversible or irreversible confusion; therefore, it is best to assume that confusion is reversible and rule out all possible causes. The nurse is only one of many who will participate in making this determination, but he or she is in a position to offer many clues.

Irreversible confusion is called dementia, organic brain syndrome (OBS), senile dementia, or, incorrectly, senility. Senility simply refers to old age. The term was popular when dementia was believed to be a normal part of aging, but unfortunately it remains in use.

The cause of **irreversible confusion** is brain damage. There are several causes of brain damage, but the most common is **Alzheimer's disease**. Other major causes are multiinfarct, or several small strokes, which accounts for 20 to 25 percent; Alzheimer's with multiinfarct, which accounts for 5 to 20 percent; and all others, such as arteriosclerosis, Creutzfeld-Jakob's disease, and adult hydrocephalus, which account for 5 to 10 percent (Table 11-4).

Multiinfarct refers to a series of small vascular accidents commonly called *strokes*. The most common cause of strokes in the elderly is a blood clot in one of the brain vessels. The clot cuts off the oxygen and glucose supply behind it. The result is death to the part of the brain denied oxygen. Hemorrhages can also be a cause of brain damage but are more apt to occur in a younger person.

TABLE 11-4 Irreversible Confusion

DISEASE	CAUSE	SYMPTOMS
Multiinfarct	Several small strokes	Abrupt onset, stepwise progression, weakness, and hemiplegia
Arteriosclerosis	Hardening of the arteries	Hypertension, dizziness, orthostatic hypotension, headaches, sleepiness
Intracranial neoplasm	Usually affects gliomas Cause unknown	Headache, convulsions, blurred vision, severe anxiety
Huntington's chorea	Inherited	Involuntary muscle movements
Hydrocephalus	Blockage in the drainage of cerebrospinal fluid	Progressive deterioration, crosses feet when walking
Creutzfeld-Jakob's	Slow-acting virus	Rapid progression, muscle atrophy
Trauma	Injury	Immediate nonprogressive deterioration
Alzheimer's	Multiple	May have been in coma, severe pain, insidious beginning, progressive deterioration
Pick's	Atrophy of the frontal and temporal lobes of the brain, associated with alcoholism	Progressive irreversible memory loss and deterioration of intellectual function

When dementia results from small strokes, the onset is abrupt. Confusion starts as soon as the blood flow to the brain is jeopardized, but it does not increase. Each time the client has a small stroke he or she becomes more confused. There can be some improvement as brain edema subsides, but the client never fully recovers. Along with the mental symptoms, the client will have the usual physical symptoms of stroke, such as weakness, paralysis on one side, or loss of speech.

Arteriosclerosis is hardening of the arteries. Because this results in less blood going through the vessels, blood supply to the brain cells is diminished. Arteriosclerosis is also accompanied by high blood pressure. If the pressure becomes high enough, brain hemorrhage can occur.

Creutzfeld-Jakob's disease is also very rare. It is caused by prions, and the course of the disease is rapid.

In adult hydrocephalus, there is a defect in the vessels that drain the cerebrospinal fluid from the brain. The fluid builds up in the skull and causes damage to the brain cells. The damage already done cannot be repaired, but future damage can be prevented by surgically placing a shunt in the brain. As long as the shunt remains open, it will drain off the excess fluid.

Alzheimer's is by far the most common cause of dementia, accounting for 50 to 60 percent. The onset is slow and gradual. It then progresses with increasing confusion until death occurs, usually from pneumonia, urinary tract infections, or other complications of immobility. The family may recall some stressful event, such as surgery, that happened shortly before the confusion became apparent. Stress does not cause dementia, but it seems to speed up the progress of Alzheimer's disease. The confusion occurring before the event may have been so slight that the family paid little attention or passed it off as normal forgetting.

There are two major changes that occur in the central nervous system. Deposits of a starchlike protein in the brain are seen on autopsy. These plaques, as they are called, interfere with transmission of impulses through the nerve cells. The nearby neurons (Figure 11-8), undergo the second change. The neuron atrophies, and the axon and dendrites then wrap around the cells and entangle them in a mass of tissue. These are actually called *tangles*. They develop mostly in the cortex and cause forgetting of the higher cognitive functions first.

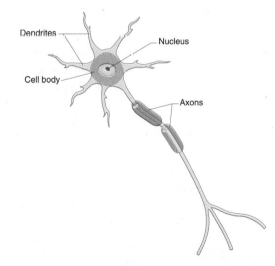

FIGURE 11-8 The neuron. In Alzheimer's disease, the axon and dendrites entangle themselves around the atrophied body of the cell.

The cause of the disease is not known, but research is on-going. Several theories have been advanced, but neurotransmitters seem to be the most promising at the moment. The possible factors associated with the development of Alzheimer's include:

- *Heredity.* A gene has clearly been identified that causes one type of Alzheimer's disease. Clients with Down's syndrome almost universally develop Alzheimer's if they live past thirty.

- *Age.* The incidence of Alzheimer's increases with age. As people get older, they seem to become more vulnerable to the disease.

- *Increased aluminum concentration in the brain.* There has been an increased aluminum concentration found in the brains of people with Alzheimer's disease. For a time it was thought an increased ingestion of aluminum might be the culprit. Further studies have shown that it is probably a result rather than a cause of dementia.

- *Slow-growing virus.* Because symptoms of Creutzfeld-Jakob's are similar to Alzheimer's disease, some studies have looked at viruses as a cause. Thus far, this theory remains unproven.

- *Neurotransmitters.* A change in the amount of the neurotransmitter, acetycholine, in a client with a familial tendency to the disease seems to be the most acceptable theory today. Within the next few years, there will be new cholinesterase inhibitors on the market. Currently, donepezil (Aricept) is the most frequently prescribed medication. In mild to moderate Alzheimer's disease, Aricept has helped to make a difference in client's participation in basic activities of daily living: toileting, dressing, personal hygiene and grooming, feeding, bathing, and walking around inside and outside the home. Shopping, using the telephone, performing household tasks, and improvement in the ability to understand situations are notable changes when the client is medication compliant. Researchers are making rapid progress in the development of an Alzheimer's vaccine.

There is no cure at present. The disease will continue to progress, with the client living from two to twelve years. The disease goes through stages, although they are not always easy to detect. The stages are not clearly defined and can overlap.

Disease Progression

In the first stage, there is memory loss (Table 11-5). As mentioned earlier, it is so slight that it can be overlooked or covered up. The client is generally disoriented, particularly to time and place. He or she may not

TABLE 11-5 Stages of Alzheimer's Disease

STAGE	CHARACTERISTICS
First	Slight memory loss; some behavior changes; may wander and get lost; disoriented as to time and place
Second	Further deterioration with increased memory loss; logic, reasoning, and judgment are diminished; neglects grooming and proper eating habits; exhibits antisocial behavior
Third	Forgetting increases; may not recognize family and self; conversation is irrelevant; may scream incessantly; unsteady gait; may be incontinent
Fourth	Not able to ambulate well or at all; incoherent speech; totally incontinent; seizures may occur

be able to find the way to the corner store where the client had been going for years. His or her ability to think logically and judgment are affected. There can also be emotional or behavioral changes.

There is further reduction in memory in the second stage. Logic, reasoning ability, and judgment are also further diminished. These people can forget social standards. They can neglect grooming and proper eating habits. They can undress in public or use profanity where they would not have used it before. In the third stage, forgetting increases. Perception changes, and clients may not recognize familiar faces or objects. They usually become incontinent of both bowel and bladder. Reading, writing, and the ability to problem solve are most likely gone. Although the client can still pronounce some words, conversation is irrelevant and, at times, can be unrecognizable. The client can scream and yell incessantly and not know why. Toward the end of this stage, there can be an unsteady gait and frequent falls may occur.

During the fourth or last stage, all symptoms become worse. Clients are probably bedridden and unable to feed self. They will have no control over their bowels or bladder. Their speech is incoherent, and, if they speak at all, it is usually only sounds. Seizures often occur.

Nursing Care

There is no cure. Drugs can be used to palliatively control specific behaviors, but they may or may not be effective. Even though the confusion is irreversible, reality orientation should be employed. Many times these clients have a reversible confusion superimposed over the Alzheimer's, making the condition appear worse than it is. Research has shown that reality orientation can slow down the progress of the confusion, even when it is due to organic reasons.

Even though the client may not answer or may answer with irrelevance, the nurse must continue to attempt to communicate with him or her (see section on reality orientation earlier in this chapter). The important points are summarized here:

1. Remain calm
2. Do not argue or speak in a raised voice
3. Break down all requests into the simplest form
4. Speak in concrete terms using low voice tones
5. Get client's attention
6. Give time to respond
7. Refer to past life experiences that a client remembers
8. Use touch frequently

These clients need skilled nursing care. They require a regular, predictable routine. They need to be kept active but not overwhelmed and receive recognition as an individual (Figure 11-9). The nurse must see that the environment is organized and safe. Because the client is already confused, he or she does not need an untidy cluttered room. Excess stimuli should be kept to a minimum. The client's physical health must be monitored and his or her physical needs tended to promptly.

Caring for the Alzheimer's client is a difficult and stressful job. The nurse needs imagination and a sense of humor and must be able to look for enjoyment in the little things they accomplish.

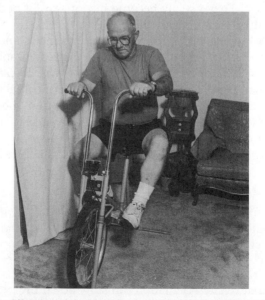

FIGURE 11-9 Clients with Alzheimer's disease must be kept active.

Nursing Care Plan:
The Client with Alzheimer's Disease

Jessica Robbins, a sixty-eight-year-old former schoolteacher, is admitted to the Shady Oak Nursing Facility with a diagnosis of stage 3 Alzheimer's disease. She is accompanied by her seventy-year-old husband, Joe, and daughter who are assisting her to walk by interlocking their arms. The daughter states that Jessica has become progressively more forgetful and confused over the last four years. She recently got lost going to the grocery store in the small town where she lives. The police found her and notified the daughter. The daughter relates that Joe reminds her to bathe and to change her clothing. When she dresses herself, she at times puts her bra on the outside of her blouse and her socks over her shoes. Two weeks ago she started wetting herself. As the daughter relates the information to the nurse, tears start rolling down Joe's face. Finally, he says "I do not want to admit her, but her care is becoming too much for me. Recently she has started yelling at me when I disagree with her." The nurse completes a thorough assessment ascertaining whether data indicate possible causes for reversible confusion. He relates his assessment data to the physician and they agree that there is no evidence for reversible confusion and the diagnosis is Alzheimer's disease.

NURSING DIAGNOSIS 1

Self-care deficit related to cognitive alterations secondary to neurological brain impairment as evidenced by husband reminding her to bathe and change clothing, inability to apply clothing appropriately, and incontinence.

Nursing Outcomes

1. Jessica will bathe herself three times a week (within three weeks).

2. Jessica will apply clothing in correct order (within six weeks).

Nursing Interventions	Rationales
Determine and continue with present habitual bathing time and manner.	By continuing with Jessica's routine bathing habits her present memory pattern will be reinforced.
Develop a reality orientation board for Jessica and state bath day on appropriate days.	A reality orientation board will assist in orientating Jessica to date, time, place, and bath day.
Assist with the bath as needed.	Assistance with the bath allows Jessica to complete as much of the bath as possible yet provides help as needed.
Ensure privacy.	Ensuring privacy preserves self-dignity.
Decrease external stimuli during bathing task.	Decreasing external stimuli assists Jessica to remain focused on the task at hand.
Keep bathroom and water temperature warm to client's preference	A warm bathroom and warm water will make bath time more enjoyable and prevent hypothermia, which could cause more confusion.

Evaluation

Jessica is bathing three times a week. The reality orientation board reminds her to bathe but the staff reminds her of bath day by taking her to the reality orientation board and requesting she look at the picture of a lady bathing.

NURSING DIAGNOSIS 2

Disturbed thought processes related to inability to process information and problem solve secondary to neurological brain impairment as evidenced by need for her husband to remind her to bathe and change clothing, inability to apply clothing appropriately, getting lost when going to the grocery store, and yelling at her husband when he disagrees with her.

Nursing Outcomes

Jessica will use intellect and problem-solving skills to the best of her ability (within six weeks).

Nursing Interventions	Rationales
Maintain a regular, pre-dictable routine yet offer appropriate stimulation and activity. Staff will ask simple, concrete questions regarding personal likes and dislikes.	A regular, predictable routine will provide continuity and stability for Jessica.
Develop, display, and utilize a reality orientation board. Encourage Jessica to partici-pate in reminiscing activities.	Giving options in personal likes and dislikes provides Jessica with some control. A reality orientation board will reinforce day, time, and place. Reminiscing activities offer opportunities to recall previous experiences, and improve communication and self-worth.

Evaluation

Jessica is adapting well to the regular, predictable routine and goes to the reality orientation board frequently throughout the day. If given an option between two choices, she usually makes a personal choice. Jessica is enjoying the reminiscing classes, and her husband attended the class with her this week.

NURSING DIAGNOSIS 3

Interrupted family processes related to admitting family member into nursing home secondary to neurological brain impairment as evidenced by daughter assisting moth-er in walking, daughter providing admission data for moth-er, and husband crying during admission of wife.

Nursing Outcomes

Family members will communicate feelings candidly and seek support from each other.

Nursing Interventions	Rationales
Invite family members to weekly conference for update on Jessica's progress and opportunity to process feelings and thoughts about personal effects of Jessica's disease.	Frequent updates on Jessica's condition will keep the family abreast of Jessica's progress and offer an opportunity for the family to vent feelings and thoughts.
Provide time for family members to be alone with Jessica and each other.	Personal family time provides opportunity to communicate thoughts and feelings.

Evaluation

Jessica and family members are attending the weekly conferences and sharing their feelings candidly with each other and the medical staff.

DEPRESSION IN THE ELDERLY

Depression is a more clearly understood term than is confusion. Everyone has been sad because of a loss. However, sadness is not considered depression unless it is prolonged or interferes with one's life.

The elderly are more prone to depression because they sustain more losses, their adaptive energy has diminished, and they take more drugs that are apt to cause the condition (see Figure 11-10). Chronic illness, more prevalent in the aged, decreases coping ability. There is also a decline in the production of hormones as people age. This reduction changes the chemical balance in the brain and predisposes the elderly to depression. The highest suicide rate of any group is found among elderly men. Salvatore (2000) reported that suicide claims more than 32,000 lives annually in the United States. More than 6200 of these deaths occur in those sixty-five years of age or older. Suicide is the third leading cause of death among the elderly and a high proportion were men, either single or divorced. Approximately 50 percent had been seen for a physical complaint in a primary care setting in the month

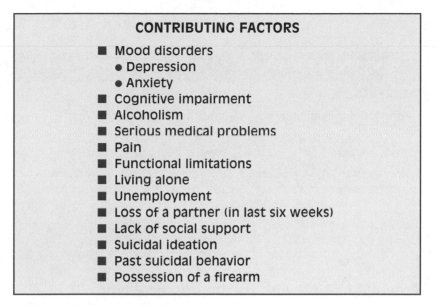

CONTRIBUTING FACTORS

- Mood disorders
  - Depression
  - Anxiety
- Cognitive impairment
- Alcoholism
- Serious medical problems
- Pain
- Functional limitations
- Living alone
- Unemployment
- Loss of a partner (in last six weeks)
- Lack of social support
- Suicidal ideation
- Past suicidal behavior
- Possession of a firearm

FIGURE 11-10 Contributing factors to elderly suicide.

before their death. Although hanging is the chief mode of death for elderly men, in the age group seventy-five to eighty-four there has been an increase in deaths due to firearms. Spousal homicide-suicide occurs with many of the perpetrators being the elderly person who has taken on the caregiver role.

Depression is probably the most common problem of the elderly and the most easily treated, yet it is the most underdiagnosed and least treated of all. Other conditions mask the depression, and symptoms, if apparent, are often not taken seriously.

Symptoms

The person who is depressed has prolonged or extreme sadness. It is a generalized sadness; that is, it is not connected to a particular loss. These clients are withdrawn and sometimes agitated, hostile, and prone to rumination. They can also be confused. Called **pseudodementia** (Table 11-6), depression involves a reduction in activity, obsessive worrying, and sleep disturbances. The client's ability to reason and remember is diminished and he or she is more pessimistic.

The elderly depressed person usually has more physical complaints. In fact, hypochondriasis is common. Physical complaints can even be the only symptom of depression. Elderly depressed clients are more apt to be constipated, and they can even be incontinent.

TABLE 11-6 Difference between Pseudodementia and True Dementia

PSEUDODEMENTIA	TRUE DEMENTIA
Depressed mood	Mood fluctuates
Impairment is inconsistent	Impairment is consistent and progressive
Onset is rapid	Onset is slow and insidious
More likely to answer questions with "I do not know."	More likely to cover up by giving an answer that may be close to correct
More likely to give up easily	Tries to stay independent as long as possible

Communicating with the Depressed Client

Communication is the major nursing tool for the depressed or withdrawn person. The focus is to improve the client's feelings of self-worth. First, trust must be established. This can entail sitting silently with the client. This lets him or her know that it is all right to be silent and puts no pressure on the client to talk. It also lets him or her know that the nurse cares enough to take the time.

After sitting silently for a time, the nurse can begin to talk about nonthreatening things. He or she can begin to build clients' self-esteem by pointing out their positive aspects. If clients voice feelings, they should be acknowledged and then reflected. The client should be allowed to talk about past unhappy experiences, because venting feelings lessens stress. Repeatedly voicing frustrations, though, reinforces them. It is important that clients be allowed to tell their stories, but there needs to be a limit on the number of times an incident can be repeated.

As with all other distressed clients, the nurse needs to remain calm. He or she uses simple, concrete sentences and does not attempt to argue, probe, or interrogate. The nurse accepts clients' anger, but, above all, he or she continually stresses reality.

Treatment

Treatment of depression depends on the cause. Depression can be the result of physical illness or drugs. It can be the result of changes in the chemicals of the brain, called **endogenous depression**. It can also be the result of abnormal grieving, called **reactive depression**.

Physical illness can act as a stress, making the person more vulnerable to depression. Illness can also cause a change in the oxygen or hormonal balance in the brain. Some diseases that do this are anemia, particularly pernicious anemia, brain tumors that cause pressure on the brain, and Parkinson's disease. A large percentage of people with Parkinson's are depressed. Parkinson's is due to a lack of a brain hormone, dopamine, which may directly cause the depression. Other illnesses associated with depression are cancer, particularly of the pancreas, and thyroid disease. Viral infections such as influenza are also associated with depression. Waste products circulating in the blood because of conditions such as kidney and liver failure can lead to depression.

As a group, the elderly take many drugs. Unfortunately the drugs most often taken by them are the very ones most apt to cause depression. These drugs include analgesics and hypnotics that lessen stimuli to the brain, antihistamines, some antibiotics, anti-Parkinson's drugs, and cardiovascular drugs such as digitalis. Hypoglycemics lower the sugar level available to the brain, anticholinergics change the chemical balance in the brain, and antihypertensives lessen the amount of oxygen supply.

The group most apt to cause depression is the antihypertensive group, the drugs taken for high blood pressure. Estrogens and antianxiety drugs can also cause confusion. If a drug is found to be the culprit, the most logical treatment is to stop using the drug.

Endogenous depression results from some chemical changes in the brain. There is no precipitating stressful event to which the client can point. The depression just occurs. These people experience guilt and self-loathing. They do not have interest in anything because nothing is enjoyable. They generally are tired all the time, have no appetite, and lose weight. They will describe their feelings as different from when they experienced a loss in the past. The depression seems to be more severe in the morning and lessens as the day goes on. There is generally a family history of depression.

Reactive depression is the most common type of depression in the elderly. It is a result of a normal grieving process becoming abnormal. Normal grieving lasts no more than six to twelve months. If it is longer and more severe, grieving is abnormal. The person experiencing loss in a normal way begins to go through the normal grieving stages immediately (see Chapter 15). When the person experiencing the loss does not react emotionally immediately, the grieving will probably be abnormal. This person may instead complain of physical symptoms or exhibit disturbed behavior.

In the elderly, depression responds better to treatment than any other mental disorder. There may not be a complete freedom from any symptoms, but clients can be reasonably happy and return to productive lives. If the depression is a result of illness, it will disappear when the disease is treated. If the disease cannot be treated, drugs may be used. Reactive depression is often self-limiting. In time, the depression will diminish. Supportive care is always indicated. Psychotherapy may be needed. If the condition is very severe, drugs are prescribed.

The client with endogenous depression is most likely to respond to treatment. This client should be given supportive care. Drugs may be indicated. If the depression does not respond to supportive care and drugs, electroconvulsive therapy may be used.

Supportive measures include: encouraging the client to talk about his or her feelings, giving information and encouragement, providing physical and mental activities, involving the client with a social group like family or friends, providing good nutrition, and providing for adequate sleep.

Electroconvulsive Therapy. Electronconvulsive therapy, (ECT), is a viable but controversial treatment for depression. Some authorities believe it is safe and effective, particularly for people with endogenous depression and depressions that do not respond to supportive care or drugs. In these situations, ECT is considered the treatment of choice. According to other authorities, however, the treatment is not safe and should not be used under any circumstances. Still others say that ECT is preferable to suicide and should be employed in the treatment of specific clients. Despite the controversy, ECT is still widely used in all parts of the country.

Treatments are generally given in three to four day intervals for the first few treatments, then the frequency is reduced to once a week. Each client is scheduled for a set number of treatments prescribed by the doctor. Though still not widely available, there are newer machines that allow a drastic reduction in the number of treatments needed.

The policies and procedures governing ECT vary in different hospitals. Many times the procedure is carried out in the surgical unit or there may be a special ECT room with a specially trained ECT staff. The client or guardian needs to sign an informed consent before the procedure. Though it is not the nurse's responsibility to initially inform the client, it is usually up to him or her to obtain the signature. Therefore, the nurse needs to ascertain that the client has been informed. The client needs information regarding the steps in the procedure, the expected results, and the possible complications. Every attempt should be made to present the material so as to inform but not frighten the client.

Besides the consent form, the nurse needs to see that certain other forms are on the chart and complete. These forms will vary in different institutions, but generally the following are included:

- Physical exam
- Routine urinalysis
- Routine blood work
- Electrocardiogram
- Brain scan
- Surgical checklist

Before the procedure, the client is given nothing by mouth, vital signs are taken and recorded, and the client is asked to void. Pre-ECT medications are ordered by the anesthesiologist or psychiatrist. They include drugs to dry secretions in order to prevent the possibility of pneumonia and drugs to relax the muscles in order to relieve anxiety and muscle spasms. In the past, jerking spasms caused by the electrical currents may have resulted in damaged muscle and bone. With current ECT machines and medications, twitches only are observed. Dentures, contact lenses, and all metallic objects are removed from the clients' body. Although the client may wear his or her own clothes for the procedure, the client is usually dressed in a gown and transported to the surgical or ECT unit by cart or wheelchair.

There is some memory loss following the procedure that is usually temporary—at least in part. Sometimes oxygen is given before and after the treatment. Oxygen seems to lessen the possibility of complications such as memory loss. However, the memory loss is thought by some to be the reason why ECT is effective—the client literally forgets to be sad. If this is true, the treatments have to be repeated periodically. On the other hand, staunch proponents of the treatment say the ECT actually changes the chemical and electrical environment of the brain, producing a more lasting effect.

Following the procedure, the client continues to need support and reassurance, particularly regarding the memory loss. Vital signs need to be monitored until they are stable or according to the doctor's orders or the policy of the institution. When vital signs are stable and the client has recovered from the effect of the medication, he or she is offered food and is encouraged to rest.

MEDICATIONS

Because elderly clients are dealing with both their mental health problems and their chronic illnesses, it is extremely important to conduct a medication review. Always review the number of medications prescribed. Prescribing multiple medications is called polypharmacy. A pharmacist needs to be consulted to assist with information about dangerous drug-drug interactions. Current dosage is important as the elderly need initial low dosing and frequent assessment of body weight maintenance or weight loss. Some clients experience paradoxical (opposite) effects from medications. Irritability, confusion, and disorientation can occur.

Working with the aged who have mental health problems is a stressful job. It can be frustrating and demands enormous patience. Mutual support among caregivers is one important ingredient in reducing job stress. A positive attitude is needed. Although this will not change the disease process, it can improve conditions and make good care more accessible to the elderly. Gerontologic nurse specialists are an excellent resource for support and care plans. Their consultation should be sought when possible. If a national priority is to reduce late-life suicides, there needs to be increased emphasis on geriatric mental health.

SUMMARY

Old age is arbitrarily defined as sixty-five years or older. It is a very diverse group in terms of economics, intelligence, and health, both mental and physical. The stereotype of the elderly as poverty stricken, cranky, and confused is simply not true.

The common mental health problems in the aged include delirium, dementia, and depression. The elderly often do not receive treatment because of certain myths and attitudes that continue to persist. The following are some examples: "The problems of the disturbed elderly are inevitable, and there is no sense in bothering with them" or "Working with the elderly is inferior to other forms of health care, and the people who work with them are either saints or stupid." Changing these myths will not help the disease process, but it will improve conditions and make good health care more accessible to the elderly.

Confusion can be reversible or irreversible. Irreversible confusion is called *dementia*. All confusion should be considered reversible. The cause should be sought out and treated. Reversible confusion can result from acute illness, stressful events, drugs, and environmental factors.

Irreversible confusion, is due to brain damage. A client can have both reversible and irreversible confusion at the same time. The majority of people with dementia have the Alzheimer's type. This is a progressive disease for which there is no cure. The disease is not caused by stress, but stress speeds up the progress. Behavior modification techniques and drugs are used to control behavior, but there is no treatment for the disease itself. Reality orientation is used to help keep all confused clients in touch with reality.

Communication is the major tool when working with the withdrawn client. Working with all distressed clients requires some rules. Remain calm; speak in simple, concrete sentences; avoid questions; and do not push the client to answer. Be very attentive to his or her physical needs. Observe nonverbal cues carefully.

SUGGESTED ACTIVITIES

▓ Volunteer to visit a client in a nursing home.

▓ Attend a reality orientation class.

▓ Contact a local Alzheimer's support group and plan to attend a meeting.

▓ With a group, discuss the effect of commonly believed myths on the care the elderly receive.

▓ Examine your own feelings about aging.

▓ Find out the current legislation affecting nursing homes in your area. Are they helpful or restrictive?

REVIEW

KNOW AND COMPREHEND

A. Multiple choice. Select the one best answer.

1. The causes of reversible confusion include
   - ❏ A. vascular accidents and brain damage.
   - ❏ B. dehydration, elevated temperature, and drugs.
   - ❏ C. Huntington's disease and arteriosclerosis.
   - ❏ D. Alzheimer's disease and cerebral infarcts.

2. The three categories of confusion are
   - ❏ A. reversible, irreversible, and chronic.
   - ❏ B. Alzheimer's, reversible, and multiinfarct.
   - ❏ C. pseudodementia, dementia, and delirium.
   - ❏ D. dementia, multiinfarct, and reversible.

3. The possible causes of Alzheimer's disease are unknown, but a clear effect of the disease is
   - ❏ A. a rapidly developing delirium.
   - ❏ B. an increased risk for intracranial hemorrhage.
   - ❏ C. an inability to cope with stress.
   - ❏ D. a change in neurotransmitters.

4. The most common mental health problem in the elderly is
   ❏ A. depression.
   ❏ B. confusion.
   ❏ C. Alzheimer's disease.
   ❏ D. dementia.

5. Reactive depression is a result of
   ❏ A. some stressful event.
   ❏ B. a change in neurotransmitters.
   ❏ C. hypochondriasis.
   ❏ D. drugs.

6. If an elderly client is depressed without a precipitating cause, is self-loathing, and feels guilty, the client probably has
   ❏ A. reactive depression.
   ❏ B. endogenous depression.
   ❏ C. bipolar disorder.
   ❏ D. pseudodepression.

7. A definite diagnosis of Alzheimer's can only be produced by
   ❏ A. a CT scan.
   ❏ B. blood chemistry.
   ❏ C. visual observation of the brain.
   ❏ D. a mental status exam with social history.

8. The pathology in Alzheimer's disease includes
   ❏ A. tangles and plaques in the brain.
   ❏ B. demyelination of the axons.
   ❏ C. destruction of the blood-brain barrier.
   ❏ d. increase in magnesium in the brain.

9. Clients who are confused need
   ❏ A. thorough directions.
   ❏ B. change and variety.
   ❏ C. simple directions.
   ❏ D. directions given in a loud, firm voice.

10. The most effective tool for helping the confused client is
    ❏ A. psychotherapy.
    ❏ B. argumentation.
    ❏ C. reality orientation.
    ❏ D. confrontation.

APPLY YOUR LEARNING

B. Multiple Choice. Select the one best answer.

1. A practical nurse contributes to the plan of care for a 79-year-old client with advanced Alzheimer's disease. It would be important to contribute interventions focused on
   - ❏ A. reducing the risk of infection.
   - ❏ B. assigning different caregivers each day.
   - ❏ C. including the client in group therapy.
   - ❏ D. isolating the client from others.

2. An elderly client is diagnosed with pneumonia and admitted to a medical unit. The client becomes irritable and restless and says to the nurse, "I need to feed my cat." A family member states the client has been living independently and managing a household. Which problem should the nurse suspect?
   - ❏ A. dementia with irreversible confusion
   - ❏ B. delirium with reversible confusion
   - ❏ C. depression accompanied by confusion
   - ❏ D. early stage Alzheimer's disease

3. The nurse gathers data to determine a client's orientation. Which question below would the nurse *not* use?
   - ❏ A. "What is today's date?"
   - ❏ B. "What is your full name?"
   - ❏ C. "What kind of place are we in?"
   - ❏ D. "Where were you born?"

4. The nurse in a skilled care facility prepares a reality orientation board. Which information would the nurse include?
   - ❏ A. today's menu for breakfast, lunch, and dinner
   - ❏ B. daily visiting hours at the facility
   - ❏ C. today's day and date, and identification of the place
   - ❏ D. name and phone number of the client representative

5. A nurse plans care for a client in the second stage of Alzheimer's disease. Which intervention(s) would be most appropriate?
   - ❏ A. assist with grooming and feeding
   - ❏ B. provide devices to aid ambulation
   - ❏ C. strategies for care of incontinence
   - ❏ D. anti-anxiety medications for hostility

6. An elderly man becomes confused after the death of his wife. Which nursing intervention would be most therapeutic?
   ❏ A. immediately begin intensive suicide observations
   ❏ B. assist the client to cope with his grief and sadness
   ❏ C teach the client about donepezil [Aricept]
   ❏ D. place a reality orientation board in the client's home

C. Briefly answer the following.

1. Name four ways the nurse can prevent confusion in his or her clients.

2. List the nursing needs of the client with dementia.

3. Describe four interventions the nurse can take to prevent reversible confusion.

4. Differentiate between dementia and pseudodementia.

D. Discussion questions. Briefly discuss the following.

1. The pros and cons of using electroconvulsive therapy in the elderly.

2. The pros and cons of treating the elderly in nursing homes rather than mental health facilities.

3. The ways in which prevalent attitudes toward aging affect the care of clients with reversible confusion.

Alcoholism

OUTLINE

KEY TERMS

alcoholism	postacute withdrawal (PAW)
DWI	replacement therapy
PI	fetal alcohol syndrome (FAS)
CAGE questionnaire	Alcoholics Anonymous (FAS)
MADD	codependency
delirium tremens (DTs)	halfway house

OBJECTIVES

After studying this chapter, the student should be able to:

■ Define alcoholism.

■ List the four progressive stages of alcoholism.

■ Describe the physiological effects of alcohol.

■ Describe the nursing care of the client with alcoholism in the hospital.

■ Describe the objectives of various community treatment programs for persons with alcoholism.

■ List six symptoms of alcohol withdrawal and the nursing care of the client with withdrawal symptoms.

■ State the treatment used for persons with alcoholism on admission to a general hospital.

■ List ten interventions of the nurse caring for the client with alcoholism.

■ Describe alcohol use and youth.

■ Identify various treatment approaches for alcoholism.

Alcohol use permeates Western society, with people consuming alcoholic beverages for purposes of religious ceremony, celebrations, medicinal therapy, pleasure, and recreation. Alcoholism is a primary, chronic disease with genetic, psychosocial, and environmental factors influencing its development and manifestation. Foroud and Li (1999) related that **alcoholism** is a common, familial yet complex genetic disorder. They documented a three- to five-fold increased risk for alcoholism among siblings and other first degree relatives of affected individuals. Estimates of inheritability ranged from 50 percent to 60 percent; thus influencing alcohol preference and leading to an increased risk for alcoholism. The role of environmental factors and genetic counseling needs to be more clearly delineated. It is often a progressive and fatal disease and characterized by impaired control over drinking, preoccupation with alcohol, use of alcohol with adverse consequences and distortion in thinking, and denial of the significance of the drinking and awareness that alcohol abuse is a problem. There are a variety of definitions for alcoholism, but most definitions include the following four elements:

- Excessive consumption of alcohol
- Psychological disturbances caused by alcohol
- Disturbances of social and economic functioning
- Loss of control over alcohol consumption

E.M. Jellinek, a pioneer in alcoholism research, defines alcoholism as any use of an alcoholic beverage that causes damage to the individual, society, or both.

The person with alcoholism is often thought of as a skid-row bum. However, only seven percent of people with alcoholism fit this stereotype. The remaining 93 percent are found in every level of society and in every occupation. The number of women with alcoholism is increasing.

Clients with alcoholism may show signs of final rejection of the world about them. They may withdraw from personal contact with others and not even attend to their needs of daily living. The client with alcoholism needs empathy and not misplaced sympathy. Innovative approaches for care are necessary for each client. The nurse should demonstrate qualities of consistency, firmness, honesty, and patience. To do this, he or she must first determine personal prejudices concerning the client with alcoholism.

Prejudice is a prejudgment. Usually, it is an unfavorable judgment based on insufficient reasons. Nurses need to examine their own prejudices because they can be reflected in nursing care. Nurses should think through their prejudices and recognize their fears and lack of information. Feelings of inferiority and insecurity need to be dealt with. Once prejudices are recognized, nurses can take responsibility for their own behavior with others. Nurses particularly need to be understanding in their interactions with all clients. They render care and do not pass judgment.

There is no single cause of alcoholism. Alcoholism is a disease, not a habit. Researchers have found that societies that induce guilt and confusion regarding drinking behaviors are more likely to produce alcoholics. It also has been found that people who develop drinking

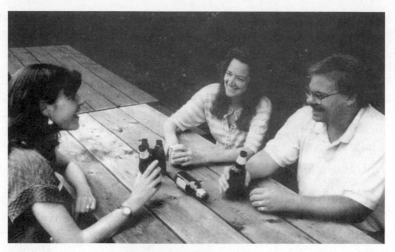

FIGURE 12-1 Fun, friends, and lots of liquor. A good—or very dangerous—trio.

problems are more likely to experience intense relief and relaxation from alcohol. The person with alcoholism usually gives a variety of reasons for drinking. The reasons may include the following:

- Relieving tension
- Helping unwind
- Drowning sorrow
- Making one feel free
- Helping one be sociable

Many people experience increased activity, laughter, and smooth-flowing speech with the consumption of alcoholic beverages (Figure 12-1). Alcohol can produce a temporary feeling of well-being, but it depresses the central nervous system. Alcohol abuse can have negative social and personal consequences. Arrest for driving while intoxicated (**DWI**) and public intoxication (**PI**) can occur, with all the complicated legal involvements. Health problems (liver disease, gastrointestinal bleeding, esophogeal varices), automobile and occupational accidents, and impaired job functioning can contribute to a disrupted lifestyle.

Alcohol dependence causes an increased consumption of alcohol and an inability to stop drinking until intoxicated. Thinking becomes confused and disorganized. Memory, concentration, judgment, and perception are dulled. Depression, frustration, and anxiety are some of the problems caused by alcohol.

HISTORY OF ALCOHOL ABUSE

The use, misuse, and abuse of alcohol is thought to date back to primitive times. During the Stone Age, humans found that chewing certain berries made their heads light. This accidental discovery brought about the international manufacture of alcoholic beverages. By 3,000 B.C., Egypt had perfected the art of manufacturing beer and wine. The making of wine also became popular in the Mediterranean countries. During the Middle Ages, grapes were cultivated throughout Europe, and monasteries began perfecting the manufacture of wines.

Distillation introduced a new and more potent alcoholic beverage. Instead of beers and wines containing 6 to 14 percent alcohol, beverages containing as much as 50 percent alcohol were made. The literature of this period reports drunkenness as a serious problem. Alcohol was available for religious and medical use when the colonists settled in America. Alcohol sometimes accompanied family meals. However, some religions scorned the excessive use of alcohol. Factors such as the diminishing family structure, the lessening influence of religion, and the dislocation of war helped cause an increase in alcohol consumption.

Alcohol became a social concern toward the end of the eighteenth century. At this time the temperance movement, which stressed moderation in the use of intoxicating beverages began. Strong support for the movement came from religious groups, legislators, farmers, businessmen, and schools. By 1919, twenty-five states participated in the Prohibition Amendment. The amendment made it unlawful to manufacture, distribute, or sell alcoholic beverages. Thirteen years later, it was repealed as a failure. Denying people access to alcoholic beverages was a simplistic way to deal with a complicated issue.

Alcoholism is a problem among all ages. It can be seen in the newborn as a result of maternal alcoholism, and in the child, adolescent, and adult. Alcohol consumption is a way that some people cope with stress. One method to screen clients who have problems with alcohol is to have them complete the **CAGE questionnaire** (Table 12-1).

There is an increasing number of teenagers who drink on a regular basis. Liquors such as vodka and tequila have become popular among teenagers because they are difficult to detect on the breath. Parents do not always recognize alcohol as a drug. When told their child has a drinking problem, many parents are extremely thankful that at least their child is not on drugs.

Parental influence can be a factor in teenage drinking. In many households, children see their parents enjoying daily cocktails before and after dinner. Peer pressure is another influence in teenage drinking. When people have equal standing within a group force or cajole

TABLE 12-1 CAGE Questionnaire

C   Have you ever felt you should cut down on your drinking?

A   Have people annoyed you by criticizing your drinking?

G   Have you ever felt bad or guilty about drinking?

E   Have you ever taken a drink the first thing in the morning to steady your nerves or get rid of a hangover (eye opener)?

(From "Detecting Alcoholism: The CAGE Questionnaire," by J. A. Ewing (1984). *Journal of the American Medical Association, 252,* pp. 1905-1907. Copyright 1984, American Medical Association. Reprinted with permission.)

another member of the group into doing something in order to gain the respect of the group, it is referred to as *peer pressure.*

Advertisements show alcohol consumption coupled with glamorous and exciting activities. If the teenager already has emotional and psychological problems, drinking can be an escape from stressors. Partying and drinking can become a way of life.

The senior citizen may hide a drinking problem. Boredom and loneliness can make a day appear endless. Poor health and inadequate income can contribute to depression, which, in turn, may lead to alcoholism. People entering old age with a well-established drinking problem should be observed for developing symptoms of alcoholism. Some families accept alcoholism or even supply the liquor in order to make the older member's life more tolerable. This misplaced affection can only lead to more loneliness and alienation.

Currently, a powerful grass-root organization exists called **MADD** (Mothers Against Drunk Driving). This organization has brought national focus on drinking and driving and mortality rates.

STAGES OF ALCOHOLISM

Jellinek conducted a study that revealed a series of stages for alcoholism. The stages do not always occur in the same order. The four progressive stages of alcoholism as described by Jellinek are

PREALCOHOLIC
Occasional drinking
Constant relief drinking
Increase in alcohol tolerance

PRODROMAL
Onset and increase of memory blackouts
Secretive drinking
Preoccupation with alcohol
Gulping first drink

Guilt feeling without drinking
Inability to discuss problem
Increase in memory blackouts

CRUCIAL
Loss of control
Rationalization of drinking behavior
Failure in efforts to control drinking
Grandiose and aggressive behavior
Trouble with family and employer
Self-pity
Loss of outside interests
Unreasonable resentment
Neglect of food
Tremors
Morning drinking

CHRONIC
Prolonged intoxication
Physical and moral deterioration
Impaired thinking
Indefinable anxieties
Obsession with drinking
Constant alibis given

PHYSIOLOGICAL EFFECTS OF ALCOHOL

The nurse should have an understanding of the physiological effects of
alcohol. A small amount of alcohol may bring about skeletal muscle
relaxation. An increased amount can impair the respiratory and cardiovascular systems. Alcohol physically depresses; while tensions and
fears appear to ease. With alcohol consumption, mental activity
changes and judgment and self-concern are reduced. With increased
levels of alcohol, a staggering gait is noted. Difficulty in standing follows. Finally the person falls and is unable to get up. A larger dose of
alcohol can produce stupor. This is a serious complication that usually follows a prolonged drinking spree. When alcohol is taken on an
empty stomach, it is absorbed immediately and the effect on the central nervous system is felt in less than twenty minutes.

THE CLIENT WITH ALCOHOLISM IN THE HOSPITAL

The majority of clients with alcoholism in medical and surgical departments of a general hospital are admitted with a diagnosis other than
alcoholism. The commonly seen diagnoses include

- Pneumonia
- Bleeding ulcers
- Multiple trauma
- Neurological injuries
- Cirrhosis of the liver
- Malnutrition
- Orthopedic injuries

The physician may or may not be aware of the client's drinking problem. The nurse may be faced with the undiagnosed alcoholic client who is admitted for elective surgery. Many times, the client with alcoholism shows an exaggerated fear of procedures or surgery. All clients should be screened for substance abuse problems. The word *alcoholic* need not be used. The nurse could say "The amount of alcohol you drink may influence the choice of medication you receive. Could you estimate your average weekly or daily intake?" The nurse should *not* ask the client "Why do you drink?" since this gives the client an opportunity to rationalize alcohol use. Adult clients tend to minimize their use of alcohol. Often questions concerning drinking habits gain the necessary information.

When clients with alcoholism arrive at the hospital, they are usually acutely ill. Even if their behavior is aggressive and abusive, the nurse's primary goal is quality care. It may be difficult to interview clients with alcoholism because their speech may be slurred and their thoughts confused. The nurse should not try to reason with disruptive, uncooperative clients with alcoholism. However, he or she should allow clients to verbalize their feelings. The nurse should speak slowly and softly. By his or her verbal responses, the nurse shows clients that he or she accepts their feelings and empathizes with their problems. The nurse should reinforce any of the clients' positive behaviors.

Underlying physical problems should be observed. Respiratory infections are common. This must be considered in the planning of care. On admission to the hospital, treatment of the person with alcoholism usually consists of

- Sedatives or tranquilizers (an example of a drug to prevent or control delirium is Librium [chlordiazepoxide]: dosage 50–100 mg for acute alcohol withdrawal, action of antianxiety; benzodiazepine (usually lorazepam), effective in fifteen to thirty minutes, peaks at two to four hours.

- Replacement of fluids and electrolytes; monitor for dehydration

- Adequate diet (high-protein, high-vitamin diet for underweight and malnourished clients)

- Vitamin therapy (the person with alcoholism usually has a deficiency of magnesium, thiamine, B complex vitamins, niacin, and folic acid)

- Monitoring for alteration in serum glucose

- Anticonvulsants (dilantin, phenobarbital)

The client with alcoholism needs to be observed closely for seizures.

Complications associated with long-term alcoholism are Wernicke-Korsakoff syndrome and Pick's disease:

- Wernicke-Korsakoff syndrome is characterized by confusion, disorientation and amnesia with confabulation.

- Pick's disease is characterized by early onset in the midfifties with presenile dementia. There is a genetic predisposition.

NURSING CARE

Many difficulties that occur with clients with alcoholism are a result of withdrawal symptoms beginning 6 to 8 hours after the last drink. Clients in mild withdrawal may suffer only trembling and agitation. A more severe withdrawal involves **delirium tremens (DTs)**. In delirium tremens the client has extreme restlessness and possibly seizures. Delirium tremens may not occur until the second or third day of treatment or later. The client must be carefully observed for any withdrawal symptoms. These may include

- Tremors

- Profuse sweating

- Nausea

- Vomiting

- Confusion

- Seizures

- Increased agitation

- Anorexia

- Hallucinations

- Increased blood pressure

It is important to note that antianxiety drugs are intended to prevent delirium tremens (DTs) and, therefore, should be used liberally. The presence of delirium tremens is a medical emergency.

Clients may struggle against attempts to feed or bathe them. The nurse must recognize the clients' need for care and be aware that their behavior is due to their illness. He or she must realize that clients are reacting in fear, possibly to hallucinations. They may see, hear, or feel things that are not there. Maintaining a relaxed environment, and talking quietly to clients are important aspects of care. The nurse's firm but gentle manner can be reassuring to clients.

If possible, the nurse should stay with clients to help keep them in touch with reality. The nurse should tell clients what is being done to them and what is expected of them. If withdrawal occurs, an explanation that they are experiencing withdrawal from the alcohol should be given to clients. The nurse should continue to speak slowly in a low, calm voice and use simple, understandable statements. Restraints may sometimes be necessary to prevent injury to clients or to others. A doctor's order is needed before applying restraints. It is desirable to keep the room lighted at night to lessen clients' fear and facilitate observation.

After the acute stage of withdrawal, clients need a nonstressful environment. They need to learn social skills in a social setting with other clients. They may need to be encouraged to eat their meals and attend to personal hygiene. Because of dehydration, clients may have dry, sore mouths. Encouraging fluids is an important nursing measure. The nurse needs to inquire what nonalcoholic fluids the clients like, and order the fluids for them. A lemon and glycerine solution is soothing for the mouth and gums. Chewing gum may also be helpful.

The nurse needs to evaluate clients' knowledge of alcoholism. The subject should be dealt with realistically. The clients' families also need support and an explanation of the facts of alcoholism.

The goal of nursing in regard to clients with alcoholism is to be nonjudgmental and understanding and to help clients to be responsible for their own behavior. The nurse should watch for such defense mechanisms as rationalization, denial, and projection. Compromise and manipulation are signs that also need to be observed. Compromising clients try to get special privileges by presenting both sides of a situation and then coming up with their own workable middle line. Manipulative clients do not want to comply with demands. They try to influence others in order to attain their needs or wants. They attempt to change their care plans to meet their own goals.

Relapse is the return to the use of alcohol (or drugs) after a period of abstinence. Observable clues include behavioral and attitude changes, (impatience, argumentativeness, and anger); changes in feelings or moods (resentment, self-pity, and cockiness); and change in thought (dishonest with increased rationalization, that is, making excuses to drink when you know you should not drink). Identifying a high-risk situation is of utmost importance to the client: When do you want to use? When do you most crave alcohol? When are you exposed to alcohol? What has led to relapse in the past? Relapse is not unusual and the client needs to pay attention to warning signs. Today, many programs include an aftercare program to help the client with the transition into abstinence and everyday life experiences. Individual, group, and couple counseling and job guidance are provided to build self-esteem and self-confidence.

POSTACUTE WITHDRAWAL

Postacute withdrawal (PAW) initially can occur seven to fourteen days into abstinence but may peak at 3 to 6 months after abstinence begins. Symptoms include

- Inability to think clearly
- Emotional overreaction or numbness
- Memory problems (short term and significant past events)
- Sleep disturbances (dreams or nightmares)
- Physical coordination problems

REPLACEMENT THERAPY

Naltrexone (ReVia) is an opioid antagonist that reduces chances that the client will drink in the future by limiting pleasurable effects. It is well tolerated by most clients, although side effects can be nausea, dizziness, headache, or an unhappy mood, hepatotoxicity risks must be considered. It is important to note that drugs with opiate-like properties (i.e., morphine, heroin) cannot be taken with naltrexone. Naltrexone therapy requires a client's informed consent, and the client needs to carry a naltrexone warning card to show to doctors and dentists.

REHABILITATION OF THE CLIENT WITH ALCOHOLISM

In 1972, the Department of Health, Education, and Welfare established the National Institute of Alcohol Abuse and Alcoholism (NIAAA). Its purpose is to help the nation gain a better knowledge of the effects of alcohol and to become aware of the responsibilities associated with using alcohol. The institute encourages public discussion of community drinking problems. Task forces were formed to study major drinking patterns of problem groups within the community. Prevention is now being recognized as essential in the battle to reduce alcohol abuse. To minimize alcohol abuse, attention should be given to the general population and not merely the problem drinker. It is important to act early in discouraging primary alcohol abuse patterns.

Nursing Care Plan:
The Client with Alcohol Abuse

Sarah Hemingway, a forty-two-year-old female executive, is admitted to the Memorial Hospital with bleeding ulcers. She is 5 feet 5 inches tall and weighs 120 pounds. She relates that she has been working long hours and experiences stress in her job. Her husband, Ray, a stock broker, accompanies her to the hospital. They have two children, ages eighteen and sixteen. Since alcohol is a cause of bleeding ulcers, the nurse tactfully asks the client to estimate her average weekly intake of alcohol. Sarah states that she has one cocktail before the evening meal.

As Ray leaves for the evening, he relates to the nurse that his wife has a bar in her office and he has noticed alcohol on her breath several times lately when she comes home from work. He also states that when the couple socializes, Sarah has been having two drinks to his one.

NURSING DIAGNOSIS 1

Ineffective coping related to increased alcohol consumption associated with stress as evidenced by Sarah stating that she has been working long hours and has a lot of stress in her job, and her husband stating that he has noticed alcohol on her breath after long hours at work and increased drinking during socialization.

Nursing Outcomes

1. Before discharge Sarah will identify stresses in her life.
2. Before discharge Sarah will identify methods she is presently using to handle stress.
3. Sarah will list three new ways to cope with stress by day four of hospitalization.

Nursing Interventions	Rationales
1a. Spend time with Sarah encouraging her to discuss her job responsibilities.	1a. Having Sarah discuss present job responsibilites will assist her in identifying present stresses.
1b. Discuss with Sarah stresses in her life.	1b. Discussing stresses will give insight to what Sarah sees as stressors.
2a. Utilize therapeutic communication and counseling skills, and discuss ways Sarah is presently handling stress.	2a. Discussing present stress management assists in identifying effective and ineffective coping strategies.
2b. Make referrals to counselors and community organizations as needed.	2b. Other resources may be able to assist Sarah in coping with stress.
3. Assist in helping Sarah find new ways to cope with stresses.	3. New coping methods will give Sarah positive outlets for handling stress.

Evaluation

Sarah is able to list present stressors in her job. She acknowlges that she is not effectively handling stress now. Sarah listens intently as the nurse shares some organizations that help people handle stress effectively.

NURSING DIAGNOSIS 2

Interrupted family processes related to stressors and increased use of alcohol is evidenced by Sarah stating that she has job stress, and working long hours, and her husband stating that he has noticed alcohol on her breath more frequently and increased consumption at social events.

Nursing Outcomes

Sarah's family will communicate concerns of job responsibilities to each other and implement effective coping mechanisms.

Nursing Interventions	Rationales
Assess family dynamics. Assist family in processing stressful situations in family life.	Assessing family dynamics assists in identifying roles and interactions of the family so that help can be obtained to meet needs.
Encourage family members to verbalize their feelings.	By encouraging each family member to share his or her perceptions of the situation, the staff gains a clearer picture of family interactions.
	Gives each family member an opportunity to share his or her feelings rather than keeping them pent up.
Inform family members that they are not responsible for Sarah choosing to drink and they cannot control the drinking.	Family clarifies ownership of drinking problem.
Make referrals as needed (e.g., to social worker, counselor, psychiatric clinical specialist, psychiatrist, stress-management class, Hope Alive, Al-Anon, Alcoholics Anonymous.)	Family learns about other resources to deal with the situation.
	Family will have freedom to interact as needed.
	A supportive environment encourages a trust relationship between the family and facility.

Evaluation

Sarah, Ray and their children candidly discuss the stress of Sarah's job. Ray has shared with Sarah his concern about her drinking as a way to cope. The family has decided to attend a stress-management class together.

Rehabilitation of the client with alcoholism should begin when the problem is defined. This is when the client with alcoholism is more vulnerable and receptive to rehabilitation. However, it is usually impossible to convince the client with alcoholism that he or she is indeed an alcoholic and needs rehabilitation. This is reinforced by families, who tend to protect persons with alcoholism and frequently deny the problem.

Tolerating stress is a problem for persons with alcoholism. Improved methods of coping must be learned. It is necessary to find a satisfactory substitute for alcohol because alcohol acts as a tension-reducing agent.

The values and customs of the community in which the individual lives influence his or her drinking behavior. For example, alcoholism is a significant problem among Native Americans. A community's attitudes, concerns, and involvement with the problem of alcoholism need to be analyzed. Community resources such as family services agencies, mental health clinics, visiting nurse agencies, police, and judicial departments must be made available to help the alcoholic. It is interesting to note that recent studies have shown that the black population is disproportionately targeted for liquor advertisements. Billboards are crammed into poor areas, and the pictures vividly connect alcohol with romance, power, and success. Cognac and malt liquor are two beverages frequently depicted. In some neighborhoods, community leaders are banding together and whitewashing billboards as a show of defiance and to deliver a forceful message to change advertising approaches.

It is important that the community offer diversified rehabilitation programs. These programs might include emergency medical care, outclient clinics, inclient facilities, and halfway houses. Outreach workers can be helpful in visiting ethnic areas of communities to identify their particular needs. The nurse can play a role in case finding, referral, and coordination of community services.

The person with a psychiatric illness and a coexisting alcohol abuse problem is a major challenge. The goal is to monitor within communities seriously dysfunctional clients, attempt to stabilize their behavior, and improve their social functioning. Careful assessment of combined alcohol and drug abuse is needed because persons with dual diagnoses can be noncompliant, and resistant to treatment. These clients will usually deny or minimize their substance use/abuse, yet an astute mental health professional will note increased psychiatric hospitalizations and exacerbation of florid psychotic symptoms.

It is important to note that the incidence of alcoholism in women has risen and has contributed to increased suicide, death from accidents, and other alcohol-related diseases. The literature describes women as drinking in response to many stressful events: marital problems, poverty and single parenting, midlife crisis, empty-nest syndrome, and unwanted pregnancy. A great concern with pregnant females who drink alchohol is **fetal alcohol syndrome (FAS)**. FAS affects the central nervous system of the fetus. Growth patterns are

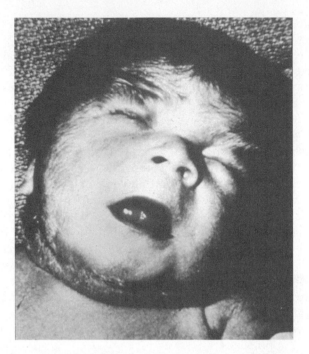

FIGURE 12-2 Infant with fetal alcohol syndrome. (Reprinted with permission. Streissguth, A. P., Landesman-Dwyer, S., Martin, J. C., & Smith, D. W. (1980). Teratogenic effects of alcohol in humans and laboratory animals. *Science, 209*(18): 353–361)

inhibited with low birth weights and small infants. Unusual facial characteristics are present, including eye slits, low placement of the ears, and a wide flat forehead with a flat nose (Figure 12-2).

ALCOHOL USE AND YOUTH

The media message to youth is that alcoholic beverages are essential in everyday life. Mini-markets even sell beer and wine, along with gasoline, food, and snacks. It is easy to obtain an alcoholic beverage to use as a reward after a sports victory or completion of a day at work or school. Studies reveal that addiction to alcohol is underdiagnosed in the young although the leading cause of death among youths fifteen to twenty-one years of age is alcohol-related motor vehicle injuries. The effects of alcohol use or abuse on youth are as follows:

- Family conflicts
- Problems with school performance
- School absences, truancy, increased dropout rates

■ Loss of peer relationships

■ Unprotected, unplanned sexual intercourse

■ Increased risk of physical or sexual abuse

■ Suicidal thoughts and possibly a plan

If the youth has a parent who abuses alchohol, studies have observed that these children are at high risk for delinquent behavior, learning disorders, hyperactivity, psychosomatic complaints, and problem drinking as adults.

Adolescents at younger and younger ages are being presented to alcohol rehabilitation centers. They are brought in by their parents, peers, or the juvenile judicial system.

The elderly are at risk for alcoholism. Many experience long periods of isolation and loneliness and drinking soothes these feelings. Family members can confuse their parent's depression and paranoia with growing old ("senility") and fail to recognize the need for alcohol treatment. The elderly frequently are excluded from intense alcohol treatment programs. However, if alcohol use or abuse is suspected it can jeopardize their geriatric health care and possibility for residential placement.

Nurses can also develop alcoholism. Impaired by alcohol consumption, they will lack sufficient insight and judgment to practice their profession. It is a moral and legal responsibility to report the impaired nurse. Many areas provide intensive therapy programs as either an inclient or outclient and the person's job position remains intact during the rehabilitation period.

TREATMENT

In contrast to the rapid response to treatment of many physical illnesses, response to treatment is generally very slow. Treatment methods for alcoholism vary. Many authorities believe that a multifaceted approach is best in meeting the needs of the client with alcoholism (Table 12-2).

TABLE 12-2 A Multifaceted Approach to Treating Alcoholism	
Alcoholics Anonymous	Hot meal programs
Rational emotive therapy	Detoxification centers
Industrial alcohol programs	Judicial rehabilitation
Antabuse	programs
Alcohol program for the aged	Transactional analysis
Halfway houses	Tranquilizers

Alcoholics Anonymous

Alcoholics Anonymous (AA) is an organization run by former alcoholics whose personal experiences with alcohol enable them to understand the problems of the person with alcoholism. They learn from direct observation of the many recovered from alcoholism in the organization. The goal of Alcoholics Anonymous is for members to abstain from drinking one day at a time. Sobriety helps to provide the person with alcoholism with a growing sense of self-control, achievement, and mastery. This provides further motivation to refrain from drinking. There is an increased awareness of self as the person begins to understand his or her problems and feelings. AA meetings use a structured group approach with a well-defined twelve-step program (Table 12-3). Each member has a sponsor and takes turns with a *lead*. A lead is a presentation of a person's struggle with giving up alcohol and the devastating effects of alcohol on his or her life. Each person defines his or her own spirituality and higher power and thereby increases self-esteem and hope. AA becomes a crucial part of successful sobriety.

Al-Anon (family groups) and Alateen (teenagers) focus on the effects of alcoholism on family and children. ACOA (Adult Children of Alcoholics) provides personal contact with others who grew up in dysfunctional family networks. This personal contact is therapeutic and provides emotional support.

Rational Emotive Therapy

Alcoholism is seen by proponents of rational emotive therapy as being a means of coping. The goal of this therapy is to help the person with alcoholism learn to tolerate the stressors that come with living and to use coping mechanisms that are less self-defeating. It teaches persons with alcoholism to recognize inaccuracies in their thinking. By changing their views of themselves and their environment, they can change their behavior. The rational emotive therapist believes that irrational thinking leads to irrational drinking.

Transactional Analysis

Transactional analysis is another therapy approach to alcoholism that has found some success. The goal of transactional analysis is to help persons with alcoholism stop playing games and to rewrite their life scripts. Alcoholism involves several games and a variety of payoffs. With the cessation of game playing, the underlying problems emerge more clearly. Clients are then able to cope with their problems more directly.

TABLE 12-3 The Twelve Steps of Alcoholics Anonymous

1. We admitted we were powerless over alcohol—that our lives had become unmanageable.

2. Came to believe that a power greater than ourselves could restore us to sanity.

3. Made a decision to turn our will and our lives over to the care of God as we understood Him

4. Made a searching and fearless moral inventory of ourselves.

5. Admitted to God, to ourselves, and to another human being the exact nature of our wrongs.

6. Were entirely ready to have God remove all these defects of character.

7. Humbly asked Him to remove our shortcomings.

8. Made a list of all persons we had harmed, and became willing to make amends to them all.

9. Made direct amends to such people wherever possible, except when to do so would injure them or others.

10. Continued to take personal inventory and when we were wrong promptly admitted it.

11. Sought through prayer and meditation to improve our conscious contact with God *as we understood Him*, praying only for knowledge of His will for us and the power to carry that out.

12. Having had a spiritual awakening as the result of these steps, we tried to carry this message to persons with alcoholism and to practice these principles in all our affairs.

Psychoanalysis

Psychoanalysis involves the direct interaction of the client with a therapist. The objective is to gain insight into behavior through talking. The therapist assists the client to clarify and work through stressful areas in his or her life. The client may be in therapy for a long time.

Group Therapy

Group therapy involves meaningful interaction among members of a group. The group members relate their personal experiences to each other. The main objective is for each group member to examine his or her impact on others through increased understanding of his or her own behavior and relationships. The group can influence change (Chapter 7).

Antabuse (Disulfuram)

Antabuse is an optional drug therapy that reinforces abstinence. Antabuse (disulfuram) is taken daily after at least a twelve-hour abstinence from alcohol. Antabuse interferes with the metabolism of alcohol and produces a toxic reaction when combined with it. Clients know they will suffer very unpleasant reactions if they do not refrain from drinking. The drug is usually well tolerated, but there are sometimes side effects. These side effects usually disappear as the body adjusts to the drug. The most common side effects include drowsiness, fatigue, acne, and a metallic aftertaste.

If clients drink alcohol while this drug is still in their systems, they experience dizziness, nausea, vomiting, and severe headaches. There may be a drop in blood pressure, a rapid pulse with heart palpitations, chest pain, and dyspnea (labored respiration). Within five to ten minutes after a drink, the face becomes flushed and the eyes red. This flushing quickly spreads over the rest of the body. All of this takes place after less than two teaspoons of alcohol is consumed. These effects may last from thirty minutes to several hours; death has sometimes occurred. During the reaction, the client is in a life-threatening situation and should be observed closely. When the reaction is over, the client is usually exhausted and goes to sleep.

No client should be on Antabuse without his or her knowledge and consent. All clients should be thoroughly warned against consuming alcohol in any form. Over-the-counter medication such as paregoric, cough syrups, and some vitamins may contain alcohol. The client should be advised to read labels carefully and be particularly watchful for foods prepared with beer or wine. Because of the severity of the reaction, Antabuse is not recommended for use by pregnant clients or clients with heart disease, diabetes, liver impairment, or mental illness. Success with Antabuse depends on a firm resolution by the person with alcoholism to abstain from drinking. However, the drug is seldom used because it is a simplistic approach to a complex problem.

Tranquilizers

Tranquilizers are drugs used in the management of alcoholism to facilitate psychotherapy and lessen anxiety. The drugs commonly used include librium, valium, thorazine, and sparine. However, substituting drugs for alcohol is not the solution to the problem.

CODEPENDENCY

Emerging from the literature on alcoholism is the concept of **codependency**. Codependency is an enabling behavior whereby someone assumes responsibility for someone else's behavior. Frisch (2002) defined *codependency* as behaviors exhibited by significant others of a substance-abusing individual that serve to enable and protect the abuse at the exclusion of personal fulfillment and self-development. Codependency blocks change and personal growth in both people. Characteristics of the codependent include

Caretaking	"I always give to others. Nobody gives to me."
Obsession	"I cannot stop worrying about _____ problems."
Denial	"I pretend I do not have any problems."
Dependency	"Why doesn't _____ make me feel happy."
Low self-worth	"I should think, feel, look, act and behave—I can't do anything right."
Controlling	"I just can't allow things to happen naturally. I fear loss of control."
Poor communication	"No one understands what I mean to say."
Lack of trust	"I do not trust my feelings."
Anger	"I feel controlled and manipulated, and I resent these feelings."
Weak boundaries	"I keep letting other people hurt me."

Codependency progresses until, in the late stages, depression, lethargy, withdrawal, and isolation occur. Serious illnesses, such as alcohol or drug addiction, eating disorders, and suicides, have been reported. Frequently, these people are seen in inclient medical units for physical problems. However, codependents can recognize their enabling behaviors and begin to look inside themselves. Individual psychotherapy may be needed to improve their own self-worth. Giving people permission to do for themselves can be difficult to put into practice. Making personal choices and developing the ability to say *no* firmly diminishes their symptoms. In recovery, the codependent must be aware of sabotaging behaviors of others and identify those people who consistently "suck them in." Monitoring passive or aggressive behaviors will assist with increased numbers of assertive encounters with others in their personal and workplace environments. Another helpful approach is the practice of daily personal affirmations. Affirmations are *I* statements chanted silently or out loud to oneself.

I deserve   satisfaction, contentment, a fulfilling relationship

I will   express my feelings today; act in an assertive manner today

Recovering codependents make their own daily choices and change their belief/value systems through action-oriented behaviors.

TREATMENT FACILITIES

Various treatment facilities are available to meet specific or general needs of the client with alcoholism. Detoxification centers are places where the client with alcoholism receives treatment and care during the withdrawal process. They comprise the first step in treatment. Later, the client participates in a continuing care and rehabilitation program. Referrals are frequently made to long-term treatment programs. Other times, the client is transferred to a residential treatment center. The **halfway house** is an intermediate residence for the client before he or she re-enters the community (Figure 12-3). Frequently, the house is located in the client's community. Individualized attention and a homelike atmosphere are just two advantages of the program. Most halfway houses are oriented to Alcoholics Anonymous and encourage participation in that program.

Hot meals programs are usually run by paraprofessionals. They are particularly geared to the person with alcoholism who has very inadequate nutrition and poor health. From these centers, referrals are made to physicians and visiting nurses. The hot meals program can be used as a detection center for disease and malnutrition. Diseases of the respiratory tract, chronic bronchitis, and tuberculosis are commonly seen in persons with alcoholism.

Each year, industry loses billions of dollars because of alcoholism. Between 6 and 10 percent of the employees in the United States have an alcohol problem. Employee alcoholism results in sporadic absenteeism and decreased quantity of work output. Unauthorized tardiness and faulty judgment are common. Some industries have begun employee assistance programs (see Chapter 16). The occupational

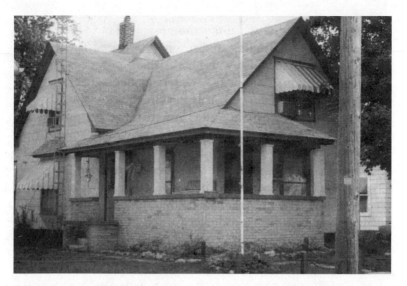

FIGURE 12-3 A halfway house may look like any other home in the community.

environment is an excellent setting for early identification and treatment of problem drinkers.

For more than 350 years, public intoxication was under the jurisdiction of criminal law. The penniless drunk revolved through a process of arrest, jail, release, and rearrest. In the past five years, progress has been made toward transferring the problem drinker from the penal system to treatment programs. It is now recognized that the person with alcoholism needs appropriate treatment and rehabilitation. Legislation is providing the framework for this needed treatment.

School alcohol programs are a preventive measure. Teenagers need alcohol education programs in the schools. The romantic idea of alcohol as seen in the media must be challenged. The real facts and pertinent literature should be presented. Alcoholism is the most-neglected health problem in America and needs to be presented to the adolescent in its true light.

Few treatment facilities care for the needs of the aged with a drinking problem. The aged need therapeutic programs geared to their underlying stressors. Treatment facilities should have an individualized approach that attempts to discover the particular problems of each aging person. Developing new friendships and a sense of well-being through group meetings helps alleviate loneliness.

Long-term goals of a program for the aged person with alcoholism are to make life worthwhile to help him or her see horizons, rather than dead ends.

SUMMARY

Alcoholism is defined as the use of alcoholic beverages that results in damage to the individual, society, or both. It is a progressive and complex disease and a serious problem in the United States. Alcoholism is found in every level of society and in all occupations.

Alcohol depresses the central nervous system; makes thinking confused and disorganized; and dulls memory, concentration, judgment, and perception. Depression, frustration, and anxiety are some of the problems caused by alcohol. Alcoholism may be a way for some people to cope with environmental stress. Many persons with alcoholism neglect their health through poor hygiene and poor diet.

Alcoholism is a problem among all age groups. Teenage drinking is on the rise. The aged are also a high-risk group for alcoholism. The four progressive stages of alcoholism as classified by Jellinek are prealcoholic, prodromal, crucial, and chronic.

Most persons with alcoholism are admitted to the hospital for reasons other then alcoholism. The nurse should have a knowledge of the physiological effects of alcohol so he or she may be aware of an undiagnosed person with alcoholism. Many difficulties that occur with alcoholism clients are a result of withdrawal. The goal of nursing in regard to the client with alcoholism is to be nonjudgmental and understanding and to assist the client to be responsible for his or her own behavior.

Some treatment methods for clients with alcoholism are Alcoholics Anonymous, rational emotive therapy, transactional analysis, psychoanalysis, group therapy, Antabuse, and tranquilizers. Treatment facilities include detoxification centers and halfway houses. Legislation is providing changes in the framework for treatment and rehabilitation of the person with alcoholism. The psychosocial aspects of alcoholism such as family disruption and economic loss cannot be overlooked.

SUGGESTED ACTIVITIES

■ Investigate the problem of alcoholism in your community. Write a report on your findings.

■ List the rehabilitation facilities available for persons wth alcoholism in your community.

■ Attend an AA or Al-Anon meeting.

■ Organize a resource file on alcoholism. Obtain information by writing for literature concerning alcoholism from

The National Council for Alcoholism Inc.
2 Park Avenue
New York, NY 10016

The National Institute of Alcohol Abuse and Alcoholism
5600 Fischer Lane
Room 11A 56
Rockville, MD 20852

REVIEW

KNOW AND COMPREHEND
A. Multiple choice. Select the one best answer.

1. The amendment forbidding the manufacture, distribution, and sale of alcoholic beverages was the
   ❑ A. Temperance Amendment.
   ❑ B. Prohibition Amendment.
   ❑ C. Distillation Amendment.
   ❑ D. Alcoholic Amendment.

2. The treatment method that focuses on changing behavior by changing the clients' views of themselves and their environment is termed
   ❑ A. transactional analysis.
   ❑ B. detoxification method.
   ❑ C. Alcoholics Anonymous.
   ❑ D. rational emotive therapy.

3. A treatment approach that tries to help the client to stop game playing and rewrite his or her life script is
   ❑ A. rational emotive therapy.
   ❑ B. transactional analysis.
   ❑ C. drug therapy.
   ❑ D. Alcoholic Anonymous.

4. Which of the following below accurately describes alcoholism?
   ❑ A. a serious problem that develops after adolescence
   ❑ B. a progressive, fatal, and complex disease
   ❑ C. an effective way to cope with stress
   ❑ D. a habit of drinking more than one intended

5. A small amount of alcohol produces which effect?
   - ❏ A. muscle relaxation
   - ❏ B. muscle tension
   - ❏ C. staggering gait
   - ❏ D. impairment of the respiratory system

6. When a client taking disulfuram (Antabuse) drinks alcohol, which response would the nurse expect?
   - ❏ A. drowsiness and lethargy
   - ❏ B. mild, transient, unpleasant reactions
   - ❏ C. hypertension and decreased pulse rate
   - ❏ D. potentially life-threatening effects

APPLY YOUR LEARNING
B. Multiple Choice. Select the one best answer.

1. A newly admitted client has a diagnosis of alcohol dependency. Which information would be most important for the nurse to gather?
   - ❏ A. When was the client's last drink?
   - ❏ B. What type of alcohol does the client usually drink?
   - ❏ C. Who drove the client to the hospital?
   - ❏ D. What time of day does the client usually begin drinking?

2. The nurse cares for a client admitted 30 minutes ago with acute alcohol intoxication. Which intervention would the nurse use during the first few hours of care?
   - ❏ A. provide the client with a pamphlet about the rules of the unit.
   - ❏ B. explain the rules of the unit to the client.
   - ❏ C. apply restraints until the client is oriented.
   - ❏ D. assign a nurse's assistant to stay with the client.

3. A practical nurse escorts a discharged client out of an alcohol treatment center. Which comment by the nurse would be most therapeutic?
   - ❏ A. "Be sure to take your disulfuram every morning to help you stay sober."
   - ❏ B. "The members of Alcoholics Anonymous will welcome you to meetings."
   - ❏ C. "Don't drink anymore. Alcohol is destroying your liver."
   - ❏ D. "I hope you've learned how to control your drinking."

4. A practical nurse talks with clients in an alcohol treatment center about their disease. Which client is in the earliest stage of the rehabilitation process? The client who says:
   - ❑ A. "I understand that alcoholism is a lifelong disease process."
   - ❑ B. "My drinking has caused problems in my family relationships."
   - ❑ C. "I've never had a problem finding or keeping a job."
   - ❑ D. "I've often felt guilty about my drinking."

5. The nurse cares for an infant with fetal alcohol syndrome (FAS). Which characteristic is most likely present in the infant?
   - ❑ A. low weight for age
   - ❑ B. narrow, pointed nose
   - ❑ C. wide, bulging eyes
   - ❑ D. edematous extremities

6. You are a nurse working on a medical-surgical unit. During the shift change report at the beginning of a new shift, you notice the smell of alcohol on another nurse's skin and breath. Based on this observation, which action would you implement?
   - ❑ A. inform the nurse of your observation
   - ❑ B. observe the nurse for impaired performance
   - ❑ C. ask a coworker if they smell alcohol
   - ❑ D. notify the nursing supervisor of the observation

C. Briefly answer the following.

1. What is the purpose of the National Institute for Alcohol Abuse and Alcoholism?

2. List the four progressive stages of alcoholism as described by Jellinek.

3. State treatments used for a client with alcoholism on admission to the general hospital.

4. List six symptoms of alcohol withdrawal.

5. List ten nursing interventions when caring for the client with alcoholism.

6. Briefly describe the objectives of each of the following community programs.

   A. Alcoholics Anonymous

   B. detoxification centers

   C. halfway houses

   D. hot meals programs

Drug Dependency

OUTLINE

KEY TERMS

drug user/abuser	cocaine
tolerance	crack
addiction	amphetamine psychosis
habituation	narcolepsy
dual-diagnosed	crank
substance abuse	barbiturates
chemical dependency	quaalude
Addiction Severity Index (ASI)	opium
caffeine intoxication	heroin
marijuana	mainlining
inhalants	skin pop
benzodiazepine	rush
hallucinogenic	nod
psychedelic	cold turkey
bad trip	methadone
flashback	detoxification

OBJECTIVES

After studying this chapter, the student should be able to:

- Differentiate among drug use, misuse, abuse, and dependence.
- Describe the historical perspectives of drug abuse.
- List six symptoms of heroin withdrawal.
- State the factors that contribute to use of drugs.
- List the effects of commonly abused drugs.
- Describe nursing care for the drug-dependent person.
- Name the treatment approaches for rehabilitation of the drug-dependent person.

Most Americans use drugs at some time during their lives. In the past two decades, there has been increasing attention given to the effects of cigarettes, alcohol, and other drugs on the individual, family, and community. Drug use is often coupled with poverty, inadequate nutrition, limited prenatal care, maternal mental health problems, and family instability. According to Public Health Reports (March 1996), the cost of addiction treatment is approximately $166 billion annually. A **drug user** is defined as a person who takes drugs according to directions for medical reasons. Drug *misuse* occurs when the directions are exceeded. When a person takes drugs for other than medical reasons, he or she is classified as a **drug abuser**. Any substance capable of altering the individual's mood or conscious state may be abused. Narcotics, depressants, tranquilizers, stimulants, and hallucinogens are the drugs most commonly abused.

Tolerance occurs after continued use of some drugs, when an increasing amount of the drug is needed to produce the desired effect. A person may be dependent on a drug either physically or psychologically. An addicting drug causes physical dependence and withdrawal symptoms if the drug is withheld. When physical dependence to a drug develops, the user is said to have an **addiction. Habituation** is the term used for psychological dependency on a drug. A habitual drug user compulsively depends on the drug as a means for coping with conflicts of daily living. It is difficult to differentiate between habituation and addiction, so the preferred term for both is drug *dependence.* However, less emphasis is being placed on the question of addiction and more on psychological and social impairment. Occupational health has looked at substance abuse and the loss of job productivity and the increase of accidental injury and death.

A special population impaired by drug dependency use/abuse is the **dual-diagnosed** client. This individual has a severe mental illness and also a substance abuse problem. Research suggests that persons with mental illness may have a biochemical vulnerability for addiction. Who provides care and management to these clients? Behavioral characteristics of dual-diagnosed persons include noncompliance and resistance. Many drug centers discourage the use of medication, expel clients who are noncompliant, and base their group work on confrontation techniques; therefore, many dual-diagnosed clients discontinue treatment and literally "fall through the cracks." Studies have reported that the tension and monotony of daily existence for persons with serious and persistent mental illness can lead to drug use/abuse with the following drugs:

Amphetamines	"It helps me to feel more normal."
Marijuana	"I can join in with my old friends."
Cocaine	"People like me, look for me, give me something, and borrow my money."

Data from Drug Abuse Warning Network, 1994	
DRUG	**RELATED EMERGENCIES**
Heroin	44 percent
Cocaine	45 percent
PCP	45 percent
Methamphetamines	61 percent
Marijuana	19 percent

FIGURE 13-1 Drug abuse and clients seen in emergency room. (From DHHS, PHS, July 1994)

It is important to note that many homeless people suffer from drug abuse.

The DSM-IV-TR states criteria for **substance abuse** and dependence with a presentation of the many different disorders related to substance abuse. They include psychoactive substance–use disorders, dependence/abuse, psychoactive substance–induced organic mental disorders, intoxication and withdrawal states (specific substance induced), organic disorder, and cocaine delusional disorder. Drug use/abuse contributes to related emergencies (Figure 13-1).

Another cogent point is that the trend nationally is to combine alcohol and drug abuse centers into one comprehensive treatment area entitled **chemical dependency** or substance abuse.

HISTORICAL PERSPECTIVES

Drug abuse has existed for many centuries. Each era had its favorite drug. Opium was used in ancient Mesopotamia, Egypt, Greece, and Rome. The effects of cannabis were mentioned by the Arabians in the 1500s. Cocaine sniffing was popular in the 1700s. Hashish was the drug of choice in the 1800s.

China was the first country to attempt to control drug abuse. Opium was transported to that country from the Middle East and India by British traders. During the nineteenth century, opium use was so widespread in China that the government banned it with an imperial edict. However, so much of the drug was smuggled in that the attempt to ban it was unsuccessful. Confiscation of large quantities of opium by the government led to the Opium War of 1839. The Chinese lost the war and as a result the British were able to force the Chinese government to legalize the opium trade. China eventually became the main source of opium and supplied the drug to the rest of the world.

Because opium could be bought legally and inexpensively over the counter, its use increased among the civilian population. Opium was also the main ingredient in many patent medicines. It was given to women and children as cough syrup, diarrhea remedies, and pain-killers. Opium and its derivative, morphine, were the most frequently used drugs following the Civil War.

America's drug problems began with the Civil War in 1861. Wounded soldiers were given morphine by injection. Its use was uncontrolled; many soldiers were given their own supply. Cocaine, a refined product of the coca plant, became popular after World War I. In 1898, heroin (a derivative of morphine) was discovered in Germany and soon was imported to America. The new drug was approximately ten times more potent than morphine. Heroin became a popular drug during World War II. Methadone headed the list in popularity immediately following World War II. Marijuana was heavily used during the Vietnam War. Today, chemicals from opium to aspirin are misused and abused. Effects of drugs on society are very complex, with medical, moral, legal, and economic consequences.

Drug controls began in 1906 when the Pure Food and Drug Act required accurate labeling of drugs. This forced many patent medicine makers to remove opium from their products. In 1909, Congress banned the importation of opium except for medicinal purposes. The Harrison Narcotic Act, passed in 1914, controlled the manufacture, importation, and sale of opium and coca leaves. Marijuana was banned in 1920. In 1930, the Federal Bureau of Narcotics imposed still more controls. By 1950, international responsibility for narcotics was given to the World Health Organization (WHO).

The 1950s brought the development of more synthetic drugs, including tranquilizers. Drugs were effectively used to treat a variety of physical and emotional problems. Successful use gave drugs the reputation of being good and beneficial. Society became conditioned to relying on drugs to alleviate distress. Drugs were thought of as an easy way to solve problems, an attitude that often leads to misuse and abuse of drugs.

The Controlled Substance Act of 1970 gave authority to the attorney general of the United States to place drugs in categories according to their effect, history, abuse potential, and scientific information gathered on them. There are approximately eleven categories. Each category carries a different penalty for violations.

COMMON ADDICTING SUBSTANCES

Addicting substances have widespread use in our society. Frequently, these substances are used habitually and compulsively. People who chronically use addicting substances feel that they are unable to function satisfactorily without them. A physiological dependency is established. When the person refrains from the addiction substance, a problem exists because the body and/or mind craves that substance.

Results of daily use of addicting substances are:

- Lack of motivation
- Lack of self-discipline
- Reduced school or work attendance
- Antisocial and violent behavior
- Increased risk-taking behaviors
- Sexual experimentation

The **Addiction Severity Index (ASI)** is a tool to assess alcohol and drug use. Medical, psychological and legal areas are explored within multiple settings: family, employment, and social. The ASI is an efficient and productive data gathering tool.

Caffeine and Nicotine

Two commonly used addicting substances are nicotine and caffeine. Caffeine is the least expensive and most abused drug in the United States. It is a central nervous system stimulant. Caffeine in large amounts causes insomnia. Over a long period of time, its use causes circulatory problems because caffeine constricts the blood vessels. People who habitually drink five to seven cups of coffee a day may suffer withdrawal symptoms if coffee is eliminated from their diets. Table 13-1 lists the caffeine content of common beverages. The DSM-IV-TR lists **caffeine intoxication** as a disorder with some of the following symptoms: restlessness, nervousness, psychomotor agitation, rambling flow of thought/speech, and tachycardia.

Smoking is a leading cause of preventable death in the United States. Approximately 20 percent of deaths annually are from environmental tobacco smoke (ETS), with 3,000 lung cancer deaths per year. The Food and Drug Administration (FDA) unsuccessfully proposed regulating tobacco as a drug-containing substance. It has been suggested that tobacco companies have long known about the harm and addictiveness of smoking and have tried to maintain the nicotine content of cigarettes at levels that would keep smokers hooked. Smokers

TABLE 13-1 Caffeine Content of Common Beverages

BEVERAGE	AMOUNT	CAFFEINE
Coffee		
Brewed, ground	8 oz	80-200 mg
Instant	1 tsp	50-66 mg
Decaffeinated	1 tsp	2-5 mg
Tea (1 regular tea bag)	—	36-46 mg
Soft drinks		
Colas	12 oz	43-65 mg
Hot cocoa	8 oz	5-10 mg
Caffeine content, miscellaneous:		
Chocolate		
Over-the-counter (OTC) medications and preparations:		
Analgesics, cold remedies, weight control		

have an increased incidence of lung and mouth cancer. Smoking during pregnancy increases the following risks: low birth weights, spontaneous abortions, premature rupture of membranes, stillborn infant delivery, intrauterine retardation, and childhood disorders.

Coffee and cigarettes are socially acceptable and easy to obtain. Unfortunately, many people use these addicting substances regularly. Next to alcohol, nicotine is the most commonly used drug in the adolescent group. Adolescents often see smoking as an initiation into adulthood. Advertising tobacco products has been restricted in an attempt to reduce the appeal to young people. It is interesting to note that as cigarette smoking has decreased, the use of cigars and other nicotine products (chews, snuff) has increased.

Marijuana

Marijuana is a mixture of dried up leaves, stems, flowers, and seeds of the Indian hemp plant (*Cannabis sativa*). Use of marijuana has become one of the biggest controversies since alcohol and prohibition. The main question is whether the drug is a sociological or an individual psychological problem. In August 1977, the decriminalization of marijuana was proposed. If marijuana is decriminalized, it would be legal to possess small amounts of it for personal use.

Marijuana is also known as grass, weed, maryjane, tea, and pot. The drug is usually crushed and rolled into cigarettes called reefers or joints. The smoke smells like burning rope. Users often burn incense to cover the odor. The effects of the drug are inconsistent and varied. They seem to depend on the user's mood and expectation and his or her interests and personality.

The effect of marijuana is immediate and lasts less than three hours. A small amount usually produces a sense of well-being, although some users experience anxiety. Light smokers appear talkative, relaxed, exhilarated, and happy. One of the most consistent effects of marijuana is an altered sense of time. Time passes very slowly for the marijuana user. Increased amounts of the drug seem to hinder memory recall. The sense of touch and hearing are enhanced, and many marijuana smokers complain of hunger after use. Larger-than-moderate doses result in impaired coordination and moral judgment. The user is easily distracted and more suggestible. Long-term use decreases sperm counts and causes respiratory changes.

Marijuana may be obtained in various strengths. The strength depends on the part of the plant used, where it is grown, the amount of the active ingredient, and whether it has been adulterated (made impure by the addition of other substances). Street marijuana is often adulterated. Marijuana may be adulterated with inactive tea, spices, grass, leaves, or parsley; it also may be adulterated with substances that are harmful to the body, such as angel dust (PCP). Many cities test street drugs and report their contents daily to prevent deaths from the use of contaminated drugs.

True tolerance does not develop in the marijuana user. However, chronic users can develop a psychological dependence on the drug and the half-life of marijuana is so long that withdrawal symptoms are masked. Although marijuana does not physically lead to hard drugs, users often experiment with other drugs. The adolescent and the young adult are frequent users. They are usually attracted to it out of curiosity and the belief that it is relatively harmless. When looking at substance use in the schizophrenic population, it was noted that marijuana was one of their drugs of choice.

Medical use of the drug is now being explored. The main active ingredient in marijuana is delta-9-tetrahydrocannabinol, or THC. In the 1800s, tincture of cannabis was used to relieve menstrual cramps. Marijuana has recently been found to be useful in the treatment of glaucoma and in reducing nausea and vomiting associated with chemotherapy. In some states, marijuana is legalized for medical purposes only.

Research on the effects of marijuana is still being conducted. Some researchers are studying the consequences of long-term use. Other researchers are examining marijuana's effects on mental and physical skills. Still others are trying to determine the drug's toxic level. Until there are more scientific facts, the debate over marijuana continues.

Hashish (hash) is a more potent form of marijuana. It is a resin from the top of the hemp plant. Because of its high concentration, it is often five or six times stronger than marijuana. Frequent use of hashish has been associated with physical, mental, and emotional deterioration.

Inhalants

According to public health authorities, the use of **inhalants** is more prevalent among the poor. However, their use crossed all sociocconomic boundaries and is especially prevalent among Hispanic and Native American children and adolescents. The peak age of usage is fourteen to fifteen years old, but some children start as early as six to eight years old. Commonly abused products are model glue, gasoline, nail polish lacquers, cooking and hair sprays, paints, aerosols, and butane fuel. Inhalants contain volatile hydrocarbons that are highly soluble in fats. The human brain is a lipid-rich organ, and chronic solvent abuse dissolves brain cells, resulting in central nervous system damage, white matter dementia and cerebral dysfunction, which includes loss of cognitive functions and coordination and gait disturbances.

Toluene abusers inhale fumes directly from a container, plastic bag, or saturated rag to produce a state similar to alcohol intoxication and usually experience a sense of floating or spinning. Occasionally the use of inhalants can result in cardiac arrest due to arrhythmia. This phenomenon, called sudden sniffing death syndrome, occurs when the fumes create strong variations in heart rhythm. Sometimes the inhalant user places a plastic bag over his or her head to prolong the effect. This is a dangerous practice because death can occur from suffocation.

Young toluene abusers exhibit failures in school, delinquency, inability to achieve, and societal maladjustments. Education in the schools may be the most effective method of prevention.

Benzodiazepines

The **benzodiazepines** most often misused are Librium, Valium, and Xanax. They can be effective in treating various medical problems, but are often abused. Benzodiazepines reduce agitation and produce a calming effect. The user thinks and behaves more rationally and frequently experiences a feeling of well-being. All benzodiazepines appear to be addictive when taken in large amounts. The effect is made stronger in combination with alcohol and sedatives. This presents a serious potential for complications such as coma or death.

Hallucinogens

A **hallucinogenic** or psychedelic drug is capable of producing hallucinations. **Psychedelic** refers to distortion of perception. In reality, hallucinogenic drugs cause a heightened and distorted perception of things. Colors become more brilliant, flat objects are seen as three-dimensional, stationary objects move, and faces are distorted. The senses are sharper and seem to merge together. The user may claim to be able to hear the grass grow. Hallucinogenic drugs include

- LSD (lysergic acid diethylamide)
- Mescaline
- Peyote (the button of a small spineless cactus)
- Psilocybin (one of the two active substances isolated from the psilocybe mushroom)
- THC (the active ingredient in marijuana and hashish)
- MDA
- DMT (dimethyltriptamine)
- PCP (angel dust)

LSD has been controversial since its discovery in Switzerland in 1943. Some say it promotes a religious experience, while others say it only distorts reality. The true potential of LSD is unknown. It causes a loss of control over normal thought processes. Serious temporary or permanent mental changes may occur. Episodes of violence and self-destruction have resulted from the use of LSD. There is evidence that it causes chromosomal damage. LSD has been used experimentally to treat psychic disorders, but its use in medicine has been limited. Even under close supervision, the behavior of users is highly unpredictable.

LSD is colorless, tasteless, and odorless. Most of it is synthetically made in illegal laboratories. LSD can be added to any food or drink. Some of the most popular items to which LSD is added are sugar cubes, chewing gum, hard candy, mints, and animal crackers. It is an extremely potent drug. An amount invisible to the eye can cause effects lasting eight to ten hours. On the street, LSD is known as 25, acid, sunshine, cubes, the big D, trips, the chief, the ghost, and the hawk. Like other street drugs, it is often adulterated. Tolerance to LSD develops quickly and is just as quickly lost, so the drug is usually taken intermittently rather than on a continuous basis.

The user's frame of mind and the environment are contributing factors to the drug's effects. A person with repressed desires, emotions, or fears may experience a **bad trip** (emotional experience that may result in panic reactions). Feelings of indestructibility or the feeling that one can fly have been reported. Serious injury and death have occurred from acting on these feelings. A **flashback**, (reexperiencing of a trip) can occur months after the drug was last taken because LSD is stored in the fat tissues and released later.

Mescaline and psilocybin are related to LSD in action but somewhat weaker. Mescaline is an active chemical ingredient found in the peyote cactus. American Indians have traditionally used the peyote cactus as a legitimate part of their religious ceremonies. Mescaline is now produced synthetically. Psilocybin is an extract of the Mexican grown psilocybe mushroom.

DMT is a hallucinogen prepared from the mimosa root. The active ingredient is N-cimethyltryptamine. DMT is found as either a liquid or a colorless crystal, which is usually mixed with other substances. Its effect comes on rapidly, producing a trip similar to LSD. The effect lasts one to two hours. Too much of this drug taken too fast can cause brain damage.

PCP, or angel dust, is an animal tranquilizer. It is important to be aware of its existence because it is often substituted for other hallucinogenic drugs on the street. PCP is an immobilizing and anesthetic agent for large animals. Its effect on humans is highly unpredictable. It may cause lapse of memory and difficulty in concentrating that can last for several days. Convulsions, partial paralysis, and death can occur.

MDA is an amphetamine-related drug. It makes the user feel very mellow. The MDA available on the street is often of low-grade quality and usually consists of less-expensive substitutes. It may in reality contain more LSD or PCP than MDA.

Psychedelic drugs are again prevalent and in a dangerous form on tattoo paper, which small children may use to ornamentally tattoo on their hands or arms and subsequently absorb the drug. Schools are distributing information to parents and children to warn them of the danger.

Some young adults attend all-night parties called "raves." New and dangerous drugs have gained popularity among this set. The following popular drugs are colorless, tasteless, and odorless:

- MDMA   Ecstasy (methylene dioxymethamphetamine)
- GHB   G (gamma-hydroxybutyrate)
- Rohypnol   Roofies (flunitrazelam)
- Ketamine   Special K

Roofie is the "forget-me" pill used in date rape or sexual assaults. The drug causes anterograde amnesia, so the victim does not remember events. Community drug alerts have been issued about these dangerous "club drugs."

Cocaine/Crack

Cocaine and crack use/abuse has reached epidemic proportions in all elements of society. **Cocaine** is implicated as impacting on illicit drug use trends more than any other substance. It is a refined product of the coca plant found in South America. It comes in the form of a pure, white crystalline powder. Cocaine is also referred to as snow, coke, or a change in form called freebase **crack.** Unfortunately, crack is inexpensive (compared to cocaine), potent, and available. Previously, cocaine was thought to be the drug of the upper-middle class and used for recreation and as a status symbol. Many studies supported the fact that there is no average cocaine user. There is an enormous variety in the type of user, including: coca leaf chewers, crack smokers, cocaine injectors, and cocaine snorters (most popular use). It appears that the socially marginalized smoke crack and inject cocaine. Cocaine can be used by several routes: nasal inhalation (sniffing or snorting), smoking, and intravenously. A language develops around the usage of cocaine:

Wired	hyper, high feelings
Coke run	consecutive days of usage
Speedball	mixture of heroin and cocaine
Lightball	approximately 1/8 ounce cocaine, with estimated cost $500
Crashing	a quick comedown physically, and psychologically when drug is not obtainable
Dealing	securing and selling drugs
Rush	euphoric feelings

Although we have increased remarkably the knowledge of cocaine use and its consequences, users/abusers possess great denial and large blinders that block their recognition of these consequences. Cocaine usage increases alertness, and heart rate, dilates pupils, produces hyperactivity, and decreases appetite.

With prolonged use malnutrition can occur. More serious side effects include schizophrenic-like symptoms with visual, auditory, or tactile hallucinations and in some cases cardiac irregularities and sudden death. Paranoid-like symptoms (fear, suspiciousness, jumpiness) can lead to impulsive or assaultive behaviors. Two serious problems that also emerge with cocaine use/abuse are how to get money to sustain a high and how to counter the crash if money or cocaine is not available. Theft, prostitution, and dealing drugs to support the habit are common practices. To avoid crashing, polydrug abuse (alcohol, sedatives) can be used to assist with the bringing-down process. Intravenous users are subject to abscesses, systemic infections, hepatitis B, and AIDS. Contamination occurs from poor injection technique, dirty equipment, dirty environment, and sharing needles.

Although our national call is for a war on drugs, the yet-unborn are not escaping addiction to cocaine because women are using cocaine and crack prenatally. The infant born is of low birth weight with subsequent poor weight gain, withdrawal, hyperactivity, tremors, and a frantic sucking mechanism. These infants need special care and their mothers need intervention for their drug abuse and assessment of their parenting skills.

Amphetamines

Amphetamines are stimulants that cause heart and other body systems to speed up. They are also known as dexies, pep pills, uppers, speed, drivers, bennies, footballs, whites, and white crosses. Amphetamines release stores of epinephrine into the body, which results in a high degree of sensitivity to stimuli and insomnia. Long-term heavy use can cause damage to vital organs. Chronic anorexia results in weight loss. Amphetamines can interfere with language control and decreased mental capability. The prolonged sleeplessness produced by the drug lead to an **amphetamine psychosis**. The user, often called a speed freak, usually suffers from acute paranoia.

During the 1940s and 1950s, amphetamines were prescribed for a wide variety of reasons. They kept truck drivers awake and college students stimulated for study. Overweight people found their appetites depressed after taking the drug. Amphetamines are now used primarily to treat **narcolepsy** (a disease characterized by brief attacks of deep sleep.). They are sometimes given to hyperactive children, persons with epilepsy, and people with Parkinson's disease. Because of their dangers, medical use of amphetamines has been diminished.

An amphetamine user is a potential abuser. Since amphetamines cause insomnia, many users resort to a depressant drug to help them sleep, thus initiating a vicious cycle. Users take sleeping pills at night to sleep and amphetamines to get them going in the morning. Tolerance readily develops. After a period of time, amphetamines may produce an opposite effect. Users may find themselves becoming drowsy instead of alert. Large doses may lead to antisocial and aggressive behavior. Sudden withdrawal of amphetamines can cause depression and suicide.

In 1972 the Drug Enforcement Administration established guidelines for production of drugs. The amount of amphetamines legally manufactured was diminished. However, amphetamines are still readily available on the street. Street users run the risk of taking adulterated drugs; amphetamines have been known to be adulterated with strychnine. Caffeine tablets also are passed off as amphetamines at a premium cost.

Methamphetamine (street names: speed, ice, chalk, meth, crystal, Crank, fire, glass) is a toxic and addictive stimulant. It is available in many forms and can be smoked, inhaled, injected, or orally ingested. Methamphetamine is a white, odorless, bitter-tasting crystalline powder that easily dissolves in beverages. It is associated with serious health consequences, including memory loss, aggression, violence, psychosis, and possible cardiac or neurological damage.

A newer potent psychomotor stimulant is N-methylcathinone, also known as cat, goob, go-fast, **crank,** sniff, star, and wild cat (when it is mixed with cocaine). Some have called it bathtub speed because of the ease with which it can be made and its similarity to methamphetamine. It can be easily synthesized in a laboratory, garage, basement, apartment, or campsite through the oxidation of ephedrine and other easily available over-the-counter chemicals. Cat can be snorted to get a hit for a four- to six-hour high. Tolerance to the drug builds quickly, and chronic abusers take the drug more often and in larger doses. Studies show that many are polydrug abusers or have abused alcohol. Cat induces the following side effects: temporary loss of memory and sense of smell, headaches, double and triple vision, stomachaches, hallucinations, powerful anorexia, and temporary blindness. Chronic users experience nervous jerks and paranoia. This drug is so addicting that the chronic user will hock anything of value to buy it. Ephedrine is a bronchial dilator used by asthmatics to ease breathing. It is also used as a stimulant, when combined with caffeine, by truck drivers and college students. Ephinedrine is an active ingredient in nasal sprays, which are sold over the counter at gas stations, truck stops, and student areas and by mail order.

Depressants

Barbiturates are the best known and most abused of the depressant drugs. Barbiturates slow bodily functions and are used medically in the treatment of insomnia and seizure disorders. All barbiturates are abused, but the most common are Amytal, Seconal, and Nembutal. The street names refer to the color of capsule such as reds, yellow jackets, or rainbows. They may also be called goofballs, downers, or barbs.

Barbiturates result in light-headedness, reduced inhibitions, drowsiness, slurred speech, and sleep. The drug produces a sense of well-being and relaxation. Tolerance is developed quickly, and increasing amounts of the drug are needed to produce the desired effects. Large doses may cause restlessness, excitability, and delusions. The user has symptoms similar to the alcoholic.

There seems to be a correlation between barbiturate addiction and age. Younger adults are more susceptible to addiction than older adults. Emotional dependence can occur at any age. Withdrawal symptoms are very severe and can result in grand mal seizures and respiratory arrest. Withdrawal should be gradual and attempted only in a hospital environment under close medical supervision.

Barbiturates are one of the main causes of accidental deaths. Bodily functions can be slowed so much that breathing and heart action stop. Barbiturates are the most common method of suicide. The potential for overdose is especially high when mixed with alcohol.

Synthetic, nonbarbiturate sleeping pills are made to eliminate the dangers of addiction and habituation. Many are on the market but none have proved completely safe. All are abused. One such drug is methaqualone, or **quaaludes**. Quaaludes are also known as ludes or soapers. This drug is addictive and has a sedative-hypnotic effect. Effects of the drug include motor incoordination, stupor, and difficulty in arousing. Severe respiratory depression can result. Quaaludes are addictive and extremely dangerous because of toxins that remain after the drug is synthesized. It is a restricted drug but reportedly available on the street as one of the current "in" drugs.

Narcotics

Narcotics are central nervous system depressants and are primarily painkilling drugs. **Opium**, its derivatives heroin and morphine, and synthetics such as meperidine (Demerol) and methadone are all classified as narcotics.

Opium is the dried milklike juice from the pod of the unripe opium poppy. It contains about 10 percent morphine. Heroin is similar to morphine but four to ten times more potent. **Heroin** is very addictive. However, heroin bought on the street has been cut many times and is usually only 2 to 10 percent pure. Heroin is also called smack, junk, horse, or skag. Its use is increasing, and there appears to be more heroin available now than ever before. Heroin usage patterns have changed. Substance abusers have discovered heroin is less expensive and produces a more prolonged "high." Initially, heroin most often was used alone then it was used with alcohol and in combination with cocaine. While cocaine was considered the drug of the 1980s, heroin was considered by many as the drug of the 90s.

Physical and psychological dependence rapidly develop from use of narcotics. The addict is strung out and may be dependent for the rest of his or her life. Heroin is usually taken intravenously. This is referred to as **mainlining**. Needle usage increases the risk of HIV infection and hepatitis B and C. The drug also can be snorted or smoked. Sometimes the addict **skin pops** (takes the drug subcutaneously). Users describe the initial dose of heroin as a **rush** (an intense feeling of well-being followed by warmth and peacefulness). The user then goes into a **nod**, which is a sleepy, drowsy state. There is no dysfunction in coordination and the addict can go about his or her regular business.

Heroin withdrawal symptoms occur four to forty-eight hours after the last dose and include

- Allergic reactions
- Sore throat
- Watery eyes
- Sweating
- Elevated temperature
- Rhinorrhea (watery discharge from the nose)
- Diarrhea
- Nausea
- Vomiting
- Leg and abdominal cramps
- Extreme restlessness

More severe withdrawal symptoms include dilated pupils, muscular twitches and elevated blood pressure.

Withdrawal without the aid of medication is called going **cold turkey**. Symptoms are uncomfortable but not necessarily dangerous. A postwithdrawal syndrome of anxiety and depression frequently occurs. Stress in daily living may lead to the desire for heroin. If the addict takes the drug, the cycle of addiction begins again. Other health problems are created by the use of heroin. Some addicts suffer from malnutrition. Death may result from an overdose.

NURSING CARE

Nurses should familiarize themselves with the street names of psychoactive drugs so that they can better communicate with the user (Table 13-2). Nursing care includes the ability to feel confident and

TABLE 13-2 Abused Drugs: Symptoms and Effects

DRUG	STREET NAME	SYMPTOMS	ADVERSE EFFECTS
Hallucinogens			
Marijuana	Grass, weed, maryjane, tea, pot, reefer, joint, hemp, hashish, hash, rope	Sense of well-being; possible anxiety; talkative; relaxed; exhilarated, happy; altered time sense	Reduced memory recall; impaired coordination and moral judgment; easily distracted highly suggestible long-term effect not known
LSD	25, acid, cubes, sunshine, the big D, trips, the chief, the ghost, the hawk	Heightened and distorted perceptions; euphoria; altered time perception; dreamy, floating state; enlarged pupils; bizarre sensations	Chromosomal damage; loss of control over normal thought processes; violence; self-destructive feelings; highly predictable behavior; slowed reaction and reflexes; personality changes; paranoid symptoms
PCP	Angel dust	Lapse of memory; difficulty concentrating; convulsions; partial paralysis	Effects highly unpredictable
Inhalants			
Glue Gasoline Spray paint Aerosols		Similar to alcohol intoxication; sense of floating or spinning; blurred vision; confusion; staggering gait; slurred speech	Brain damage; lead poisoning; damage to liver, heart, kidneys, and bone marrow; death

comfortable with the drug-dependent person. Nurses must have insight into their personal attitudes and value systems. They must develop sensitivity to the feelings and reactions of others. They need to have some understanding of the influences that led to the problem. Skill in assessing the mood and attitude of the client is necessary. The drug addict is very persuasive and tends to manipulate the behavior of others. Nurses may have to limit visitors and mail and possibly do body searches; they need to deal with the addict in a straightforward, honest manner.

Nurses must watch for and report the danger signals of drug abuse. The symptoms and treatment vary with the type of drug. With heroin and barbiturate overdose, the symptoms are muscle flaccidity, respiratory depression, and coma. Time spent searching for needle marks or constricted pupils is wasted. Multiple drugs may have been taken.

The most important action for the nurse to take with an overdosed client is to assure a patent airway. The mouth must be cleared of any obstructions. The nurse should be sure that a flaccid tongue is not obstructing the airway. Respiratory resuscitation or mechanical ventilation may be needed. If possible, assistance of another person should be obtained.

It must be remembered that barbiturate withdrawal is dangerous; abrupt withdrawal from barbiturates may be fatal. Withdrawal should be attempted only in a hospital situation and under close medical supervision. Researchers have found that misuse of barbiturates causes interference with the rapid eye movement (REM), or dream cycle, of sleep. The user, being deprived of dreams, becomes less stable.

If the overdose is with amphetamines, the client is irritable, hyperactive, and suspicious. He or she should be kept in a quiet environment and not touched. The user's feelings of persecution and suspicion may lead to violent behavior. Judgment is impaired because of the delusional state. No attempt should be made to administer injections because the needle may be misinterpreted as a knife.

Under the influence of LSD, the user is apprehensive and suspicious. He or she needs a quiet environment and calm reassurance. The room should be darkened and free from external stimuli. If a friend has accompanied the client to the hospital, it is important to encourage the friend to remain quietly at the client's bedside. The presence of an understanding friend can help establish a working relationship.

This client needs to be talked down. *Talking down* is softly and calmly helping the client to fully experience and complete his or her trip. It is very important that the trip not be interrupted. The client should be told what is being done and reassured that he or she is in a safe place with sympathetic people. The client is very suggestible, so his thoughts should be guided gently, keeping in mind the goal of a good trip. Do not attempt to talk down a person on PCP as this will increase agitation.

Since many drugs are not pure, it may be difficult to identify the drug that has been taken. The client withdrawing from drug use requires special nurse monitoring, including the following:

- Vital signs; particularly respiratory function
- Level of consciousness (orientation and alertness)
- Reaction of pupils to light
- Patent airway
- Stage of withdrawal
- Nutritional needs
- Fluid intake
- Urinary output

If PRN medications (medications that are ordered to be given as needed) are ordered for the client, they should not be withheld. Withholding medications may cause the client to convulse.

Care of the Child and Adolescent Drug Abuser

The National Institute on Drug Abuse in 1985 recognized the magnitude of the problem of drug dependence in the adolescent. The drug-dependent adolescent presents a special concern because adolescents at younger ages are moving through different treatment modalities, with their first appearances occurring in the juvenile justice system. Thus, a focus for the future needs to be on the systems serving these minors and the ramifications of adolescent drug abuse.

The drug-dependent adolescent presents a special challenge for the nurse. Many adolescent drug users have low self-esteem, which may have been the problem leading to the use of drugs. These clients are frequently hostile and negative. Accusations may be shouted at the nurse and tears of frustration may be seen. Coping mechanisms are often ineffective. The nurse must remain calm, supportive, and reassuring. As the adolescent's physical condition improves, the environment may need to be manipulated to increase external stimuli. The nurse should take time to talk to the client about the issues that led to his or her drug involvement.

Schools have a great potential for preventive programs for the adolescent. Sound education can establish pathways in which students clarify values and improve their self-images. School nurses can help by assessing the problem in their schools. They may observe students for symptoms of drug misuse such as emotional instability, sluggishness, shakiness, and evasiveness. They also may watch for students who suddenly lose interest in school, sports, and other activities. School nurses can provide students with factual information. They can be understanding listeners and agents for referral to community agencies if needed.

Women and Drugs

Recent studies have documented that an increasing number of women of childbearing age use licit and illicit substances. One out of ten infants have been exposed to illicit drugs in utero, and exposure occurs in all racial and socioeconomic groups. An increasing number of infants are being admitted to special care nurseries for complications caused by intrauterine exposure to alcohol and other drugs. These infants are at increased risk for a complex of medical and social problems, including neglect and abuse. All illicit drugs reach the fetal circulation by crossing the placenta and can cause direct toxic effects on the fetus. At birth, depending on the drug used by the mother, the infant may be irritable, tremulous, and lethargic with a possible abnormal crying pattern. Drug-treatment programs designed to meet the needs of women, especially pregnant women and those with small children, are an important multidisciplinary approach to early intervention.

TREATMENT APPROACHES

Rehabilitation of a drug-dependent person is a long-term project. The drug user must be motivated and willing to cooperate. Treatment approaches include

- Group therapy
- Maintenance programs
- Narcotics Anonymous
- Psychotherapy
- Self-help programs

Live-in drug rehabilitation centers run by former drug addicts have proved effective in treatment of the drug addict. At the center, the addict withdraws without the support of any drugs. The addict must voluntarily decide to eliminate his or her drug habit. To be admitted to the homelike atmosphere, addicts must recognize that they have a commitment to themselves and to the people at the center. The new resident is given the opportunity to relate to former addicts, who have achieved success and act as role models. New members soon become involved in sharing and caring family-like groups. Group therapy and behavior modification are used. The members are rewarded for good behavior and punished for infractions.

One of the chief problems with a live-in drug rehabilitation center is follow-up care. When former addicts leave the center, they no longer have the reinforcement of the center. Addicts go back to their old towns, friends, and possibly drug habits.

Methadone is an opiate substitute taken orally that is used in the treatment of opiate addicts. It is classified as a synthetic narcotic and has painkilling properties. Methadone is legally dispensed by approved treatment centers. It is given once a day. An average dose lasts twenty-four to forty-eight hours. Randomized blood or urine specimens are collected to secure drug screens. Methadone maintenance programs have specific guidelines to stringently follow for obtaining urine samples and maintaining active participation in the program.

Methadone relieves withdrawal symptoms and has no secondary effects. However, it is addictive. Many people are critical of treatment with methadone. They point out that the addict is only changing the drug on which he or she is dependent. When the heroin habit has become too expensive, the user may turn to methadone simply to lower his or her heroin tolerance. Some peddle methadone received at free clinics to purchase heroin for their own use. Methadone maintenance, however, has returned addicts to their communities as functioning adult members. LAMM (1-alpha acetyl-methadol) is a longer-acting derivative (taken every three to four days) of methadone (taken daily) that is used for long-term maintenance and provides for home dosing ("take homes").

Narcotics Anonymous holds group meetings similar in format to Alcoholics Anonymous. The meetings are held in the local community. Members include addicts and former addicts (see Chapter 12, Table 12-3).

Many believe that psychotherapy and social therapy are very important treatment approaches to drug dependency. Since anxiety and depression are difficult to cope with during physical withdrawal, the client is encouraged to participate in occupational therapy, recreational therapy, physical therapy, and social activities.

Some communities offer the drug-dependent person help through drug hot lines, drug crisis centers, and drug treatment centers. These are considered self-help programs. Centers are located in target areas of the community where paraprofessionals assist the addict. The nurse may act as a liaison between the traditional hospital setting and the community.

Addicts have a great deal of time on their hands. They need to learn new patterns of living and to expand their interests. Some type of employment is advocated. Classes on current events or encouraging personal opinions are often successful. Vocational classes are a form of therapy. Members of addicts' families should be sought out for possible group meetings and discussions. The family members may also be in need of counseling or referrals.

Rehabilitation of the drug-dependent person requires long-term management (Figure 13-2). The addicted person must be motivated and willing to stop abusing drugs. Rehabilitation should include adequate follow-up care in the client's own community and referrals as needed. Social skills training needs to be initiated, and alternate means of coping must be investigated. An open support line is necessary.

Community-wide, culturally specific interventions need to assess for risk resiliency. The tendency toward relapse develops out of abstainers' experiences in social situations in which they may see themselves as different. They are constantly re-examining the meaningfulness of their nonaddict world. Watch for personal sabotage as the abstainers search for their identities. Support for abstinence must come from policy makers, community groups, private agencies, school districts, health and social service providers, and family members.

OUTPATIENT TREATMENT

Outpatient **detoxification** rather than twenty-four-hour inpatient observation is more cost-effective for a client who has not had serious withdrawal histories. Efforts to control addiction treatment costs by limiting reimbursements to inclient services help expand rather than contain overall treatment costs. Higher costs reduce access to care and diminish benefits or treatment to the entire population that need help. Ongoing treatment promotes reduction in a wide range of symptoms that gradually decline over a course of multiple episodes, or "treatment career." According to public health statistics, untreated alcohol and drug users fill 10 to 50 percent of hospital and emergency room beds for the treatment of illnesses secondary to the addiction. Capture sites for alcohol/drug abusers would be hospital emergency rooms, courthouses, jails/prisons, vocational rehabilitation programs, and job training programs.

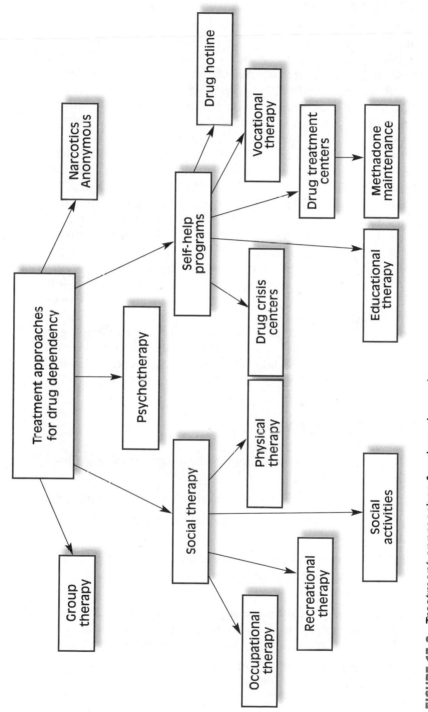

FIGURE 13-2 Treatment approaches for drug dependency.

SUMMARY

When a person takes drugs for other than medical reasons, he or she is classified as a drug abuser. Drug abuse dates from ancient times. All drug users are potential abusers. People who are dependent on drugs are found in every level of society and in all age groups. The effects of drug abuse on society are complex, with medical, moral, legal, and economic consequences. Legislation has been passed in an effort to control the drug problem.

Caffeine and nicotine are two common sources of addicting substances. Frequently abused drugs include the hallucinogens (marijuana, LSD, mescaline, peyote, psilocybin, MDA, DMT, PCP); inhalants (glue, gasoline, spray paint, aerosols); tranquilizers; stimulants (cocaine, amphetamines); depressants (sedatives, barbiturates); and narcotics (opium, morphine, heroin). Withdrawal symptoms range from uncomfortable to deadly. Physical and/or psychological dependency occurs with the use of most drugs.

Rehabilitation of the drug-dependent person requires long-term management. Treatment may include group therapy, social therapy, psychotherapy, Narcotics Anonymous, and self-help programs. Rehabilitation centers have proven effective in helping the drug abuser give up drugs and return to a normal life. The nurse must be aware of the conditions to watch for and report concerning the drug-dependent client.

SUGGESTED ACTIVITIES

- Have a group discussion about current legislation regarding drug use and abuse.
- List your community resources available to the drug abuser.
- Write a report on your local hospital's method of treating the drug abuser.
- Role-play a mental health professional nurse assisting a client who has been admitted to the hospital while experiencing a bad trip from LSD.
- Learn how local schools are supporting a zero-tolerance policy against alcohol, tobacco, and other drugs at school and at school-sponsored and school-sanctioned activities.
- Obtain and review pamphlets from the National Clearinghouse for Drug Abuse Information, P.O. Box 1635, Rockville, MD 20850.

REVIEW

KNOW AND COMPREHEND
A. Multiple choice. Select the one best answer.

1. Select the term that refers to making a drug impure by adding other substances.
   - ❑ A. adulteration
   - ❑ B. drug abuse
   - ❑ C. tolerance
   - ❑ D. mainlining

2. Drugs that cause heightened and distorted perception are classified as
   - ❑ A. amphetamines.
   - ❑ B. barbiturates.
   - ❑ C. hallucinogens.
   - ❑ D. tranquilizers.

3. Breathing difficulties caused by a deviated septum may develop from abuse of
   - ❑ A. amphetamines.
   - ❑ B. barbiturates.
   - ❑ C. cocaine.
   - ❑ D. heroin.

4. Speed is another name for
   - ❑ A. amphetamines.
   - ❑ B. barbiturates.
   - ❑ C. cocaine.
   - ❑ D. LSD.

5. What is the most abused stimulant in the United States?
   - ❑ A. amphetamines
   - ❑ B. heroin
   - ❑ C. caffeine
   - ❑ D. nicotine

6. Select the most likely reason toluene abuse is on the rise.
   - ❑ A. inhalants are not addictive when used in small quantities
   - ❑ B. the "high" from inhalants lasts longer than from alcohol
   - ❑ C. inhalants are inexpensive and easy to obtain
   - ❑ D. there are no lasting physiologic effects from inhalant use

7. What drug is classified as a narcotic?
   - ❏ A. crack cocaine
   - ❏ B. N-methylcathinone
   - ❏ C. methadone
   - ❏ D. alcohol

APPLY YOUR LEARNING
B. Multiple choice. Select the one best answer.

1. The nurse cares for a client who abuses ephedrine. Which finding would the nurse expect?
   - ❏ A. difficulty breathing
   - ❏ B. lethargy and sleepiness
   - ❏ C. complaints of hunger
   - ❏ D. rapid heart rate

2. A client admitted six hours ago has a history of cocaine dependency. The client says to the nurse, "I'm crashing." The nurse would anticipate which finding?

   The client is
   - ❏ A. feeling discomfort from a drop in the drug level.
   - ❏ B. undergoing a frightening, phobic reaction.
   - ❏ C. experiencing elation and euphoria.
   - ❏ D. fearful of a possible drug overdose.

3. The nurse prepares to teach a class to school age children. The goal of the class is drug abuse prevention. Which topic would be most important to include?
   - ❏ A. cocaine
   - ❏ B. barbiturates
   - ❏ C. amphetamines
   - ❏ D. inhalants

4. The nurse interviews a pregnant adolescent. The client states she has smoked two packs of cigarettes per day for the past year. What would be the nurse's first concern at this time?

   Increased risks for:
   - ❏ A. complications of pregnancy.
   - ❏ B. ineffective coughing.
   - ❏ C. sub-clinical tuberculosis infection.
   - ❏ D. lung cancer.

5. The nurse cares for a client who has abused amphetamines for the past two years. Which intervention would be most important?
   - ❏ A. note the client's respiratory rate and sounds
   - ❏ B. include a high-fiber diet in the plan of care
   - ❏ C. monitor weight and encourage a nutritious diet
   - ❏ D. help the client recognize when the dependency developed

6. A client with a newly diagnosed cardiac problem is trying to reduce caffeine intake. Which substance would the nurse teach the client to eliminate from the diet?
   - ❏ A. fruit juices
   - ❏ B. herbal teas
   - ❏ C. ginger ale
   - ❏ D. bottled water

C. Match the drugs in column II with the statement in column I.

Column I

1. Produces a talkative, relaxed, exhilarated, happy feeling

2. Associated with retarded intrauterine growth of the fetus

3. Causes insomnia and circulatory problems

4. Causes lungs to become coated, which impairs air exchange

5. Hallucinogen that produces highly unpredictable behavior

6. Animal tranquilizer that causes lapses of memory and difficulty in concentrating for several days

7. Produces a sense of alertness and wakefulness

8. Depressant drugs that are one of the main causes of accidental deaths

9. Highly addictive narcotic that may cause lifelong dependence

Column II

a. Barbiturates
b. Caffeine
c. Cocaine
d. Heroin
e. Inhalants
f. LSD
g. Marijuana
h. Nicotine
i. PCP

D. Define the following.

1. Drug abuse

2. Drug use

3. Drug misuse

4. Tolerance

5. Habituation

6. Addiction

7. Chemical dependency

8. Dual diagnoses

E. Briefly answer the following.

1. List six symptoms of heroin withdrawal.

2. List six nursing observations required for the chemically dependent client experiencing withdrawal.

3. List three treatment approaches to rehabilitation of the drug-dependent person.

4. What is the most important action of the nurse when a client has taken an overdose of drugs?

5. List four factors that contribute to the widespread use of drugs in American society.

Human Sexuality

OUTLINE

Masturbation
Homosexuality
Acquired Immune Deficiency Syndrome
Abortion

KEY TERMS

sexuality

impotence

neuropathy

retrograde ejaculation

dyspareunia

Viagra (sildenafil)

premenstrual dysphoric
   disorder (PMDD)

fetishism

voyeurism

exhibitionism

pedophilia

transvestism

transsexual

cross-gender identification

masturbation

sensory deprivation

gay

lesbian

acquired immune deficiency
   syndrome (AIDS)

human immunodeficiency virus
   (HIV)

abortion

OBJECTIVES

After studying this chapter, the student should be able to:

- Name three surgical procedures that may threaten sexuality
- State three aspects of sexuality
- List three medical problems that may affect sexuality
- Describe premenstrual dysphoric disorder (PMDD)
- Describe networks for HIV assistance
- Name four psychosexual disorders

The nurse who accepts the concept of total care must consider human sexuality as a significant part of the client's identity. Sex is not an isolated activity; it involves many aspects of the client's life, such as identity, social role, and physical functioning. **Sexuality** is a facet of personality and is self-affirming. It encompasses the individual's personal value system and philosophy of life. Sexuality is an integral part of self-concept. An individual is a sexual being at birth. However, sexuality is not just the difference between male and female.

Sexual behavior includes how a person acts regarding sexual intercourse, reproduction, and childbirth. This is based on boundaries set by a particular culture. The basic identity, however, is taught by society as children learn what roles are expected of boys and girls. Sexual roles are taught and reinforced throughout life. Boys and girls are frequently given toys that are traditionally considered gender specific, such as trucks for boys and dolls for girls (Figure 14-1). Sexual identity and the behavior that goes with it are part of the total being. Thus sex is part of what a person is, as well as what the person does.

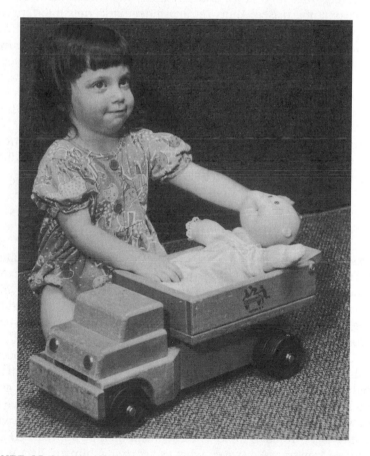

FIGURE 14-1 Toys that were once considered gender specific are a playful combination for this little girl.

Sexual well-being can contribute to a positive attitude. The person who is able to accept himself or herself is better able to maintain a level of wellness. Remember, the chief source of sexual desire is in the mind.

Historically, sexuality and the physical acts of sex were seldom discussed openly in our cultures. These subjects were shrouded in secrecy and embarrassment. Some types of sexual activity brought punishment. Today, in spite of the more permissive attitudes toward sexuality, society still condemns many aspects of sexual behavior. Fear and embarrassment still add to the general lack of knowledge. People with questions about sex are often reluctant to seek help or advice. Hospital clients with such questions may be hesitant to seek answers. Nurses may have problems responding to such questions.

Nurses must reevaluate their attitudes about sexual matters. They should recognize any biases and any areas that make them uncomfortable or embarrassed. Angry or sarcastic remarks only interfere with the nurse-client interaction. Nurses must learn to cope with their own fears and anxieties. Their attitudes, beliefs, and behavior either curtail discussions with clients or create an atmosphere that contributes to open and spontaneous discussion.

There is a great deal of controversy surrounding sexual behavior and personal rights. A person's social and religious background helps to determine his or her attitudes. Nurses need to investigate their own value systems in relation to these and other controversial issues involving human sexuality. They must be able to care for people with differing values. This requires a nonjudgmental attitude.

PHYSICAL ILLNESS AND SEXUALITY

Illness brings about a disturbance of physical and emotional equilibrium. This affects all aspects of the person, including his or her sexuality. Clients may not need in-depth counseling. They may only need someone with whom they can talk. An empathetic ear might be enough. Having a knowledgeable person give reassurance or assistance in problem solving may be a great help.

Clients often avoid mentioning sexual problems or concerns because they feel embarrassed. However, they may give nonverbal and verbal cues that they are worried. The nurse who wishes to be of assistance should look and listen for these cues. The nurse must give the client permission to talk about this subject because the client may view sexuality as a forbidden topic. The client can then be approached, and the nurse can try to discover what is worrying him or her. When encouraging clients to express their feelings, an open, nonjudgmental approach is important. Really listening to what the client is saying can show the nurse if the client seems uninformed or misinformed. The nurse can then offer correct information and respond with facts and not opinions. Good communication skills are essential. Nurses need to know when they have met their own limitations and should seek qualified assistance. Nurses cannot be expected to do highly specialized counseling. An appropriate referral to counselors, gynecologists, or urologists in the community may be necessary.

The nurse may encounter other communication problems. Older clients may resent younger nurses giving them sexual instruction. Male clients may be hesitant to discuss sexual concerns with a female nurse. Adolescents especially need sexual education.

Although it is good practice to use anatomical terms in teaching, nurses should make sure the client understands their message. It may be necessary to avoid using technical words. Nurses also need to be aware of street language the client may use and not overreact to it. Nurses should assume nothing and seek clarification as necessary.

Clients may have questions or problems concerning sexual intercourse or reproduction. At times, their problems are broader and may encompass the client's total relationship with his or her sexual partner. For example, illness can be a threat to a sexual relationship. Illness, as well as medications, can decrease the sex drive and sexual performance. The hospital environment lacks privacy, and marital or romantic partners sense a loss of intimacy. Hospital gowns tend to alter body image, making the client feel unattractive.

Because of dependency and loss of physical strength following illness or surgery, many clients fear sexual inadequacy. Mass media advertising and entertainment impress upon the public the importance of being young and attractive. The message received is that happiness is being sexy. Sick people do not usually see themselves as sexy. They feel "bad all over," not sexy.

Nurses may also encounter situations in which clients make sexual advances. The best approach to this situation is to confront the client with his or her behavior. If nurses go about their nursing care and pretend the sexual advance did not occur, clients may interpret this as encouragement. Nurses should verbalize that the sexual advance is inappropriate and may interfere with clients' needed nursing care. This statement should be made in a calm, objective manner and not in judgmental tones. It is important for nurses to assess their own dress and behavior.

When dealing with clients' sexual problems, nurses should be objective, sensitive, and empathetic. They must reach out to clients who need help.

MEDICAL PROBLEMS AND SEXUALITY

Some medical conditions can have a direct effect on the client's sexuality, including cardiopulmonary conditions, diabetes, hypertension, arthritis, and spinal cord injuries. These conditions can alter the client's strength, range of motion, sexual desire, and body image. The nurse should watch for hidden fears and unasked questions. An open and accepting approach is necessary to encourage discussion and reassure the client.

Sexuality is an important part of an intimate relationship; it contributes to total well-being. A client with a medical condition that affects sexual functioning requires extra sensitivity. The meaning and importance of sex to the client should be explored. An honest discussion of the severity and permanence of any sexual impairment is needed. Personal fears and anxieties must be verbalized. It is vital that the feelings of the client's sexual partner be considered. With the understanding and cooperation of the client and partner, solutions may be found.

Cardiopulmonary Conditions

With a cardiopulmonary condition, such as a myocardial infarction or chronic obstructive pulmonary disease (COPD), the client may have to assume a dependent and passive role. Many of these clients have a fear of sexual intercourse. Sexual activity may be perceived by the client, sexual partner, or both as too much strain on the client's heart. Either partner may be afraid of a recurrence of the chest pain or may fear an inability to function; therefore, all sexual advances of the other partner may be discouraged. Some clients are in need of sexual counseling.

These clients may be advised by their physician to refrain from intercourse for two to four months. It has been shown, however, that sexual activity does not put an excessive strain on the heart. Clients should be instructed to check with their physicians before engaging in sexual intercourse. They should watch for fatigue and take special note of chest or arm pain during or after intercourse. Extreme fatigue the following day is a symptom that should be reported. Alternate positions for intercourse may prevent overburdening the cardiovascular and pulmonary systems. A stressless environment is encouraged, along with sexual expressions that are less fatiguing such as hugging, cuddling, and kissing.

Before resuming sexual activity, the clients and their partners must first accept the clients' conditions and limitations. They can then set realistic goals for a satisfactory sexual adjustment.

Diabetes

Diabetes is a chronic disease that can cause sexual problems. Many men with diabetes suffer from **impotence** (the inability to have an erection). Some problems may be caused by **neuropathy** (disease of the nerves), which may occur in the later stages of diabetes. One physiological problem of men with diabetes is **retrograde ejaculation** (a sexual dysfunction in which semen ejaculates into the bladder) and other disorders due to microcirculatory changes. Men with these sexual difficulties may need professional counseling.

Women with diabetes have an increased incidence of vaginal infections. **Dyspareunia** (painful intercourse) may occur. The vaginal infection requires treatment. Many diabetic women express a fear of pregnancy. This is because there is an increased incidence of stillbirths among persons with diabetes. However, modern technology has improved the chances for a successful pregnancy. The woman with diabetes should be encouraged to express any fear and anxiety she feels about sexual matters.

Hypertension

Sexual problems associated with hypertension are sometimes brought on by treatment measures. Impotence can be a side effect of certain drugs prescribed for hypertension. Reserpine, a common antihypertensive medication, decreases sexual desire. Ismelin, another often-used drug, can cause ejaculatory dysfunction. Since uncontrolled hypertension can lead to more severe medical conditions, use of the proper medication is vital. The physician should inform the client of any possible sexual dysfunction resulting from medication. If a problem occurs, the client should be encouraged to consult the physician. A combination of medications can be tried, which may relieve the problem. Sexual counseling may also be advantageous.

Arthritis

Arthritis is a chronic disabling and deforming disease that affects more women than men. The disease causes inflammation of the joints of the hands, wrists, and knees. In a more advanced stage, all joints may be very painful. The joints, particularly the hip joint, become stiff and immobile. The appearance of the joint changes. If surgery is done, there are scars. With these deformities, the client's self-image may change, or he or she may feel more vulnerable.

Rehabilitation of the client with arthritis should include restoring sexual functioning. It is best if both members of a sexual partnership are involved. They should be helped to realize the importance of sex in their relationship. Sexual counseling should include a frank discussion of potential problems.

Relaxation exercises may be helpful. Motion exercises done daily are an important part of routine care. Partners may need to develop their communication skills so they can better understand each other's needs.

Much practical advice can be offered. For example, variations of sexual positioning might be considered. A discussion of family planning may be of value. Family planning encompasses social, psychological, economic, physical, and religious concerns of the couple and their decision regarding children. Information can be given in an objective and nonjudgmental way.

The client needs to know that corticosteroids may decrease sexual desire. The timing of intercourse is also important. Early morning may be a poor time for intercourse because of stiffness and pain of the joints. By evening, the arthritic person may feel too tired for sexual activity.

Adequate sexual counseling can dispel some of the client's psychological stress. It could prevent a divorce or the partner's seeking pleasure elsewhere. A loving, understanding response from a partner and a feeling of sexual fulfillment can decrease the incidence of depression in the client with arthritis.

Spinal Cord Injuries

The functioning of the genital area may be altered by a spinal cord injury. If the male client's bladder empties spontaneously, he is probably capable of an erection. The client with an injury to the lumbar and sacral segments of the spinal cord is least likely to have an erection. Penile erection may be unpredictable and of short duration. Few clients are capable of an ejaculation. When clients realize they have these problems, they usually feel angry and depressed.

Some clients, both male and female, suffer from bladder spasms. The client can take antispasmodic medication to control the spasms. Some clients must wear urinary catheters. This need not limit sexual intercourse. Most catheters can be removed before and reinserted following intercourse or folded and taped over the penis. The client or partner can be taught to do this.

Because of possible bowel and bladder dysfunction, both the client and his or her sexual partner need to be included in frank discussions. Alternatives to coitus may need to be explored. There are a variety of body sensations and possible responses that can give sexual pleasure. The partners need to discuss what is satisfactory to each of them. It is important that each knows the types of lovemaking with which the other feels comfortable. Emotional closeness is a satisfying element in loving.

Clients who have suffered spinal cord injury also need sexual counseling. Group discussion with other victims of spinal cord injuries can provide a much-needed opportunity for sharing problems, especially sexual ones.

SURGERY AND SEXUAL PROBLEMS

Sexual procedures can represent a threat to the client's sexuality (Table 14-1). Some procedures, such as mastectomy and amputation, subject the client to body distortion. Clients may feel undesirable. These clients need to be able to explore their feelings. They also need to be reassured of their sexual attractiveness and capability.

Although the nurse should be concerned with the sexual adjustment of all clients, some need special consideration. These include persons who have undergone ostomy surgery, a hysterectomy, a mastectomy, or a prostatectomy.

Colostomy and ileostomy surgery have a physical and emotional impact on the client's self-esteem. It is difficult to accept bowel elimination through a stoma on the abdomen. Counseling of the sexual partner is important because the partner's attitude and understanding influence the client's adjustment.

Sexual intercourse does not injure or damage the stoma. Psychic problems, however, especially those concerning continuous fecal draining, can contribute to impotence or a nonorgasmic response. The nurse should reassure the client that a colostomy does not drain con-

TABLE 14-1 Medical and Surgical Procedures
That Can Affect Sexuality

MEDICAL PROBLEMS	SURGICAL PROCEDURES
Cardiopulmonary conditions	Ostomy
Diabetes	Hysterectomy
Hypertension	Mastectomy
Spinal cord injuries	Prostatectomy
Arthritis	

tinuously and sexual encounters can be timed accordingly. The ileostomy client can be reassured that the appliance he or she wears does not come loose during intercourse. A client who has had an abdominal perineal resection may in some cases be impotent if nerves have been severed.

Many clients worry about how their partners will react to seeing the stoma. The nurse should try to prevent a possible avoidance and denial syndrome. If the client remains uninformed and fearful, becoming a desirable sexual partner will be difficult. Some clients worry about possibly becoming pregnant. Frequently, a member of the local ostomy association can be of great assistance in helping the client achieve a healthy approach to living and loving.

Hysterectomy

A hysterectomy is one of the most common surgical procedures for women. Many women suffer postoperatively from an identity crisis and exhibit depression. They feel they have lost their femininity or their sexuality. Misconceptions about hysterectomy abound. The client may have heard the following: "You turn old because the vagina dries up" or "you get fat when the uterus is gone." However, changes in hormonal levels may affect libido or sexual responsiveness.

The client should be encouraged to discuss her anxieties. Misconceptions should be accepted as the client's point of view. Refusing them usually does not persuade the client that the notions really are wrong. Instead, the observant nurse should listen for remarks that may lead to discussion. The nurse should remember that the client is going through a time of heightened emotional sensitivity. The nurse's interest, concern, and willingness to listen will help the woman see her body in proper perspective.

The nurse should help the client to think positively. Some women like the idea of not having a menstrual cycle following a hysterectomy. Other women are pleased to be free of the risk of pregnancy. Focusing attention on positive aspects decreases the woman's preoccupation with the hysterectomy.

Prostatectomy

Many men must undergo surgery for removal of the prostate gland. These men may fear that the surgery will affect their sexual functioning. A prostatectomy usually does not cause impotence. However, sexual activity should be delayed for six to eight weeks until healing has occurred.

Potency is retained when the prostate is removed by one of the usual procedures. If a perineal incision is made, the client may have difficulty with retrograde ejaculation and sterility. He is likely to become impotent if there is a radical excision due to cancer. Preoperative preparation and counseling aid the client in postoperative adjustment.

Mastectomy

The client who undergoes a mastectomy needs a competent nurse who can promote a favorable body image. Television, movies, and stories are constantly emphasizing the female breasts. The mastectomy client needs reassurance that she is still sexually attractive despite removal of a breast. This client needs preoperative counseling and postoperative support. Her sexual partner also should be involved in the counseling. Even with counseling, the client should be allowed to adjust to the surgery at her own pace. She usually starts the adjustment by looking at the scar. If the client is reluctant to look at the incision site, however, her resistance must be respected. She will eventually work up to touching the scar.

Nurses should demonstrate that they care about the client through talking, listening, and encouraging the client to verbalize her feelings. The mastectomy client usually has many questions. The best person to suggest answers is another woman who has adjusted to a mastectomy. Women from the group Reach for Recovery, sponsored by the American Cancer Society, are available to visit the client. They offer reassurance and suggestions concerning clothing. These women share their own emotional adjustment phases to their mastectomy and altered body image with the new mastectomy client.

Many types of breast prostheses are available. These include the fluid-filled type, the air-filled type, and those made of sponge rubber. The fluid-filled type is the most satisfactory. This type of prosthesis is filled with a thick, slow-flowing fluid. In order to have any prosthesis fit well, a properly fitted brassiere is necessary. Prostheses may be made specifically for the individual, or they may be purchased ready-made. Many department stores now have mastectomy boutiques.

Breast reconstruction is possible after the initial procedure. If biopsies of the nipple are negative, the nipple areolar complex can be temporarily attached to the client's anterior abdominal wall. Six months to one year later, surgery can be scheduled for reconstruction of the breast utilizing the pectoralis major muscle and an inflatable prosthesis. The client's own nipple is then attached to the reconstructed breast. Other innovative surgeries are available to help the mastectomy client regain a positive body image.

PHARMACOLOGICAL INTERVENTIONS

Sexual dysfunction has become a topic of media coverage. **Viagra (sildenafil)** is taken in pill form approximately one hour before sexual activity and results in smooth muscle relaxation, flow of blood into the penile shaft, and an erection. Viagra potentiates the hypotensive effects of nitrates. Another medication used for male sexual dysfunction is MUSE (alprostadil), a urethral suppository. It is reported that medication will soon be available for female sexual dysfunction.

Many third-party reimbursement providers do not pay for these medications. This loss of a pharmacological intervention can be overwhelming, especially to the older adult on a fixed income.

PREMENSTRUAL DYSPHORIC DISORDER

Premenstrual dysphoric disorder (PMDD) comprises a group of intense emotional and behavioral changes reported by some women during the premenstrual phase of their menstrual cycle. Characteristics of this syndrome include depression, increased irritability and variability of moods, tension, impulsivity, and distractibility, and impaired concentration. It is important to note that these symptoms are time limited and go away soon after the menses start. Diagnosis may be difficult. It is important to assess the timing of symptoms in regard to the menstrual cycle (e.g., "I shout at my children and hit them five to seven days before my period occurs"). Physical symptoms such as abdominal bloating, headaches, and breast swelling and tenderness are also reported. Many outpatient clinics are providing support groups for women with PMDD.

- ■ Communicate with sexual partners.
- ■ Consistently use condoms for oral and vaginal sex.
- ■ Consistently use condoms for anal intercourse.
- ■ Avoid abusing substances in sexual situations.
- ■ Use HIV antibody counseling and testing services.
- ■ Notify a partner of STD or HIV exposure.
- ■ Indicate whether an intravenous drug user (IVDU) participates in needle exchange programs.

FIGURE 14-2 Program of sexual education.

ADOLESCENT SEXUALITY

Over the past twenty years, there has been a downward shift in the age of onset of sexual intercourse among adolescents. Early onset increases problems with sexually transmitted diseases (STDs) such as HIV/AIDS, and increased pregnancy rates, abortion rates, and precocious childbirths. Figure 14-2 shows some safe sex strategies for preventing the spread of HIV.

SEXUALITY AND THE AGED

Aging is a phase of human development. As in all other phases of life, loving and giving are important for the elderly (Figure 14-3). Sexual desire and ability do not end with old age. Anxiety, depression, and irritability may occur during menopause. These symptoms are usually

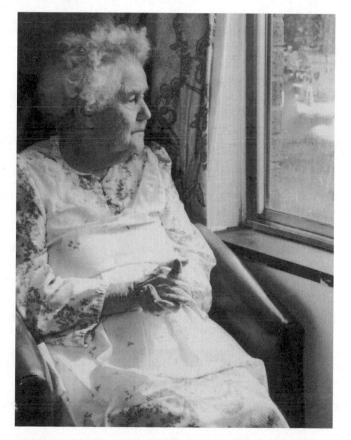

FIGURE 14-3 The elderly need love and affection.

related to hormonal imbalance and the woman's acceptance of the new phase. Men often experience similar feelings. They may feel less sexually responsive. Emotional and adjustment problems may also occur.

It is most important for nurses to reevaluate their ideas concerning sex and the aged. Deterioration of the body due to age need not mean an end to sexual activity. Because people associate youthfulness or the ability to reproduce with sex, it is difficult for some people to see the elderly as sexual beings. Nonetheless, the elderly need love. The aged need to touch, to be close to someone, and to express affection. They should be encouraged to assess their needs realistically. The elderly should never be considered abnormal for choosing intercourse.

Some elderly men have difficulty with erection. The vagina is drier in the aged woman. The application of a water-based lubricant by either sexual partner makes penetration easier. Chronic illness and vascular insufficiency also can cause sexual difficulties. Suppression of sexual needs may lead to frustration and depression. As in any other age, the sexual drive can be satisfied in nongenital ways.

If the aged person is living an independent life, he or she may feel free enough to develop a relationship. In the nursing home environment, the elderly need privacy. A judgmental, negative approach by the nurse can only contribute to lower self-esteem for the client. Full and satisfying lives for the elderly should be among the nurse's goals.

PARAPHILIAS

The nurse should be aware of the following psychosexual disorders.

- **Fetishism:** sexual excitement and gratification from touching or fondling certain objects or clothing. It occurs primarily in men and is a substitution for a normal love object.

- **Voyeurism:** sexual pleasure derived from secretly watching people involved in sexual acts, or by looking at their bodies and sex organs without their knowledge. This person is known as a Peeping Tom. This disorder occurs mainly in men.

- **Exhibitionism:** a sexual desire to display the genital area to the opposite sex in socially inappropriate situations. The exhibitionist usually does not talk or touch his or her victim; he or she gets gratification from the shock of the opposite sex. Exhibitionism occurs primarily in men.

- **Pedophilia:** unnatural desire for sexual relations with children.

- **Transvestism:** adopting the dress and often the behavior of the opposite sex. There is no desire to change sex or to be homosexual. Men dress in women's clothing and women dress in men's clothing. An example of transvestism is a man wearing a bra and garter belt under his business suit. This is usually done in a private and secretive manner.

- **Transsexual:** a person who is biologically one sex but has a psychological urge to be the opposite sex. A transsexual may seek help through requesting a sex-change operation.

GENDER IDENTITY DISORDER

Gender identity disorder (GID) is a DSM IV-TR sexual disorder whereby an individual feels a persistent and marked distress related to gender. They desire to be a member of the opposite sex and seek **cross-gender identification** by dressing as the opposite sex and developing mannerisms and voice inflections of the opposite sex. The usual short-term goal is cross-gender identification, with the long-term goal being sexual reassignment surgery. There are gender-identity clinics that deal with hormonal replacement and emerging issues. A referral is usually made to a speech therapist to assist the client in developing an appropriate pitch and spontaneous voice production during conversation. In this way, a feminine voice is optimized over the physiological male voice, and vice versa. Support groups are available for transgender individuals.

Nurses assigned to care for a client with a psychosexual disorder may feel afraid or uneasy. They should not let their personal feelings about different sexual behavior affect the care they give the client. This client has health needs apart from his or her sexual preference. Fellow employees also should be evaluated on work performance and not sexual preferences.

Nurses should be aware of their own feelings, values, and beliefs regarding unconventional sexual behavior. Do they feel that clients with psychosexual disorders are queer or perverted? Nurses must be able to develop a tolerant attitude toward clients with unconventional sexual behaviors.

MASTURBATION

Masturbation is manipulation, by fondling or touching, of one's own genital area for sexual gratification. Although masturbation is considered normal, there are some cultural taboos forbidding the practice. Some people at a young age are warned by a parent that masturbation leads to serious illness, even insanity. People masturbate to meet their own needs.

The nurse may come upon a client who is openly masturbating. The best approach is to leave the client and then provide privacy. The nurse should be prepared for the possibility of such a situation occurring in all age groups. In the hospital environment, this behavior may be a response to sensory deprivation. **Sensory deprivation** is a lower level of sensory input than what that individual requires to function at an optimal level. The nurse can intervene by offering a variety of stimulation, such as a radio or television. Music enhances sensory awareness. Personal contact with other people is very therapeutic. The nurse should discover the client's interests and provide pictures, posters, or books about those subjects.

HOMOSEXUALITY

Homosexuality is engaging in sexual relations with a person of the same sex. The term **gay** usually refers to men whose sexual desire is directed toward men only. The term **lesbian** refers to women whose sexual desire is directed toward women only. The American Psychiatric Association has stated that it no longer considers homosexuality a mental disorder. Some people experience a strong, yet irrational fear of their own homosexual feelings and do not seek out a professional counselor to work through these issues. Instead they speak in a disparaging manner about those who seek a variation in sexual expression.

It is a myth that all homosexuals are promiscuous. They are not all unhappy, guilt-ridden individuals. Some have committed themselves to lasting, effective relationships. Homosexuals are now working toward understanding and acceptance through a movement called Gay Liberation.

ACQUIRED IMMUNE DEFICIENCY SYNDROME (AIDS)

Since 1983, a serious challenge for the health profession is the client with **acquired immune deficiency syndrome (AIDS)** and **human immunodeficiency virus (HIV)**. The World Health Organization (WHO, 2000) reports on HIV/AIDS global epidemic with an estimated 34.3 million people currently infected. Approximately 5.4 million are newly infected each year with 620,000 being children under the age of 15. Many of these people will develop AIDS. Although there have been medications developed to slow the disease process, AIDS is fatal; there is no cure. All are at risk. Higher-risk populations are male homosexuals and intravenous drug users (IVDU). IVDU shoot drugs, share and reuse needles, and frequently use other drugs (e.g., alcohol, amphetamines, marijuana in combination with cocaine, crack, or heroin). Judgment is impaired, and risky sexual behaviors are practiced. These behaviors are shown in Figure 14-4.

According to the CDC, the proportion of women (adults and adolescents) with AIDS has increased from 7 percent in 1985 to 18 percent in 1994. The report further states that these women acquired AIDS through intravenous drug usage (41 percent) and through heterosexual contact with at risk partners (38 percent). The most rapidly increasing transmission route is heterosexual contact. A large percentage of these women are African-American and Hispanics. In 1993, more than 7,000 HIV-infected women delivered infants, with prenatal HIV transmission being as high as 30 percent. Public hysteria has caused much media coverage and this has generated increased public education for safe-sex practices. Safe sex is sex with the use of a latex condom with a germicidal gel (oxy-9). In reality, safe sex minimizes your chances of contacting the HIV virus by contact with semen, blood, or vaginal cervical secretions. Latex condoms when used properly will reduce the risk of transmitting HIV infection and other STD such as chlamydia, genital herpes, genital warts, gonorrhea, hepatitis B, and syphilis. Current epidemics of syphilis with its ulcerative lesions compound the issues of HIV. However, one is always at risk. Sweat, tears, and urine contain the AIDS virus but in such decreased concentrations that transmission is extremely unlikely.

As life is prolonged with new drugs, more long-term facilities will be treating persons with AIDS. Inpatient psychiatric units will admit clients with the psychiatric complications of AIDS: stress responses, depression with suicidal ideation, and organic or delusional syndromes. Problems will exist in providing care for these clients. Standard precautions need to be strictly followed and enforced by facilities and by the Occupational Safety and Health Administration (OSHA). Areas of concern include needle disposal, disposal of certain

---

- Number of sexual partners
- Number of drug-injecting sexual partners
- Number of times sexual relations occur while abusing alcohol or other drugs
- Number of times sex is traded for drugs and/or money
- Number of sexual acts performed without protection

FIGURE 14-4 Sexual risk factors.

contaminated equipment and linens, blood spills, and securing protective barrier equipment. For the staff, education programs must include discussion of stigmatization and information concerning transmission. Health care providers express fear of infection, and many relate pressure from their families and friends to actually change jobs. Support groups that allow verbalization of these fears are important and will decrease the incidence of burnout, with its emotional exhaustion and job dissatisfaction.

The professional will have to develop ease at sexual counseling because explicit questions may be asked and changes in sexual behavior may need to be recommended.

Currently, respite care programs are providing relief to families caring for loved ones with these special needs (Figure 14-5). Respite care gives a family member a break from the twenty-four-hour-a-day job and much needed time-out. There are AIDS counseling, testing sites, and hot lines. HIV testing needs to be done anonymously. If the first test is positive, the second test should be done confidentially. If testing was done through the client's place of business, the result becomes a matter of record for insurance companies; therefore, the client may want to go to a community health testing center. Some literature is geared specifically toward cultural communities such as African American and Hispanic communities. Remember that the AIDS client lives in a world of uncertainty because he or she does not know when the time bomb might explode and an opportunistic infection set in. They are dealing with a terminal disease process and multiple losses: employment, the right to privacy, intimate relationships, questionable insurance benefits, and eventually the loss of life itself. We need to deal with our own strong reactions in order to approach the client with care and compassion and not with fear or prejudice.

- ■ Street outreach
- ■ Risk-reduction counseling
- ■ Prevention Case management
- ■ National AIDS hot line
- ■ Pastoral care
- ■ AIDS action networks, which deal with legal problems associated with confidentiality, rights to privacy, job discrimination

---

FIGURE 14-5 Networks for HIV assistance.

ABORTION

Abortion is a very controversial issue. The nurse may be assigned to the client undergoing an abortion either before or after the procedure. A nurse who is assigned to care for the client who has undergone an abortion may need to explore his or her own feelings and values about abortion. Some nurses who oppose the procedure have a great difficulty relating to such clients. The abortion client should be viewed by the nurse as a person who needs health care. Refusal to give care has been tested in some courts. Nurses who refuse to give care may, in some states, jeopardize their jobs.

There are many reasons for choosing abortion. Each client is unique, but the decision is seldom easy. Some women who undergo abortion have little choice, since it may be a therapeutic necessity. The abortion may be necessary to preserve the life of the mother. Before an abortion is performed, the pregnant woman should receive counseling. Counseling should help the woman voice her concerns. A counselor will help her to understand the pros, cons, and alternatives to abortion and explain the types of abortion.

The client who has an abortion frequently experiences loneliness, depression and alienation. She needs the understanding, acceptance, and caring of the staff. Postabortion care is important. The nurse may need to explain contraceptive methods. A follow up visit to a doctor or psychologist (if emotional problems develop) is essential.

SUMMARY

Human sexuality must be considered when caring for the whole person. Sex is not just an isolated activity; it includes identity, social role, and physical functioning. The nurse should become knowledgeable in discussing human sexuality.

Illness may affect sexual functioning. Clients may be worried about intercourse or reproductive stability. Usually the client's concerns are broad and encompass the total relationship with the sexual partner. The nurse who deals with sexual problems must be objective, sensitive, and empathetic.

Some medical conditions may have a direct effect on the client's sexual functioning. These conditions include cardiopulmonary conditions, diabetes, arthritis, spinal cord injuries, and hypertension. These conditions can alter the client's strength, range of motion, sexual desire, and body image. Counseling and help with problem solving are important aspects of nursing care.

Surgical procedures can present a threat to the client's self-image. Clients having ostomy, hysterectomy, mastectomy, or prostatectomy surgery are in need of special help. These procedures alter the body image and may make the person feel undesirable.

It is important for nurses to reevaluate their ideas concerning sex and the aged. Sexual closeness is a realistic need of the elderly. An empathetic nurse who recognizes this need can help the elderly to a fuller and more satisfying life.

Some clients evoke negative reactions from the nurse. Nurses who feel fearful or uncomfortable in caring for a client must clarify their own feelings and moral values. Nurses should accept the client as a person who needs their help and a great deal of psychological support.

SUGGESTED ACTIVITIES

- Find out what information sex education programs in your community have to offer clients with particular problems.
- Write for literature from
  Reach for Recovery
  American Cancer Society
  777 Third Avenue
  New York, NY
- Role-play the following:
  a. Counseling a man, age thirty-five, who has suffered a myocardial infarction, to consider his sexual functioning. The nurse is twenty years old and unmarried.
  b. Counseling a woman with arthritis, age thirty-five, concerning her sexual functioning.
  c. Counseling a young woman who has recently discovered her husband is an intravenous drug user.

REVIEW

KNOW AND COMPREHEND
A. Multiple choice. Select the one best answer.

1. When a cardiac client expresses concern about sexual intercourse, the nurse should offer which response?
   - ❏ A. refrain from sexual activity for six to eight months to allow the cardiac rate to stabilize
   - ❏ B. consider alternate means of sexual pleasure, such as hugging
   - ❏ C. check with the doctor, but inform the client that sexual activity does not usually put added strain on the heart
   - ❏ D. avoid discussing the subject with anyone until the client's prognosis is clear

2. A male client with diabetes mentions to his nurse that he does not "feel like a man." The nurse should
   - ❏ A. conclude the client is talking about intercourse and refer him to counseling.
   - ❏ B. refer the client to his physician for discussion of the complaint.
   - ❏ C. tell him it is a temporary problem and will resolve in six to eight months.
   - ❏ D. encourage more discussion about his feelings and offer professional counseling.

3. What type of sexual problems usually affects the client with arthritis?
   - ❏ A. immobility of the joints
   - ❏ B. dyspareunia
   - ❏ C. impotence
   - ❏ D. retrograde ejaculation

4. Spinal cord injury results in what type of change to one's sexuality?
   - ❏ A. the client may participate only as a passive partner
   - ❏ B. spinal cord injury results in an inability to be sexually active
   - ❏ C. clients must use alternatives to intercourse
   - ❏ D. the level and extent of the injury determine the client's physical abilities

5. A client who has had a mastectomy states that her husband will probably divorce her now. Which response by the nurse would be the most helpful?
   - ❑ A. advise her to wear a bra under her nightgown
   - ❑ B. suggest that she discuss this with her husband
   - ❑ C. encourage her to express her fears
   - ❑ D. refer her for psychiatric counseling

6. Which statement is true?
   - ❑ A. impotence is only psychological in nature
   - ❑ B. masturbation is an abnormal activity
   - ❑ C. incest is an accepted practice in many cultures
   - ❑ D. sexuality includes a person's value system and philosophy of life

7. An HIV-positive client expresses worry about having sex with a new partner who has tested negative. The nurse's best response would be to
   - ❑ A. advise the client not to have sex with anyone who is not infected with HIV.
   - ❑ B. instruct the client to seek the advice of a primary care physician.
   - ❑ C. discuss strategies for safe sex and encourage the client to discuss these fears with the new partner.
   - ❑ D. advise client to stop seeing the person, "You are HIV positive!"

APPLY YOUR LEARNING
B. Multiple choice. Select the one best answer.

1. After discovering her eight-year-old child masturbating, the mother tells the nurse she's afraid the child is mentally ill. Which response by the nurse is most appropriate?
   - ❑ A. "How often has the child been masturbating?"
   - ❑ B. "Has the child used foreign objects to masturbate?"
   - ❑ C. "Masturbation is a normal part of human behavior."
   - ❑ D. "We need to refer your child to the sex therapist."

2. The nurse interviews a fifteen-year old adolescent girl at the family planning clinic. Which comment would be most appropriate to begin the interview?
   - ❑ A. "I'd like to talk with you about your sexual relationships."
   - ❑ B. "When did you start having sexual relations?"

    ❏ C. "Are you using protection during sexual activities?"

    ❏ D. "How many sexual partners have you had?"

3. A male client, hospitalized for 21 days, comments to a female nurse, "Why don't you crawl in the bed with me? You could really take care of me if you'd do that." Which response by the nurse would be most appropriate?

    ❏ A. "How can I take care of you when you talk to me like that?"

    ❏ B. "I'm your nurse and sex is not part of our relationship."

    ❏ C. "I can hold your hand if that would make you feel better."

    ❏ D. "Your comments are unwelcome and offensive. Stop now."

4. The nurse gathers data for a newly admitted client with a long history of diabetes and congestive heart failure. The nurse asks the client about recent sexual activity and the client responds, "Oh well, there's not much point in us talking about that." Which response by the nurse should follow?

    ❏ A. "Everyone with diabetes and heart problems experiences sexual difficulties."

    ❏ B. The nurse should move on to the next topic. The client does not wish to discuss sexuality.

    ❏ C. "Of course we should talk about it. Sexuality is part of the nursing admission form."

    ❏ D. "What do you mean when you say 'there not much point in us talking about that.'"

5. The nurse interviews a client who had surgery to create a colostomy six months ago. The nurse asks the client about sexual intercourse since the surgery. The client says, "I haven't had sex because I'm afraid I'll hurt the stoma." Which comment by the nurse would be most helpful?

    ❏ A. "It's safe for you to have sex now. You should resume your usual activities."

    ❏ B. "Your fears are not warranted. The stoma has healed; so, you have no excuses."

    ❏ C. "Your stoma has healed but sexual activity is often emotionally difficult after a colostomy."

    ❏ D. "Talk to your surgeon about this problem. The surgeon can give you the best advice."

C. Briefly answer the following.

1. Name three medical problems that may affect the client's sexual functioning.

2. List three surgical procedures that the client may view as a threat to sexuality.

3. Name three aspects of sexuality.

4. List four psychosexual disorders.

5. Describe safe sex and the use of alcohol and drugs.

Grieving and Pain

OUTLINE

KEY TERMS

grief	meditation
grieving survivors	guided imagery
denial	relaxation
anger	humor
bargaining	massage
depression	therapeutic touch
acceptance	music
palliative care	aromatherapy
hospice	mindfulness
pain management	art
sensory overload	thought-field therapy (TFT)
breathe	divorce

OBJECTIVES

After studying this chapter, the student should be able to:

- Identify stages of the grief process.
- State ways the nurse can help the dying client and his or her family through the grief process.
- State the importance of completing the grief process.
- State three reasons why children need added help to cope with death.
- Name three concerns of the dying client.
- Identify three reasons for pain being established as the fifth vital sign.
- Compare two alternative/complementary methods to assist clients coping with chronic pain.
- List the objectives of a hospice program.

Grieving is a major stressor that most people experience at some time in their lives. Many people experience difficulty working through loss and grieving. **Grief** occurs after many different types of losses: divorce, loss of a job, amputation of a limb, or loss of a loved one. Special circumstances can affect the grieving, including death of a child, mourning and dying teenager, widowhood in early life, death after a lingering illness, and long vigils at the bedside of a friend in an advanced stage of AIDS. Throughout the life span, there are loss experiences. The grief process must be successfully coped with and completed for good mental health. If the individual is unable to do so, anxiety and depression may result. Depression is a stage of grieving. People often need help completing the grief process. Since many loved ones die in hospitals, the function of helping the family becomes a responsibility of the nurse. To help the client and family cope with impending death, nurses must first be aware of their own feelings about death. Some questions nurses may ask themselves to determine their attitudes about death are found in Figure 15-1.

Years ago, death was considered a natural phenomenon. An elderly family member became very ill and was cared for in the home. When death came, the viewing (wake) was also held at the home. Dying was a familiar and accepted sight. Today, we have moved dying to hospitals and wakes to funeral homes. We have become uncomfortable with the thought of death. Our present life styles effectively shield us from the finality of death. Phrases such as "now that she is gone" or, as nurses frequently state, "he has terminated" avoid actually verbalizing death.

1. Does a dying client make me very uncomfortable?
2. Do I have difficulty controlling my feelings when I know a client is dying?
3. Am I afraid of dying because I fear the unknown?
4. Should children be shielded from death?
5. Does being with someone who is dying frighten me?
6. Is pain the most difficult part of dying?
7. Do I believe that death is the end and that there is nothing more?
8. If a person has lived a good life, should he or she fear death?
9. Should time be spent on the dying client when there is nothing more that can be done?
10. Is taking care of a dying client satisfying?

FIGURE 15-1 Questions nurses may ask themselves to determine their attitudes about death.

Death has become a controversial issue in the millenium. Natural death occurs as a natural (inevitable) response to aging or a disease process. However, much discussion now evolves around euthanasia and mercy killing. Euthanasia is the withdrawal of therapeutic means allowing death to occur. Mercy killing is an act of taking another's life. Debates have occurred in hospital settings over criteria and ethical issues surrounding DNR (do not resuscitate) orders for terminal clients. A document called a living will has evolved. In a living will a person gives direction about the use of life-prolonging medical procedures. The statement usually reads that no heroic or artificial means are to be taken in the event of terminal illness.

Reactions to death are influenced by cultural and religious beliefs. Nurses are conditioned by their own background and experiences with the deaths of others. Nurses who have come to terms with the thought of their own deaths are better able to help the dying client. Some nurses tend to ignore the dying person because they do not know what to say. This is made more difficult when the client has not been told about the prognosis.

Nurses are taught that one of their goals is to save lives. In spite of what is done for the client this goal cannot always be met. Because of this, some nurses feel anger; others become discouraged or depressed. In working with the dying client, the nurse must set different goals. Satisfaction must come from knowing that the client has been helped to a more peaceful death and that needed support, care, and attention to the client and family have been given.

THE GRIEF PROCESS

Grief is the process of coping with a loss. The loss may be one's own imminent death, the death of a loved one, or the loss of a limb, prized object, or image. The grief process must be completed (Figure 15-2). A person who is unable to complete the grief process often has difficulty coping with the simple stressors of living.

Families of servicemen killed overseas sometimes experience anxiety until the bodies are returned. Even though it may take years, the grief process continues until the family sees to the burial themselves. Mothers who have stillborns or who place their infants for adoption without contact with them often have anxiety and guilt feelings for the rest of their lives. They are unable to complete the mourning process because they were never allowed to see and touch their infants.

It is always difficult to decide whether clients should be told they are dying. Some doctors and families request that the client not be told.

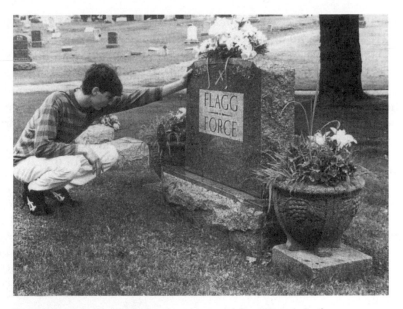

FIGURE 15-2 The grief process must be completed.

They feel the individual is unable to cope with the truth. Some clients respond to such news by giving up. They become so overwhelmed by fears that they cut off all stimuli and become unfeeling. They cooperate but no longer care. Other clients who are told they are dying choose to discuss their deaths openly. They struggle with their feelings and fears but continue to participate actively and to maintain control over their lives.

Nurses may find that clients suspect their prognoses even if they have not been told. Clients recognize nonverbal cues. They can also feel the changes occurring in their bodies. It may be very difficult to care for clients who have not been told of their diagnoses or prognoses. Because death is unspoken, there is no sharing of grief. The client, the family, and the nurse all grieve alone.

According to Kyes and Holfing, the **grieving survivors** of the deceased adjust to the loss in gradual steps.

- Total preoccupation with the deceased. This preoccupation may last three months. It includes normal grieving behavior.

- A period of redistribution of emotions. There is a marked detachment from the deceased, with a gradual letting go of emotional ties. Much of the bereaved person's time may be spent with projects or organization.

■ A period of gradual reattachment of emotional ties to an activity or to significant others. The grief process is completed and the loss has been accepted.

Most people need assistance to complete the grief process. Nurses need to understand and respect the importance of grieving for themselves and others. To avoid feelings of isolation and abandonment, people experiencing grief need outlets and emotional support. Some people need to cry; others feel better by shouting. Emotional stability may be supported by religious faith. A social network of family and friends with whom problems can be discussed and possible solutions verbalized is an important facet of the grief process. As the reality of death penetrates, this sharing network helps the grieving person attain security, self-confidence, and a sense of well-being. Without a sharing network, a person can become detached and unfeeling because of emotional depletion. Many people express a feeling of numbness. Nurses who work with the terminally ill need to establish support groups so that communication networks are open to them on a daily basis.

Stages of the Grief Process

Dr. Elisabeth Kubler-Ross describes five stages in the grief process when a person experiences loss or death. Although not absolute, the stages serve as a basis for understanding the process. The stages are **denial, anger, bargaining, depression**, and **acceptance** (Table 15-1). A person may experience all five stages in rapid succession. He or she may move back and forth between stages or remain for some time within a single stage. Stages should be recognized but never rushed.

TABLE 15-1 Nursing Interventions for the Stages of Grief

STAGE	INTERVENTION
Denial	Use reflective responses
Anger	Give understanding and support; listen; meet needs and requests immediately
Bargaining	Act upon requests, if possible; listen
Depression	Avoid reassuring clichés; demonstrate caring
Acceptance	Remain close to the client

Denial. Denial begins when the person is made aware that he or she is going to die. Initially, there is shock. People feel numb. They are unable to allow the information to be processed further. Later, they begin to deny the information. They may state, "This is not happening to me" or "doctors have been wrong before." The client may turn to quackery that promises a cure or look for another doctor.

When clients are in the denial stage, they know they are dying. They do not want confirmation. It would not help for the nurse to say "Yes, I am afraid you are dying" or "I am awfully sorry." It also does not help to say "No, you are not going to die." Instead, the nurse might reflect the statement, for example, "Do you think you are?" or "You must be pretty frightened." Clients' statements such as, "I cannot have cancer; I am too healthy" or "I am too young to die" may be indications of denial. As health deteriorates, denial becomes more difficult.

Anger. Eventually, clients are no longer able to deny that they are dying. They then become angry. Clients are desperate because they realize they are losing their hold on life and fearful of what will happen to them. They are frustrated because they cannot change events. Their anxiety and frustration are turned into anger toward anyone around them. Even small added stressors are difficult to handle.

When clients become angry, they may lash out at the nurse by saying "It is all your fault. You made me sign for the biopsy and now they found I have a malignancy." The nurse must understand the source of the anger. Clients require understanding and support. Their needs and requests must be met immediately because they cannot handle added stressors. The nurse must take time to listen to their frustrations. Clients should be allowed and encouraged to vent their anger. Attempts should be made to convince them that their anger is acceptable.

Bargaining. During the third stage, people accept the fact that they are dying but bargain for more time. They may bargain with God or with the staff: "God, if you will let me live just a little longer, I will donate all my money to the church" or "you have to let me go home to finish this task before I die." The requests are for more time: "I am ready to die but not yet."

If it is possible to do as the client requests, it should be done. If the client is bargaining with God, the nurse can only listen quietly as the client attempts to work through this stage.

Depression. Depression marks the fourth stage. There is a full realization that death is near. People are sad because they realize that they will no longer be able to see their family or friends and that they will not be able to do things that were planned. This is a lonely time for clients.

The nurse should avoid using reassuring clichés with depressed clients. There is a real cause for depression, and the client needs to be depressed. Things are bad and depression is appropriate. The depressed client needs to know that someone else cares that he or she is dying. Touching the client and even crying in his or her presence are ways of letting the person know the nurse cares.

Acceptance. When people begin to prepare for death, they are in the stage of acceptance. They may complete unfinished business and comfort those they will leave behind. They have accepted that they are to die. Even when clients have accepted their fate, they are still afraid. They need someone with them until the end.

Although our lives may not be as rhythmic as the following biblical passage, throughout life we must accept the presence of change.

> For everything there is a season, and a time to every purpose under heaven:
> a time to be born and a time to die;
> a time to plant, and a time to pluck up what is planted;
> a time to kill, and a time to heal;
> a time to break down, and a time to build up;
> a time to weep, and a time to laugh;
> a time to mourn, and a time to dance;
> a time to cast away stones, and a time to gather stones together;
> a time to embrace, and a time to refrain from embracing;
> a time to seek, and a time to lose;
> a time to keep, and a time to cast away;
> a time to rend, and a time to sow;
> a time to keep silence, and a time to speak;
> a time to love, and a time to hate;
> a time for war, and a time for peace.
>
> Ecclesiastes 3:–18

Helping the Family

The family that has lost a loved one goes through the same stages as the grieving client. If the death is sudden, the grief process begins after the death. If the illness has been long and death anticipated, the family may be helped in the grief process before the death actually occurs. Anticipatory grief occurs when one is preparing for the death.

The family should be allowed to help in the care of the client as much as possible. Becoming involved in the client's care helps the family members express love. It increases their self-esteem and lessens guilt. Being able to stay with the client, even during the night, helps the client and the family. The nurse must be watchful that the family is not overtaxed because fatigue lessens the ability to handle stress. The nurse should make the family aware that the client's hearing is commonly the last sense lost and that even whispering frequently can be heard.

Like the client, the family members need an opportunity to express their concerns and vent their feelings. Observe for the absence of grief. Some people see tears as weak. Those who repress their emotions may experience physical symptoms, such as chest pain, nausea, headaches, and depression. Relatives do not see themselves as nurses' responsibility, so nurses must recognize their needs. Nurses must seek them out and encourage communication. Nurses should not say "Oh, you are so strong." The family member should not feel the need to maintain constant composure. Crying can be a desirable emotional release. Some people have difficulty expressing their grief publicly. Nurses may convey more caring through a gentle touch than through words. The fact that nurses care is important to the family.

After the death of a loved one, the family members need comfort and guidance. There are immediate decisions that can be difficult such as a possible autopsy or locating the name of a mortician. Telephone calls need to be made and the family's privacy maintained. If family members are extremely distraught, it may be necessary to arrange for transportation home. Optimally, a follow-up call is made to the family within the next few weeks. Encourage family members to reminisce and verbalize feelings and remind them that anniversary times and holidays can reactivate grief feelings. Planning time with family and other supportive people can be helpful.

Children need added help to cope with the death of a loved one. Parents tend to shield their children from death. The more parents avoid talking about it, the more children fear it. When children are told about death, they are usually not told the truth. Statements such as "Daddy has gone to sleep," "God has taken Mommy away," or "Aunt Liz has gone on a long trip" confuse the child.

Children require special attention because they need a concept of death in order to grieve. Most children do not understand the finality of death. The young child has difficulty differentiating death from sleep. Children are often forgotten as the adult members work through their own grief. A child needs open, relaxed communication concerning death. Many excellent books explaining the meaning of death are available for children. These books help to open further discussion about death.

Nursing Care Plan:
The Client Experiencing Grief

The nurse practitioner has been counseling Jamie Oswald on a regular basis since the sudden death of her husband. Jamie finds it difficult to manage the responsibilities of home and work. On her last visit she stated "My emotions are bouncing all over the place. I cry at the drop of a hat. I still miss being with him after work and sharing the events of the day. Yet, the next minute, I am angry because he left me with this mess. I also miss going out with friends, yet there never seems to be enough time to do everything."

NURSING DIAGNOSIS 1

Dysfunctional grieving related to loss of husband secondary to death of spouse as evidenced by crying easily, missing husband and sharing events of the day together, and verbalizing anger.

Nursing Outcome

Jamie will continue to share feelings of grief.

Nursing Interventions / Rationales

Nursing Interventions	Rationales
Encourage a trust relationship.	A trust relationship gives Jamie freedom to share her thoughts and feelings.
Accept Jamie's expressions of grief. Explain the grief process to Jamie.	Open acceptance of Jamie's grief feelings encourages her to share and not keep them pent up.
Encourage Jamie to express enjoyable times and disappointing times in her relationship with her husband.	Encouraging Jamie to review her life with her husband will enable the process of grieving feelings in a healthy manner.
Reinforce Jamie's strengths.	Emphasizing Jamie's strengths provides support and encouragement.

Evaluation

Jamie is openly sharing her feelings of grief with the nurse practitioner. She and the children also are supporting and encouraging each other. Jamie has started reviewing life events with her husband.

NURSING DIAGNOSIS 2

Impaired social interaction related to change in social interactions secondary to death of spouse as evidenced by busy schedule and decreased social life.

Nursing Outcomes

Jamie will review her schedule and identify ways she can have time for one social event each week by the next counseling session.

Nursing Interventions	Rationales
Assist in finding alternative ways for socialization.	By assisting in socialization ideas, the nurse practitioner is demonstrating support while encouraging Jamie to make personal decisions and choices.
Role-play situations that seem difficult.	Role-playing will assist Jamie in feeling more comfortable in situations perceived as difficult.

Evaluation

On Jaime's return visit she had planned a weekly social event for an entire month. She smiled when describing the events to the nurse practitioner.

The Dying Child

Society tends to protect children even from their own deaths. When children are seriously ill, they may not be told the seriousness of their illness. However, nurses who work with these children say that children, like adults, sense the truth. Many seem to want open communication. Secrecy is an added burden; it means the child must die alone without the support of his or her family.

The death of a child is not easily accepted in American society. For this reason, it is much more difficult for family members to watch a young person die. Children withdraw from their parents in the latter stages of the death process. This is difficult for parents to understand, and they often see it as rejection. It is really the child's attempt to let go. Parents fear the suffering of their child even more than death. They feel guilty in not being able to relieve pain.

The nurse must consider the child's concept of death. Toddlers usually have none. They may hurt and feel anxiety about their pain, but have no idea of what is happening to them. Preschoolers begin to consider death. It may be seen as a long journey, going to sleep, or going to heaven. Their concept depends on what they have heard about death. They do not understand it. Children have a great deal of faith in their parents. They look to them to solve all problems. They tell themselves that their parents will see that they get better.

To school-age children, death becomes more permanent. They seem to be more concerned with death and violence. Death is more frightening to this age group. There may be a concept of the soul leaving the body. There is often a fear of what will happen to the body, along with fear of being abandoned and alone.

Preteens are frightened at the thought of death. Unable to cope with the fears, they may joke, tell ghost stories, or act brave. The preteen's fear also seems mostly concerned about what happens to the body when it is buried. Adolescents seem to have a need to prove their immortality. They seem to take risks just to prove that death cannot take them. Adolescents need open, relaxed communication networks.

Dying children must go through the same grief process as adults. The ease with which they go through this process depends on many factors. Some of these factors are their concept of death, their religious beliefs, and their families' support. Children's desire to voice their fears should be encouraged. They should be given as much information as possible. They should be allowed the amount of activity they want, even though they may not seem capable of handling it.

Children are sometimes taken home to die. This seems like an added burden on the family, but it actually helps them in the grief process. The family seems better able to cope with the death if the child has died within the family unit because they know they have done all that is possible for him or her.

NURSING INTERVENTIONS

The most frequently voiced concerns of the dying are pain, isolation, and the fear of the unknown. The dying person should be made as physically comfortable as possible. Physical comfort can be offered through oral hygiene, repositioning every two hours, and good skin care. Hair and nail care, shaving, shampooing, and applying makeup contribute to a sense of well-being. The nurse's touch conveys caring. A steady, smooth touch is therapeutic; jerky movements should be avoided. The nurse's goal is to maintain the client's optimum level of functioning, comfort, and dignity until the time of death. This is called **palliative care**.

Fear of the unknown is common in most people. One cannot adequately prepare for the unknown. Ideally, the dying person should never be left alone. Family and close friends should be encouraged to stay with him or her. The nurse should plan time for extended visits to the client. A satisfying and productive interaction is very comforting. Frequently, the client enjoys reminiscing. The nurse can facilitate this review of the client's life.

Spiritual needs should be considered. The nurse can offer to call the chaplain, priest, minister, or rabbi. Some clients find comfort in prayer or bible reading. Nurses should ask the client whether they would like him or her or to pray or read to them. Be certain to ask the client's preference. Expressions of human need can be found in the Bible, Torah, Koran, etc. Spiritual readings can be an excellent source of comfort.

One method of offering skilled, compassionate care for the dying client is the **hospice** movement. Hospice means refuge. The hospice may be in a facility in the hospital or a home care program. The goals of the hospice movement are to increase the dying client's quality of life, to develop pain-control methods, and to help the family actively participate in the client's care. Hospice services are available twenty-four hours a day. However, hospice does nothing to treat the illness.

THE CONCEPT OF PAIN

Pain is a subjective sensation ranging in intensity from mild discomfort to intolerable agony. Pain is a private experience. It is experienced by the individual; only its effects can be seen by the observer. Effects of pain are both physical and psychological in nature. The primary purpose of pain is protection. It serves as a warning that tissue damage is taking place in the body.

Pain is caused by stimulation of special nerve endings. A stimulus is picked up by the nerve endings and transmitted to the brain, where it is interpreted. The brain's interpretation of the stimulus depends on many factors, including prior conditioning concerning acceptable responses to pain. Previous experiences with pain, fatigue, and the state of health of the client are contributing factors.

People learn about pain from families and experiences. They learn which stimuli to call pain, which to call discomfort, and which to call annoyance. They learn what are acceptable responses to pain in their culture. Prior experiences also teach people how to cope with pain. Perception and interpretation of pain vary with different individuals and even within the same individual. What is painful at one time may not be painful at another.

Perception and interpretation are affected by anxiety. The more frightened a person is, the more he or she is apt to interpret stimuli as pain. Anxiety leads to tension. Muscle tension results in fatigue. When a person is tired, he or she is more apt to interpret a stimulus as pain. The ability to cope is also an important influence. The more stressors the person has, the more pain he or she feels. To ignore pain is inexcusable. Whether or not pain has a physiological basis, the pain is real to the client who has it and should be accepted by the nurse. A common misconception about pain is that if you do not report pain, you do not have pain. Cleeland (1998) stated that unrecognized pain is untreated pain.

The Child and Pain

Small children's perception of pain is often confused; they do not understand it. Their reactions are as varied as those of the adult. Some children rock rhythmically. Others become hostile and aggressive; many do not cry. Some children are restless, and some quietly deny their pain. Anxiety and pain seem to be confused in the child's mind. Fear is often felt as pain. Pain is increased by anxiety. Many children confuse pain with dying.

Adolescents are struggling for independence. They see pain as a hindrance to that independence. Pain is something they cannot control.

A loss also may be experienced as pain. The loss may be a loss of privacy, self-control, or a personal relationship. Children in pain must cope with these losses. At the same time, they must cope with the uncertainly that accompanies pain.

To help the child in pain, the nurse must know the meaning of pain to that child. Separation from parents increases anxiety. Feeling abandoned or unloved increases pain. Measures to relieve anxiety should be employed. Massages, warm baths, and relaxation exercises help relieve tension. Storytelling helps distract the small child. Nurses must be warm, understanding, and caring if they are to help the child who is in pain.

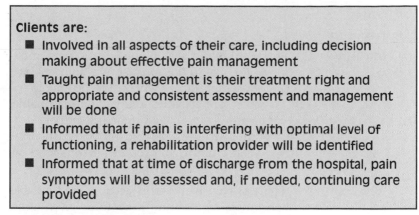

Clients are:

- Involved in all aspects of their care, including decision making about effective pain management
- Taught pain management is their treatment right and appropriate and consistent assessment and management will be done
- Informed that if pain is interfering with optimal level of functioning, a rehabilitation provider will be identified
- Informed that at time of discharge from the hospital, pain symptoms will be assessed and, if needed, continuing care provided

FIGURE 15-3 Standards for pain management.

PAIN ASSESSMENT AND MANAGEMENT

The Joint Commission on the Accreditation of Healthcare Organizations (JCAHO) (2000), revised pain standards for the assessment and management of pain for all clients in health care settings. **Pain management** is the priority, and facilities will be expected to have processes in place to assess and manage pain appropriately in all clients (Figure 15-3). The Veterans Administration (VA) has incorporated pain as the fifth vital sign. The documentation of pain is on the vital signs graphic record: temperature–pulse–respirations–blood pressure–pain rating. All areas of the hospital (admissions, emergency room, psychiatry) ask the following question: "Do you have pain and how would you rate it?" Every client has the right to an appropriate, thorough assessment and management of pain in a nonjudgmental manner. McCaffrey (1999), in pointing to the critical role of pain management, reports that 90% of clients should experience pain relief; however, 50% of clients continue to have moderate-to-severe pain.

Nurses play a critical role in pain management. There is an unrelenting aspect to pain because it is difficult for a client with pain to remember when pain was absent. Pain usually comes in waves, and excruciating pain becomes an unsurmountable obstacle that leaves the client feeling dispirited and impotent. Sirloin (1995) found that pain rated above 4 significantly interferes with mood and activity levels. Pain is assessed for the following characteristics:

- Location — A drawing of the entire body (front and back) is used
- Quality — Stabbing, burning, searing, gnawing, shooting, knife-like

- Onset
- Frequency
- Intensity   0-10 rating with 0 equal to no pain and 10 equal to the most severe pain; ask at what level the client would be able to perform activities and be at a reasonable comfort level. Picture boards of pain intensity are available and are particularly useful for children or persons who do not understand the pain scale.

The client's self-report of pain is the most accurate and reliable tool for medication intervention. Medication needs to be given at an adequate dosage and titrated within a safe range to relieve pain without causing unacceptable side effects, such as: confusion, dizziness, poor concentration, fatigue, and constipation. Constipation needs to be anticipated as an untoward effect of medication and prevented. Stool softeners (Dulcolax, Senokot) may be given. Alternatives offered in the diet may be senna tea and prunes. It is important to maintain regular bowel elimination, usually daily.

Breakthrough pain must be monitored. Assess and analyze unrelieved pain and respond quickly to the client's need, thus placing the client in as much control as possible. It is now recognized that morphine and hydromorphine are safer in the treatment of pain than meperidine (Demerol) which has an active metabolite that accumulates, resulting in renal dysfunction (Pasero & McCaffery, 1996).

With the mandate to improve pain management in health care facilities, a Pain Care Committee should be established that is interdisciplinary (pharmacy, nursing, psychiatry, physician). The goals of the committee are to promote improved outcomes for the client with pain while educating staff that may have inaccurate knowledge, insufficient education, or negative pain attitudes that influence their perception, judgment, and care of the client with pain. Remember, the goals are client comfort and function.

Jon Kabat-Zinn (1993) presented a ground-breaking documentary entitled *Healing and the Mind* that depicted chronic pain clients choosing to live with pain while adjusting their attitude and practicing new techniques. This has led to an increase in group work with clients who experience pain. The group is a safe place to uncover emotions and feelings and begin to heal. Self-discovery and personal growth can occur in a supportive, affirming environment. A "Coping with Chronic Pain Group" can consist of twelve psycho-educational sessions where teaching, education, demonstration, and practice of new techniques occurs. (Table 15-2).

TABLE 15-2 Coping with Chronic Pain Group

12 Sessions at 1 1/2 hours each; meets weekly

1. Orientation: beliefs, attitudes

2. Breathe and breathing: (based on distress tolerance work of dialectical behavioral therapy [DBT, M. Linehan, 1993])

3. Relaxation: guided imagery

4. Cognitive behavioral therapy (CBT): Part I–negative beliefs versus alternative positive beliefs

5. Cognitive behavioral therapy: Part II–cognitive distortions and mood log

6. Meditation and mindfulness

7. Anger and forgiveness

8. Rest, conservation of energy, and humor

9. Nutrition (presented by dietician)

10. Sexuality

11. Spirituality (presented by chaplain)

12. Volunteering options at hospital and in community

Nursing Intervention

Realizing that the person is in pain is the first step in helping. Observation and listening are essential. Because of prior conditioning clients may not be able to complain of pain; they may feel that it is a sign of weakness. Clients feel they must cope in silence. This type of person expresses pain in nonverbal ways. Restlessness, increased pulse rate, withdrawal, sadness, grimacing, and clenched fists are some of the signs of pain. The client's statement of "Nurse, I have a terrible pain" should be believed.

Many things can be done to relieve pain. The nurse should check for tight dressings, wrinkled sheets, and uncomfortable positioning. If the pain is mild or moderate, distraction methods can be used. Distraction focuses the client's attention and concentration on other stimuli and prevents concentration on pain. Backrubs and repositioning can be effective. Music, reading, and hobbies are other diversional activities. If medication is given, it is helpful for the nurse to say to the client "Mr. Jones, I have something to give you for your pain."

TABLE 15-3 Coping with Pain	
RELAXATION TECHNIQUES	**EMOTIONAL SUPPORT**
Lessening of stimuli	Gentle touch
Quiet room	Attentive look
Soothing bath	Genuine concern
Dim lights	Encourage verbalization
Distraction activities	Conversation
Position change	Communicate caring

Methods used to relieve anxiety also can be used to relieve pain. When the reason for the pain is unknown, anxiety is increased. The more severe the anxiety, the more difficult it is for the client to cope with pain. Relaxation techniques and emotional support lessen anxiety and increase the client's ability to cope. Acknowledging that clients have pain and allowing them to voice their frustrations may be helpful. The nurse should reinforce that he or she will protect them from unnecessary pain (Table 15-3).

Sensory overload can increase the perception of pain. Lessening the number of stimuli the client must handle may also help to relieve pain. A quiet room, soothing bath, and dimmed lights all help to contribute to a restful atmosphere. It is important for nurses to communicate their caring to the client. Nurses' touch, attentive looks, and genuine concern give support to the client. Nurses should take time to sit with the client experiencing pain; he or she may need to verbalize feelings of sadness, anger, frustration, or loneliness.

Today, there are many alternative or complementary approaches that are utilized with chronic pain clients. Examples are:

- **Breathe** and breathing—basic breathing exercises with a rhythmic base to enhance circulation and relaxation through listening to the breath sounds

- **Meditation**—setting aside time to focus and clear the mind

- **Guided imagery**—with relaxation breathing, focus and concentrate on using the imagination to go to special places remembering sights, sounds, and smells

- **Relaxation** (Benson, 1987)—tensing each large muscle group in a progressive manner while doing relaxation breathing

- **Humor**–jogging the internal cells through laughter
- **Massage**–producing relaxation through skin stimulation and improved circulation
- **Therapeutic touch** (Kreiger, 1987)–touch based on working with energy fields
- **Music**–choosing specific kinds of music that soothe the mind-body-spirit
- **Aromatherapy**–scents and fragrances chosen to enhance emotional well-being (such as lavender, bergamot, chamomile)
- **Mindfulness** (Thich Nhat Than, 1987)–spiritual practice of staying focused in the present moment through breath control and bringing the mind back to a central focus; listening to your breathing; inner peace and stillness occur as you let things go.
- **Art**–self-expression through shape and color
- **Thought-field-therapy (TFT)** (Callahan, 1988)–a powerful technique that resolves psychological problems by directing the client to tap on specific energy points on the body in a specific sequence while thinking about a specific problem to which a subjective rating is given (0 to10, with 10 being severe), and continuing with TFT until a subjective rating of zero is obtained.

Many of these therapies require therapists who have had further education and are specialists governed by state licensure laws (for example, certified music therapist, certified massage therapist).

Care Providers

On units where death, dying, and pain are everyday experiences, special attention must be given to the care providers. As care providers offer comfort and strength to clients and families, they may begin to recognize feelings of hopelessness and helplessness within themselves. Watch that the care providers are not reverting to inactivity on their days off, with decreased contact with friends and family. Care providers are survivors, and hospitals, hospice centers, and so forth would do well to provide them with support groups so they can express their grief and address their anger, depression, and sense of failure.

GRIEVING AND DIVORCE

Divorce is a termination of the family characterized by painful losses that reemerge at holidays, birthdays, and special events. Grieving occurs not only in the partners who have severed their marital bond

TABLE 15-4 Children's Ages and Responses to Divorce

AGE	RESPONSE
Toddler	Irritability, crying, fear, separation anxiety, sleep problems, aggressive behavior, and developmental skills regression
Pre-school	Self-blame, high vulnerability, and decreased self-worth
School age	Moody, pre-occupied, increased daydreaming, and tantrums
Adolescents	Anger, aggression, anti-social behavior, substance abuse, increased peer influence, and increased sexual relationships

but also in the children (Table 15-4). Ways to work through individual grief are honoring your experience and taking care of yourself through rest and sleep, good nutrition, exercise, meditation, and seeking out nurturing people. Each year, more than 1 million children experience divorce of their parents.

Single parenting and divorce result in approximately 61 percent of all children living in a single-parent environment. Custodial parents usually work longer hours, and it becomes more difficult to focus on their children's feelings and needs when they are working through their own personal anger and loss. Children often become overly aggressive and experience problems with divided loyalties as parents are working out visitation arrangements and discipline strategies.

SUMMARY

Grieving is a major stressor that most people experience at some time in their lives. If it is not successfully completed, anxiety and depression may result. Reactions to death are influenced by cultural and religious beliefs, background, and experience with death. Dr. Kubler-Ross describes five stages of grief: denial, anger, bargaining, depression, and acceptance.

Pain and isolation are two concerns of the dying. The dying person should be made as comfortable as possible and never left alone. The family of the dying client also needs the support of the nurse. Because family members often do not feel they are the nurse's responsibility, the nurse usually must seek them out and encourage communication. Children need added help to cope with death because their concept of death is often confused.

Pain is a subjective sensation that ranges in intensity from mild discomfort to intolerable agony. Effects of pain are both physical and emotional. Perception and interpretation of pain vary with different individuals and even within the same individual. Anxiety and fatigue increase pain. The nurse needs to observe for nonverbal signs of pain and record the client's perception of their pain, when pain is recorded as the fifth vital sign. Both emotional measures and medication can be used to relieve pain. When pain cannot be relieved, the client must be helped to accept the discomfort. Psychoeducational groups and ongoing pain support groups can enhance coping and encourage personal growth.

SUGGESTED ACTIVITIES

- Think about your first experience with death (it may have been an animal, relative, or friend). How did you feel? How did you resolve your feelings?
- Discuss the following questions with your classmates:
  a. Which type of dying client would you consider the most difficult to care for?
  a five-year-old with leukemia
  a mother, age twenty-seven, with two preschool children
  a retired gentleman, age sixty-eight
  b. Should the dying person be told he or she is dying?
  c. How do you expect to react to your own death? Would you want to know you are dying?
- Investigate religious beliefs on death by talking to various clergy.

REVIEW

KNOW AND COMPREHEND

A. Multiple choice. Select the one best answer.

1. To help a client cope with death, the nurse must first know
   - ❑ A. the meaning of death.
   - ❑ B. how the client feels about dying.
   - ❑ C. how the family feels about death.
   - ❑ D. how the nurse feels about death.

2. Dying clients are sometimes ignored because the nurse feels
   - ❑ A. they do not need as much care as other clients.
   - ❑ B. unsure of what to say or do.
   - ❑ C. time is needed for clients who can be helped.
   - ❑ D. nursing efforts would be wasted.

3. Grief is the process of
   - ❑ A. coping with loss.
   - ❑ B. feeling sorry for oneself.
   - ❑ C. mourning the dead.
   - ❑ D. depression.

4. When a client begins to prepare for death they are probably in the
   - ❑ A. denial stage.
   - ❑ B. bargaining stage.
   - ❑ C. depression stage.
   - ❑ D. acceptance stage.

5. A client says "Please, doctor, help me to live just one more year." What stage of grief is most likely occurring?
   - ❑ A. shock stage
   - ❑ B. bargaining stage
   - ❑ C. depression stage
   - ❑ D. acceptance stage

6. If a client diagnosed with metastatic cancer looks for another doctor, which stage of grief is most likely occurring?
   - ❑ A. denial stage
   - ❑ B. bargaining stage
   - ❑ C. depression stage
   - ❑ D. acceptance stage

7. When the dying child withdraws from his or her parents, it is an indication of
   - ❏ A. pain.
   - ❏ B. withdrawal from reality.
   - ❏ C. rejection of the parents.
   - ❏ D. an attempt to let go.

APPLY YOUR LEARNING
B. Multiple choice. Select the one best answer.

1. A military pilot dies in a plane crash during a training exercise. Which reaction would the nurse expect from the family when they are first notified of the accident?
   - ❏ A. "That can't be true. You have notified the wrong family."
   - ❏ B. "How could God let something like this happen to us?"
   - ❏ C. "We knew this was a possibility in such a hazardous occupation."
   - ❏ D. "It's the military's fault. They don't safely maintain the planes."

2. A military pilot dies in a plane crash during a training exercise. Which statement from the family indicates acceptance and resolution of grief?
   - ❏ A. "That can't be true. You have notified the wrong family."
   - ❏ B. "How could God let something like this happen to us?"
   - ❏ C. "We knew this was a possibility in such a hazardous occupation."
   - ❏ D. "It's the military's fault. They don't safely maintain the planes."

3. An uninsured family loses all their possessions in a house fire. Which response would the nurse expect?
   - ❏ A. a severe mental illness
   - ❏ B. a grief reaction
   - ❏ C. a critical response
   - ❏ D. effective coping

4. A six-year-old child, admitted with a fractured femur from a motor vehicle accident, says to the nurse, "I think I'm dying." Which response by the nurse is most therapeutic?
   - ❏ A. "When you say 'dying,' what does that word mean to you?"
   - ❏ B. Check the child's vital signs and notify the physician.
   - ❏ C. Tell the child, "You'll be just fine as soon as your leg heals."
   - ❏ D. Offer the child a recreational activity, such as a video game.

5. The nurse cares for a client diagnosed with metastatic lung cancer. In addition to administering analgesic medications, which intervention would be best for pain management?
   - ❏ A. turn on the lights and open the curtains
   - ❏ B. keep the client very still in bed
   - ❏ C. invite some of the client's friends to visit
   - ❏ D. keep the lights dim and the room quiet

6. A client says to the nurse, "My pain is 9 on a scale of 10." The nurse knows there is no medical diagnosis that would cause this pain. Which action by the nurse is indicated?
   - ❏ A. confront the client with information about the diagnosis
   - ❏ B. accept and believe the client's perception and description
   - ❏ C. challenge the client's perception and description
   - ❏ D. medicate the client promptly with a placebo

C. Briefly answer the following.

1. Name the three reasons children need added help to cope with death.

2. Why is it important for the grief process to be completed?

3. Name three concerns of the dying.

4. List five characteristics assessed in pain management.

5. List three objectives of the hospice program.

CHAPTER 16

Facilitating Mental Health and Reentry into the Community

OUTLINE

KEY TERMS

health

prevention

culture

acculturation

traditional

homeless

persons with serious and
   persistent mental illness

incarcerated

trauma

drop-in facility

outpatient services

residential treatment center

sustaining care center

day-treatment center

mental health units

rehabilitation

reentry

prevention

primary

secondary

tertiary

OBJECTIVES

After studying this chapter, the student should be able to:

- Name five ways that modern society contributes to mental illness.
- State four stressors that make the poor a high risk for mental illness.
- State how culture affects mental health.
- Describe the mental health issues of the growing prison system.
- Name four ways that the family can help to improve the mental health of children.
- List four needs of the client who is reentering the community.
- Explain why it is more difficult to establish identity today than it was in the past.

Health is defined by the World Health Organization (WHO) as a state of complete, physical, mental, and social well-being. Health is not merely the absence of disease or infirmity. Mental well-being involves functioning with emotional equilibrium in everyday life. People must function adequately within their roles in society. They must adapt to their environment, and the environment must continually adapt to their needs—it is an ongoing, continuous process. The stresses of life create problems for individuals and society as a whole. Social, economic, and cultural factors that influence behavior can be complex. The nurse needs to develop a deep understanding and awareness of the complicated network that surrounds each individual's life.

Prevention is the ultimate goal in dealing with the problem of mental illness. In an effort to prevent mental illness, personal happiness and the ability to deal with stress must be enhanced. This is not an easy task in the vastly complex society in which we live today. Modern society has greatly increased the stress that precipitates mental illness. Our world has become impersonal and highly technical. The rapid changes that society is undergoing have contributed to social disorganization, disrupted family units, and disturbed parent-child relationships.

This rapid change is enhanced by the mobility in today's society. Fast travel, new opportunities, and changing jobs move people from place to place on a national and international scale. Each move is a new stress. Adaptation to the new environment includes family, friends, schools, and community resources. Feelings of alienation and loneliness become prevalent as people are separated from loved ones.

Everyone needs significant others in their environment. Hostile feelings can develop when the basic need of belonging is not satisfied by a support system. A significant other may be a parent, husband, wife, teacher, or friend. These significant others accept the individual with his or her own limitations and strengths and offer encouragement to take responsibility for his or her own actions. Significant others are the individual's support system; they frequently influence the person's behavior. These people are a necessary part in the creation of autonomous, satisfying lives.

Unemployment is another stress in society. It places a strain on the entire family unit. Long-term unemployment can erode the self-concept. Many who have jobs are bored with them and feel no sense of pride or accomplishment. They often feel unfulfilled. A feeling of being powerless to control the environment or change events is common. Meaningful work contributes to a sense of well-being. Financial stability enhances personal status.

In an effort to obtain fulfillment, people often turn to materialistic objects. Finding no lasting satisfaction in objects, they constantly strive for bigger and better things—a new car, new home, or expensive jewelry. The constant striving and lack of lasting satisfaction tend only to increase stress and frustration.

Lack of identity is a large problem in today's society. Years ago, America was an agricultural nation. Extended families that included grandparents and relatives usually lived in the same community. There was a closeness and support that is seldom seen today. Children felt confident in their place in society and often worked along with their parents. Today, children usually do not see their fathers or mothers at work and may not know the nature of their occupations.

In the past, children accepted their parent's values and grew into their adult role with little questioning. Today's children are constantly confronted with choices. There is no single way of looking at situations. However, learning to choose from alternatives can give direction to a person's life.

Modern society has brought with it more freedom. Although there are several advantages to this, freedom also increases stress. Life is no longer simple. Families are constantly on the move and therefore may become fragmented. Roots are uncertain, and support systems may not be readily available. Family, religious, and political structures that once provided security have been weakened. One out of every five families is disrupted because of divorce, separation, death, imprisonment, or institutionalization. Even in two-parent families, approximately 75 percent of mothers work outside the home. Parental employment and youth activities leave little time for family experiences. The child has more freedom but less help in learning to use it wisely.

Although radio and television broaden individuals' worlds by exposing them to greater learning and enjoyment, they also expose individuals to greater stress. Television can be both entertaining and disruptive. Some people watch television or play with their computer to the exclusion of all other experiences. Although television and computers provide an awareness of world difficulties, they limit family interactions and detract from personal development. Spending absorbing hours before the television set or computer divests people of valuable reading, writing, and talking time.

CULTURE AND MENTAL HEALTH

Culture is defined as the customary beliefs, values, and ideas held by a racial, religious, or social group of people. There seems to be a correlation between culture and mental health problems. More research is needed to understand why this is true. There is more violence in the ghetto, fewer role conflicts among Mexican-Americans, and a problem of increased alcoholism and suicide among Native Americans. If mental illness is to be prevented, consideration must be given to cultural influences. Culture affects an individual's total way of life because customs are passed down from one generation to the next. Culture is a complex phenomenon that is learned through interactions with others.

Cultural differences can cause problems in health care because a person's attitudes toward health and illness are influenced by cultural background. The language of a culture may contain words and phrases that have meaning only to the culture because of background, problems, or interests. This may make communication difficult between groups of different cultures. There are important steps in developing a culturally sensitive practice. Two areas deal with ourselves. Do we have an awareness and acceptance of our own racial/ethnic group? What are the cultural experiences that have influenced us (as child/adolescent/adult)? A culturally competent person understands the dynamics in the helping process and assists the client by recognizing the reality of the client. We adapt our practice skills to fit our clients and not the reverse—our client is expected to adapt or fit into our mold. Affirming our culturally different clients' problem-solving skills and their survival instincts reflects our caring and gives them power.

The nurse should also be aware of subculture differences. A subculture is an ethnic, regional, economic, or social group having similar behavior patterns that distinguish the group from others within the culture. For example, separating the aged from the rest of society creates a subculture. Singling out and discriminating against an ethnic group also contributes to the growth of a subculture. People within a subculture interact chiefly among themselves.

Dealing with mental health problems must include a concern for the cultural and subcultural backgrounds of the client. What may seem to be maladaptive behavior to the nurse may be normal behavior within the client's subculture (Table 16-1). Nurses only create more stress for the client if they try to impose their own values on him or her. They must, instead, be attuned to the client's expectations, needs, and lifestyle. Empowerment is the key word. Areas of empowerment include families and effective support systems, problem solving techniques, communication skills, and family rules and roles. Identifying blocks in their power diminishes feelings of oppression and enhances therapy. Clients feel understood. When appropriate, bicultural and bilingual professionals need to be sought.

TABLE 16-1 Culture Variations

Acculturation	Uncomfortable with own cultural identity
	Join dominant culture*
Bicultural	Pride in racial identity
	Seeks racial diversity
	Experiences reflect both cultures
	Integrated setting for work and home
	Sense of being between cultures
	Result can be pain and discord
Culturally immersed	Rejects dominant cultural norms and values
	Pro their culture
	Attempts to meet all needs in culture*
	May blame society for all problems
Traditional	Dominant culture is not accepted or rejected
	Community is church

Adapted from the writings of Peter Bell, 1981
* Language, music, art, entertainment

POVERTY AND MENTAL HEALTH

The environment plays an active role in determining stress factors and the individual's ability to cope. There is also a definite correlation between socioeconomic levels and health. A low socioeconomic level often leads to poor nutrition, crowded living conditions, maternal deprivation, and a lack of self-esteem. Mental illness can develop as the person becomes more oppressed and more vulnerable. Frisch (1995) reports that the Federal Task Force on Homelessness & Severe Mental Illness found that every third **homeless** person in the United States suffers from severe mental illness.

The poor are a high risk for mental health problems because they are exposed to many more stressors than the average person (Figure 16-1). Their biggest problems concern finances, employment, and social isolation—all of which limit their access to health care. Lack of adequate housing, schools, and available living space and a high crime rate also contribute to mental health problems. If the health care is provided, the clinics may be far from home. Even though health care is often free or inexpensive, there may be no money for transportation or baby-sitters. Transportation and baby-sitters may even be unavailable. Seeing a different health care person at each clinic visit only adds to the client's stress. The questions and paperwork at the clinic may be frustrating and overwhelming.

Lack of stable employment is a particular stress for the poor because it blocks efforts to provide basic needs of food, shelter, and clothing. Many who have tedious, task-oriented jobs become frustrated and bored. There is no sense of pride or accomplishment. Having no

■ Social isolation
■ Maternal deprivation
■ High crime rate
■ Lack of adequate
     Employment
     Finances
     Housing
     Nutrition
     Schools
     Living space
     Child care
     Health care
     Transportation

FIGURE 16-1 Stressors of poverty.

power to control the environment or to bring about change can be devastating. Continued frustrations often cause people to withdraw and become apathetic. This is a way of initially warding off stress, but it also causes added stress. Health care workers often turn away from the apathetic poor because they feel the poor do not really care or want the help themselves. This type of attitude places more stress on the already overburdened person. Shives (1998) relates that unemployment of recently discharged psychiatric clients is as high as 70 percent.

Persons with serious and persistent mental illness have severe and chronic symptoms of mental or emotional disability. Recent studies have pointed to a serious problem of the lack of medical treatment for persons with chronic mental illness. There is a diminished level of functioning in regard to their daily living skills. Some primary aspects include personal relations, living arrangements, and work skills. An isolative approach and the avoidance of minimal stresses can enable them to remain in their homes and in the community. Persons with serious and persistent mental illness are sometimes referred to as the wanderers of cities and can be characterized as highly impulsive, reactive, and frustrated.

They are found in many areas: the YWCAs–YMCAs, boarding houses, soup kitchens, bus stations, skid row, and jails. Approximately one third of nursing home (intermediate and personal care) residents have a psychiatric diagnosis. If the person with mental illness is in residential housing, what is the quality of the neighborhood? Do the neighbors accept this population, and are they viewed as contributing to a neighborhood blending? Some of these live-in board and care homes are also segregated, removed from the community, and therefore similar to the state hospitals. Before admission to residential housing, the following data should be collected: Is the client able to maintain personal hygiene and physical activity; shop, cook, and clean; and seek out and use public transportation? If we can identify the people's strengths, we can help them cope with their limitations.

In New York state, a project called Community Link-Up Experiences (CLUE) is under way that consistently works with persons with mental illness on job abilities, money management, job seeking, interviewing, and filling out job applications. This approach creates successful experiences for the chronic client. Social and economic changes have rapidly increased the number of homeless in our country–approximately 350,000, or a very high 2,000,000 when families and children are included. Innovative programs have begun for the homeless. In Portland, Oregon, an inner-city residential facility provides a continuum of medical, psychiatric, and rehabilitative services in a homelike atmosphere. The Department of Veterans Affairs has initiated programs for the homeless veteran with serious and persistent mental illness. A provision is made for aggressive outreach services and on-site assessments and referrals to homeless veterans. The Department of Housing and Urban Development (HUD) supports Shelter-Plus Care. It provides permanent supportive housing for homeless people who are severely mentally ill or chronic alcohol or drug abusers, and those who have AIDS. Supportive services are linked to rental assistance through the Affordable Housing Act 1990. Supportive care is also matched to culture with consideration for traditions, lifestyle, identity, standards, and values.

Some people with mental illness who are living in the community attend day care four days per week. It provides a structured environment, daily group therapy, and educational activities. This program fosters and encourages noninstitutional living patterns.

To pay for and facilitate placement in these areas, the person with mental illness needs Supplemental Security Income (SSI). SSI is available to people certified as having a psychiatric disability. The applicant must have a specific mental disorder that is expected to last a minimum of twelve months and will result in an inability to work.

HOMELESSNESS

A major problem with homelessness has been a useful, accurate, operational definition of homelessness. There is a wide variety of homeless people, from marginally housed to literally homeless, and they live in hotels, motels, friends' houses, apartments, rooms, halfway houses, jails, prisons, hospitals, institutions, detoxification facilities, shelters, parks, vehicles, abandoned buildings, subways, trains, buses, street encampments, underpasses, and woody areas along creeks and rivers. Homelessness can be transient, episodic, or ongoing. Seven areas determine problem severity: medical condition, employment status, drug use, alcohol use, illegal activity, family relations, and psychiatric conditions. Victimization, social isolation, and vulnerability are risks to the quality of life of the homeless. Increased emphasis on early intervention and prevention of homelessness is extremely important to our society.

PRISONS/JAILS

The prison population has quadrupled since 1980. Kupers (1999) reports that according to the U. S. Department of Justice, more than 250,000 prisoners suffer from mental illness; frequently, a dual diagnosis. There has been an increase in the rate of violence, mental deterioration, and suicides in prisons and jails. Today in the prison system there is a higher incidence of victimization of prisoners with mental illness through assaults and rapes. These forms of violence are under-reported and underinvestigated. Problems with safety, cleanliness, and privacy continue to exist. Jails are overcrowded, and there are many facility deficiencies. Solitary confinement is becoming a way of isolating difficult prisoners; frequently, the prisoners are psychotic or developmentally disabled or both.

With the recognition of the fact that many **incarcerated** (those confined to jail or prison) people have experienced lifetimes of **trauma** (physical, emotional, and/or sexual) and have witnessed or been victimized by violent behaviors, an increased collaboration with mental health providers prior to release from prison and jail is crucial. Many people who are released from prison will remain on probation or parole. Preparation for prison release requires job training, acquisition of social skills, and specific ways to cope with the transition to family and community. A millennium goal is the upgrading of adolescent and adult correctional services for clients with mental illness.

PREVENTION OF MENTAL HEALTH PROBLEMS

Primary prevention of mental health problems is aimed at lessening stress and developing improved coping mechanisms. Prevention must begin in the family. Studies show that parent–child relationships influence all future relationships. It is through the parent–child relationship that the child develops self-concept. A higher self-concept is associated with a close family bond that has been established at birth. This bond must be fostered throughout life. Ways must be found to strengthen the family unit and to support family members. Families must see the importance of being together; family discussion and positive interaction increase the self-concept of each member (Figure 16-2).

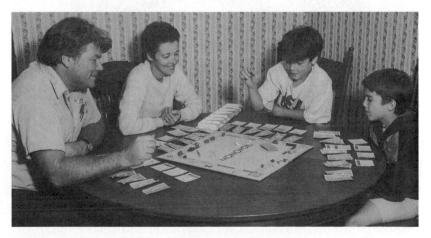

FIGURE 16-2 This family enjoys being together.

Parents are the child's most important teachers. Parents cannot effectively delegate their responsibility to teach children about themselves to anyone else. The family is still the most effective place for strengthening its members. It is within the family that sensitivity to others is learned. Coping mechanisms and values are also acquired within the family. Children need to learn responsibility and to make decisions within the family in order to properly prepare them for adulthood. Children who are given reasons for restrictions are more apt to accept themselves as worthwhile.

Children, like adults, feel frustration, anger, insecurity, and a need to express their feelings (Figure 16-3). They need to know that these feelings are normal and acceptable. Seeing children as people, listening to them, and considering their ideas are new concepts. Talking with children instead of at them is difficult for many parents. Some communities have recognized this difficulty and have instituted programs to help parents communicate with their children.

Many of these programs are based on Thomas Gordon's *Parent Effectiveness Training*. Gordon believes that the child must feel accepted. He teaches parents to listen to and hear what the child is saying and to accept the child's feelings. Solutions to problems should not be imposed. Greater growth is accomplished if solutions are mutually

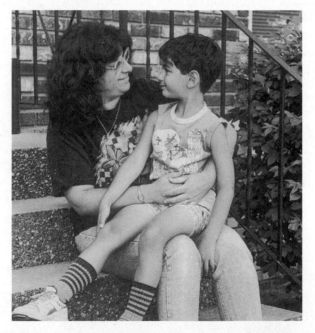

FIGURE 16-3 Communication between adult and child is important.

sought and agreed on. A child's problems are important to the child, no matter how insignificant they may seem to others. The child should never be belittled.

Open communication between parent and child at any age is essential. Blocks to communication should be avoided. Openness and honesty are important. Reasons should be given for demands or restrictions. Sometimes a parent cannot compromise and cannot give a reason. In these instances the parent might say "I may be wrong, but this decision is my responsibility. You will just have to accept it this time." Parents sometimes are under too much stress to cope with a child's problem immediately. The child should be told honestly "I cannot cope with it right now." Sincere honesty does not hurt the child's self-concept but helps the child to understand. Honesty contributes to a realistic perspective.

Support services for families are available and should be used if needed. These services include crisis counseling, hot lines, drug counseling, suicide prevention centers, abortion and antiabortion counseling, child and family services, family service agencies, and runaway services. Many people do not contact mental health agencies. They feel more comfortable seeking help from family members, clergy, or friends.

Single parents may require more help, because they must cope with day-to-day problems alone. As problems accumulate and multiply, the person may become more vulnerable. Day-care centers, the Big Brother and Big Sister organizations, and Parents without Partners are groups that provide support for single parents. These supportive services can cushion the effects of a crisis and help the family feel a part of community.

A new idea in prevention of mental illness is home care. Mental health workers work with high-risk families by initiating discussions and problem solving in the home. This is thought to be effective because the problems are viewed within the actual home setting. This facilitates working out available alternatives. Positive areas and strengths are reinforced, and feedback can be received. By talking through a situation, obstacles that may cause a potential crisis can be more easily seen and thus averted.

Small **drop-in facilities** have been established throughout the country in areas such as shopping centers, airports, and bus terminals. Individuals can stop by at any time and find an empathetic and receptive listener. Mental health problems require creative solutions. Some judicial/court systems have implemented a mental health diversion program to emphasize and encourage the treatment of persons with serious and persistent mental illness. Defendants, in lieu of criminal prosecution when charged with a misdemeanor criminal offense, have the opportunity to seek mental health treatment. A treatment plan is developed by a mental health professional, who follows the defendant for a period of six months to a year. If the defendant is compliant with the treatment plan, including counseling, medication when indicated, and probation visits, all charges are eradicated from their records.

Because the majority of clients with mental illness return to their families, family approaches that attempt to decrease the tremendous physical, mental, and emotional family burden need to be carefully considered. The following can prove to be beneficial: family therapy, interpersonal skill improvement, client/family education (especially concerning medication regimen and monitoring), and home visits by professionals. Major questions include: How do we prevent a family from feeling very depleted? What additional social supports are available? Is there an extended family, financial support, religious affiliations, or community contact people? What is the quality of this family's life?

TREATMENT FACILITIES

Treatment facilities for persons with mental illness include **outpatient services**, **residential treatment centers**, **sustaining care centers**, **day-treatment centers**, and **mental health units**. Outpatient services are usually available through the local mental health department. Community centers provide therapy through psychiatrists, social workers, psychologists, and nurses. The services vary according to the financing available to the community. Fees for services are based on the individual's ability to pay. Appointments are made at the convenience of the client.

After a period of hospitalization, a client may be placed in a residential treatment center, which provides for the individual's day-to-day living. The treatment center may be a private home or a foster home that has met state guidelines for the care of persons with serious and persistent mental illness. Clients must be evaluated and their condition stabilized before being placed in a residential treatment center.

A sustaining care center is similar to a nursing home environment. Individuals reside at the center. They have some functional skills and are further guided by professional personnel. There is usually a structured program of social activities.

Day-treatment centers are concerned with clients who are emotionally dysfunctional. This includes clients who experience daily living problems and are in need of an intermediate step toward independent functioning. The goal is to increase the client's self-responsibility and self-esteem. The client comes to the center during the day to learn basic living skills. Educational and vocational training may be provided. Functional living skills are explored. Assertiveness training, problem solving, goal formulation, and decision skills are reaffirmed. Any of the psychotherapies may be used. Day-treatment centers attempt to help individuals manage themselves in a way that is meaningful to them. Acceptance into the program is on a referral basis.

Mental health units are frequently located in the local community hospital. The care is usually geared toward short-term or emergency needs. Self-direction and personal initiative are among the goals. Care is given until the individual can return to the community.

Take time to assess your client's financial status. Many clients may need assistance to file for social security benefits. The client who has worked long enough may be eligible for SSDI (Social Security Disability Income) and if not may meet federal disability criteria for SSI (Supplemental Security Income). It is estimated that one half of all persons with serious and persistent mental illness have not applied for these benefits because of feeling overwhelmed by the severity of their problems and their inability to work through all the laborious details required to file a claim.

REHABILITATION

Before reentry into the community, the client may need rehabilitation. **Rehabilitation** is a process that enables an individual to return to the highest level of functioning. Brief stays at intermediate facilities can be helpful. Intermediate facilities include foster homes and halfway houses. Clients need time to discuss and reevaluate basic living skills. They must be able to adapt and survive in a new environment and function adequately. If they seek employment, their ability to file an acceptable application needs to be evaluated. Interviewing techniques should be reviewed. To be independent in the activities of daily living, the client may need assistance with budgeting, shopping, menu planning, and cooking.

Good health habits contribute to vitality. The client needs to have adequate diet and exercise. Exercise and relaxation help the person avoid fatigue and are essential components for good mental health. Exercise leads to better physical health and is a way of working out frustration. Relaxation techniques could be demonstrated and practiced. The physically healthy person is better able to handle stress. Adequate sleep is essential. Some people who have suffered a mental health problem escape from stress by sleeping. This is not recommended. Adequate sleep at night with an afternoon nap during the immediate reentry period is sufficient. Effective use of leisure time is important. Enjoyable activities should be encouraged. Hobbies and interests need to be cultivated (Figure 16-4). Making leisure time productive adds to positive life experiences.

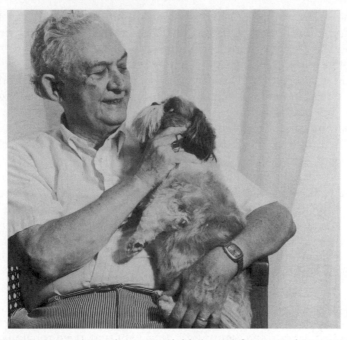

FIGURE 16-4 A pet can be a special interest for an aging person.

All clients should receive some medication education. Drug dosage and possible side effects must be explained. Careful compliance to medication times needs to be evaluated. If family members must administer the medication, teaching sessions should be scheduled.

Clients and their families should be instructed to watch for overwhelming stressors. Too much stimulation can cause irritability. The individual will probably be better off with limited stimulation for a time after returning home. People also require a certain amount of space for privacy in their environment. However, private moments need to be balanced with satisfying interactions. Satisfying interactions relieve feelings of loneliness and isolation. Community resources, such as museums, YWCA or YMCA, library, parks, and modes of transportation should be discussed. A brochure that covers these areas of interest in the community, times of availability, modes of transportation, and possible fees is an excellent method of making the client aware of community resources.

During the rehabilitation phase, employment becomes an issue. We need to recognize that work can add great stress to the lives of psychiatric clients and they will need adequate support and help with motivation. A wider array of vocational options that considers the variety of skills, personal wishes, and talents of these individuals is needed. Expecting all persons with mental illness to engage in the same kind of employment is a denial of their individuality. One must reflect: Does the failure of persons with mental illness at job sites reflect the restrictiveness of the offerings and the lack of additional provisions for support and motivations? Creative rehabilitation efforts are looking at greater flexibility and new ideas (i.e., shared jobs and shortened work schedules). With increased realistic expectations about what a particular person with a mental illness is able to do, a more satisfying experience can result. Rehabilitation should prepare the individual to enter the community as a worthwhile, confident participator.

REENTRY

A person who has been confined or isolated for a period of time must go through a process called **reentry**. This is a difficult process because of stigma and stereotyping. Many former clients are regarded as mentally ill or "crazy" for the rest of their lives. They are often feared or ignored, which adds to their stress. Returning home can be very stressful. Neighbors and friends often avoid the former client. They do not know what to say or how to act. This only makes the person's self-concept more negative. Families need assurance that the individual's behavior has changed and that the maladaptive behavior need not return. They should be informed of factors that may have contributed to the problem and how they can help the person cope in the future. Initial symptoms of maladaption or relapse need to be explained so that early intervention and treatment can be provided. Community reception can be a factor in a return to maladaptive behavior. People who are reentering need an adequate support system to offset these negative aspects. Hospitalization greatly disrupts the person's lifestyle, and a difficult period of readjustment begins after discharge from the hospital. Lines of communication must be kept open. Communication occurs when talking to, not at, a person. Listening encourages frankness; people feel free to express their fears, insecurities, and disappointments. Social agencies, schools, churches, health care workers, and families need to work together to provide a support system. Professionals in both the private and public sector must be more aware of the full range of available community services and resources.

The person reentering a community needs an adequate problem-solving approach. The person's problem-solving approach should be evaluated and alternatives discussed. General guidelines for approaching a problem include the following:

1. Place attention on the immediate problem.

2. Write down possible solutions.

3. Look at personal strong points.

4. Determine the support system.

5. Choose an appropriate action.

6. Act.

Effective problem solving strengthens coping and adds to the individual's self-confidence and self-acceptance. This helps to make his or her life more consistent and stable.

If the person is going directly into the home situation, some type of home visit might be needed. The extent of burden on the family extends to many areas. Research points of five specific areas of burden: financial, family routine, leisure, interaction, and the health of other family members. There is a disruption of routine in the family and home and increased arguing over the client and the client's irrational demands. A financial burden becomes evident because there is loss of the client's income, increased expenses of the illness, and dipping into family funds to expand financial needs. Often family members miss important activities (school, work, outings) because they are designated to stay home and "watch" their family member. Fun and play are abandoned or postponed, and the family's life becomes more absorbed in the client. Frequently, families become isolated because friends refuse to drop by or families now are not comfortable entertaining at home. These stressors can have an adverse effect on the physical and mental health of all family members.

Weekly group meetings are sometimes arranged to reinforce new behaviors. Discussion groups can be excellent reinforcers of self-growth. Giving individuals the opportunity to voice their own opinions can increase their sense of confidence and competence. Group therapy can assist in resocialization and allow clients to test out new behaviors safely. Sharing with others through group therapy helps people learn to cope. It is also a way to develop new friendships and practice new social skills. Adequate support and encouragement help to motivate clients toward recovery.

Returning to a previous work environment can be stressful. Sometimes fellow workers who pitched in to get the job done during the person's absence resent his or her return. The former client may be discriminated against when it comes time for salary increases and promotions. Nurses who work in industry can act as liaisons among the hospital, home, and work environment. They can do much more to promote healthful attitudes among the workers. Industrial nurses can arrange seminars that contribute to positive well-being, such as stress-reduction or retirement seminars. Some companies and business have developed employee assistance programs (EAP) to offer help to the troubled employee. The employee can be supervisor- or self-referred. An assessment is done of personal problems and their degree (i.e., absenteeism, substance abuse, family/marital conflicts, financial difficulties, or legal problems). The assessment can also include recommendations and referrals for help.

The elderly reentering the community especially need frequent home visits. Reentry can mean return to the same stressors the person left. The elderly should be reintroduced to drop-in centers, Golden Age Clubs, or Foster Grandparents.

Retirement and preretirement counseling are a new dimension to mental health for the aging. At these counseling sessions, the continued usefulness of the individual is reinforced. Various activities and future prospects can be explored through utilizing therapeutic communication techniques and community resource people. Areas to be explored include increased leisure time, decreased income, personal attitudes toward retirement, adaptability, community resources and activities, and support systems. A meaningful reorganization of the individual's life can help the retired person to adapt and adjust to this new stage in the life cycle.

The nurse in the community health setting needs to approach the client through the nursing process. The nurse should observe the client's behavioral patterns, interpersonal relationships, family role, communication skills, coping mechanisms, and social skills. Anticipatory counseling prepares the individual for problematic situations in his or her particular setting. The goal is to prepare the person for future coping. The nurse helps the person look at new ways of resolving problems. Social skills may require further developing. Adequate feedback is a necessity.

Intervention

Appropriate interventions must be developed, since a crisis could be overwhelming. If the person is thoroughly prepared, crises can be avoided. Times of potential crisis should be anticipated. For example, adolescence, menopause, and aging are times with added stressors. Other situations that need to be carefully observed include

- Completion of school
- Changing residence
- Starting a new job
- Sudden loss (death of a loved one, loss of income)
- Childbirth
- Retirement

The rapport nurses establish with the client provides the client with a significant other that he or she can turn to when problems arise. During the nursing process, nurses need to constantly reevaluate both the long- and short-term goals. Individual needs of the client must always be taken into consideration. All aspects of people and their individual situations must be considered to make their environment as problem free as possible.

Community Programs

Special community programs geared to contemporary services are a necessity. More research needs to be done to explore innovative programs and methods of service. The evaluation of community needs should include the following:

- Residential care
- Centers for the aged
- Custodial care
- Home visitation programs
- Acute treatment centers
- Effective leadership
- Youth seminars and services

A problem in some communities is the lack of centralization of available services. People must be properly referred to the service that will coordinate and facilitate resolution of their unmet needs (Figure 16-5). The goal of prevention is a fully alive, healthy person who can become a satisfied, functioning member of his or her family and community.

The levels of **prevention** can be described as **primary**, **secondary**, or **tertiary**. In primary prevention, an intervention occurs before the health problem disrupts the person's life. In secondary prevention, an intervention occurs promptly when a health problem is present; this intervention decreases the severity and duration of the problem. Tertiary prevention limits the disability related to the illness.

The National Advisory Mental Health Council of the National Institute of Mental Health has formulated a national plan and research strategy to improve services for people with serious mental illness. Money allocations were estimated at $47 million in 1990, with an increase to $369 million by 1997. Systems of care that will benefit the client are being explored. Two areas of study are clinical services and service systems. Assessment for serious and persistent mental illness includes the characteristics of severe mental illness; outcomes (good

What type of care is given in the local hospital?
Does the staff identify with the client?
Is work output hindered by stereotyping?
Is there a problem working with ethnic or racial groups?
How often is the client seen by the doctor?
How is cost controlled?
Are there consultant services to schools and courts?
Is the public educated concerning mental illness?
What is the usual mode of care?
What is the method of treatment?
How effective is the method of treatment?
What is the method of rehabilitation?
What is socially accepted in the community?

FIGURE 16-5 Questions that can be used to assess how well a community is meeting the needs of its residents.

and bad); diagnosis; and physical, social and vocational functioning across cultural groups. Specific interventions in areas of treatment and rehabilitation will be observed and outcome studies done to assess effectiveness. Special interest areas are risk factors, complications caused by physical health problems, preventive techniques, and the risk of HIV infection. Services needed by communities and their various populations will be identified and swift referrals implemented.

Models of care management, continuous treatment teams, and the strengths and weaknesses of the community mental health centers are observed and documented. Research priorities include

- Quality of care
  Assessment
  Treatment and rehabilitation
- Financing of care
  Coordination
  Continuity
  Mental health laws
  Stigmatization
- Research
  Capacity (skilled researchers—multidisciplinary) method of knowledge exchange

We are finally facing the extraordinary, complex problem of the person with serious mental illness and focusing attention on this problem. *The Surgeon General's Report on Mental Illness* (1999) and *Healthy People 2010* are federally designed, comprehensive roadmaps to promote and improve health and prevent illness, disabilities, and premature death of all people in the United States during the first decade of the millennium. Mental health is viewed as fundamental health. It regards mental disorders as real health conditions that have an immense impact on the individual and families. By setting priorities and developing strategies based on scientific research, the care, services for, and quality of life of persons with mental illness will improve.

SUMMARY

Prevention is the ultimate goal in dealing with the problem of mental illness. Personal happiness and the ability to deal with stress are important factors in preventing mental illness. Modern society has greatly increased the stress that precipitates mental illness. Mobility, unemployment, culture, poverty, and broken homes are all stressors that add to the probability of mental illness. Primary prevention is aimed at lessening stress and improving coping mechanisms.

Prevention begins in the family. Positive family interactions are necessary for a positive self-concept. Parents cannot effectively delegate their responsibility for their children to others. Open communication between parent and child is essential. Many support services for families are available in the community. These support services include crisis counseling, hot lines, drug counseling, suicide-prevention centers, abortion and antiabortion counseling, child and family services, family service agencies, and runaway services.

Treatment facilities for the client with mental illness include outpatient services, residential treatment centers, sustaining care centers, day-treatment centers, mental health units, and mental hospitals.

Reentry into the community after mental illness is difficult because of stereotyping. Many former clients are often feared and ignored. The person reentering the community needs an adequate support system to offset these negative aspects. Families of the former client should be informed of factors that may have contributed to the problem and be advised how they can help the person cope in the future. Before reentry, the client may need some rehabilitation at an intermediate facility such as a foster home or halfway house. Referrals to special community programs should be coordinated.

SUGGESTED ACTIVITIES

■ Discuss how modern society contributes to mental health problems.

■ Make a list of stressors and acceptable ways to relieve stress within your culture.

■ View a popular television program and determine its negative and positive aspects.

■ List several ways your family has influenced your coping mechanisms.

■ Obtain a brochure of community-sponsored activities.

■ Visit a local community resource center to gather information concerning "helping agencies" within the community.

REVIEW

KNOW AND COMPREHEND
A. Multiple choice. Select the one best answer.

1. Select the goal of primary prevention of mental illness.
   ❏ A. lessening stress and developing improved coping mechanisms
   ❏ B. working with rehabilitation centers
   ❏ C. early detection and treatment of symptoms
   ❏ D. prevention through genetic counseling

2. Reentry refers to the client's
   ❏ A. return to the community.
   ❏ B. return to the hospital.
   ❏ C. return to reality.
   ❏ D. acceptance of his or her illness.

3. Select the therapeutic benefit of discussion groups for persons with mental illness who live in the community. They provide:
   ❏ A. answers in learning how to cope.
   ❏ B. a low-cost way to continue treatment.
   ❏ C. reassurance that others are in bad shape, too.
   ❏ D. support and encouragement.

4. A nurse cares for a client who speaks little English. After the second time explaining a procedure, the nurse realizes the client still does not understand the treatment. Select the nurse's next intervention.

❏ A. Explain the procedure again until the client understands.

❏ B. Seek an English-speaking member of the client's family or an interpreter for assistance.

❏ C. Discontinue the verbal interaction and begin the procedure.

❏ D. Ask another nurse to take over the care for this client.

APPLY YOUR LEARNING

B. Multiple choice. Select the one best answer.

1. A nurse helps a client make discharge plans after a three-month hospitalization for mental illness. Which resource would best support the client's successful return to the community?

❏ A. an intact support system

❏ B. a job opportunity

❏ C. a means of transportation

❏ D. emergency phone numbers

2. A nurse helps gather admission information for a newly hospitalized adult female. The client says, "I must ask my husband before any procedures are done to me." Under which section of the admission form would the nurse record this information?

❏ A. discharge planning

❏ B. legal issues

❏ C. cultural preferences

❏ D. financial needs

3. A nurse plans parenting education classes for a public housing community with high poverty rates. Which factor would be most important to consider when choosing a place for the classes?

❏ A. heating, ventilation, and air conditioning in the classroom

❏ B. means of transportation to and from the classes

❏ C. wide entrances and exits from the building

❏ D. access to video equipment and overhead projectors

4. A nurse volunteers four hours per month at a free clinic for migrant farm workers. Select the intervention which would be focused on mental health promotion.
   - ❏ A. encouraging strong family relationships
   - ❏ B. offering nutritious meals daily
   - ❏ C. scheduling religious services weekly
   - ❏ D. explaining local community health services

5. In the infirmary of a federal prison housing dangerous felons, the health care team plans topics for health education classes for the prisoners. Which topic would be most important to promote the prisoners' mental health?
   - ❏ A. "Improving Your Communication Skills"
   - ❏ B. "Exercise and Physical Fitness"
   - ❏ C. "Coping with Memories of Violence"
   - ❏ D. "How to Interview for a Job"

6. A school-age child steals $5 from a coach's wallet. The school nurse meets with the child's parents to discuss responses to the child's behavior. Which parental comment would the nurse encourage?
   - ❏ A. "We give you an allowance every week. Why did you steal money from your coach?"
   - ❏ B. "We've taught you not to steal. You may not play Little League baseball as punishment for this behavior."
   - ❏ C. "We are so embarrassed by your behavior. You will get a spanking when we get home."
   - ❏ D. "Did you offer to return the money to the coach? Maybe you would be forgiven for stealing."

C. Briefly answer the following.

1. Name the five ways that modern society contributes to mental illness.

2. Why is the parent–child relationship so important?

3. Why is it more difficult to establish identity today than it was years ago?

4. List four stressors of the poor that make them a high risk for mental illness.

5. Name four ways the family can help improve the mental health of children.

6. Why is it important to be aware of problems in the prisons and jails?

7. List four needs of the client who is returning to the community.

National Federation of Licensed Practical Nurses (NFLPN) Code for Licensed Practical/Vocational Nurses

- Know the scope of maximum utilization of the LPN/LVN as specified by the nursing practice act and function within its scope.
- Safeguard the confidential information acquired from any source about the client.
- Provide health care to all clients regardless of race, creed, cultural background, disease, or lifestyle.
- Refuse to give endorsement to the sale and promotion of commercial products or services.
- Uphold the highest standards in personal appearance, language, dress, and demeanor.
- Stay informed about issues affecting the practice of nursing and delivery of health care and, where appropriate, participate in government and policy decisions.
- Accept the responsibility for safe nursing practice by keeping oneself mentally and physically fit and educationally prepared to practice.
- Accept the responsibility for membership in NFLPN and participate in its efforts to maintain the established standards of nursing practice and employment policies that lead to quality client care.

NFLPN NURSING PRACTICE STANDARDS
Introductory Statement

Definition: Practical/Vocational nursing means the performance for compensation of authorized acts of nursing that utilize specialized knowledge and skills and that meet the health needs of people in a variety of settings under the direction of qualified health professionals.

Scope: Practical/Vocational nursing comprises the common case of nursing, and, therefore, is a valid entry into the nursing profession.

Opportunities exist for practicing in a milieu where different professions unite their particular skills in a team effort for one common objective—to preserve or improve an individual client's functioning.

Opportunities also exist for upward mobility within the profession through academic education, and for lateral expansion of knowledge and expertise through both academic and continuing education.

Standards

Education. The Licensed Practical/Vocational Nurse

1. Shall complete a formal education program in practical nursing approved by the appropriate nursing authority in a state.

2. Shall successfully pass the National Council Licensure Examination for Practical Nurses,

3. Shall participate in initial orientation within the employing institution.

Legal/Ethical Status. The Licensed Practical/Vocational Nurse

1. Shall hold a current license to practice nursing as an LPN/LVN in accordance with the law of the state wherein employed.

2. Shall know the scope of nursing practice authorized by the Nursing Practice Act in the state wherein employed.

3. Shall have a personal commitment to fulfill the legal responsibilities inherent in good nursing practice.

4. Shall take responsible actions in situations wherein there is unprofessional conduct by a peer or other health care provider.

5. Shall recognize and have a commitment to meet the ethical and moral obligations of the practice of nursing.

6. Shall not accept or perform professional responsibilities which the individual knows (s)he is not competent to perform.

Practice. The Licensed Practical/Vocational Nurse

1. Shall accept assigned responsibilities as an accountable member of the health care team.
2. Shall function within the limits of educational preparation and experience as related to the assigned duties.
3. Shall function with other members of the health care team in promoting and maintaining health, preventing disease and disability, caring for and rehabilitating individuals who are experiencing an altered health state, and contributing to the ultimate equality of life until death.
4. Shall know and utilize the nursing process in planning (assessing [data gathering]), implementing, and evaluating health services and nursing care for the individual client or group.

■ **Planning (Assessing [data gathering]):** The planning of nursing includes:

- assessment of health status of the individual client, the family and community groups.
- an analysis of the information gained from assessment
- the identification of health goals.

■ **Implementation:** The plan for nursing care is put into practice to achieve the stated goals and includes:

- observing, recording and reporting significant changes which require intervention or different goals.
- applying nursing knowledge and skills to promote and maintain health, to prevent disease and disability and to optimize functional capabilities of an individual client.

NANDA Nursing Diagnoses: 2001–2002

NANDA nursing diagnoses that are pertinent to mental health:

adjustment, impaired

anxiety

anxiety, death

attachment, risk for impaired parent/infant/child

body image, disturbed

caregiver role strain

caregiver role strain, risk for

communication, impaired verbal

conflict, decisional

conflict, parental role

confusion, acute

confusion, chronic

coping, defensive

coping, ineffective

coping, disabled family

coping, compromised family

denial, ineffective

diversional activity, deficient

falls, risk for

family processes: dysfunctional, alcoholism

family processes, interrupted

fatigue

fear

grieving, anticipatory

grieving, dysfunctional

hopelessness

identity, disturbed personal

loneliness, risk for

memory, impaired

noncompliance

nutrition: imbalanced, less than body requirements

nutrition: imbalanced, more than body requirements

pain, acute

pain, chronic

parenting, impaired

parenting, impaired, risk for

post-trauma syndrome

post-trauma syndrome, risk for

powerlessness

powerlessness, risk for

rape-trauma syndrome

rape-trauma syndrome: compound reaction

rape-trauma syndrome: silent reaction

relocation stress syndrome

relocation stress syndrome, risk for

role performance, ineffective

self-care deficit, bathing/hygiene

self-care deficit, dressing/ grooming

self-care deficit, feeding

self-care deficit, toileting

self-esteem, chronic low

self-esteem, situational low

self-esteem, risk for situational low

self-mutilation

self-mutilation, risk for

sensory perception, disturbed

sexual dysfunction

sexuality patterns, ineffective

sleep deprivation

sleep pattern, disturbed

social interaction, impaired

social isolation

sorrow, chronic

spiritual distress

spiritual distress, risk for

spiritual well being, readiness for enhanced

suicide, risk for

therapeutic regime management, effective

therapeutic regime management, ineffective

therapeutic regime management, ineffective community

therapeutic regime management, ineffective family

thought processes, disturbed

trauma, risk for

violence, risk for other-directed

violence, risk for self-directed

wandering

Adapted from North American Nursing Diagnosis Association (2001). *Nursing Diagnoses: Definitions & Classification, 2001-2002.* Philadelphia: Author.

Appendix C

DSM-IV-TR Classification

NOS = Not Otherwise Specified.

An *x* appearing in a diagnostic code indicates that a specific code number is required.

An ellipsis (. . .) is used in the names of certain disorders to indicate that the name of a specific mental disorder or general medical condition should be inserted when recording the name (e.g., 293.0 Delirium Duc to Hypothyroidism).

Numbers in parentheses are page numbers.

If criteria are currently met, one of the following severity specifiers may be noted after the diagnosis:

      Mild

      Moderate

      Severe

If criteria are no longer met, one of the following specifiers may be noted:

      In Partial Remission

      In Full Remission

      Prior History

(Reprinted with permission from *Diagnostic and Statistical Manual of Mental Disorders*, 2000.)

Disorders Usually First Diagnosed in Infancy, Childhood, or Adolescence (51)

MENTAL RETARDATION (52)
Note: These are coded on Axis II.
317 Mild Mental Retardation (52)
318.0 Moderate Mental Retardation (52)
318.1 Severe Mental Retardation (52)
318.2 Profound Mental Retardation (52)
319 Mental Retardation, Severity Unspecified (52)

LEARNING DISORDERS (53)
315.00 Reading Disorder (53)
315.1 Mathematics Disorder (53)
315.2 Disorder of Written Expression (54)
315.9 Learning Disorder NOS (54)

MOTOR SKILLS DISORDER (55)
315.4 Developmental Coordination Disorder (55)

COMMUNICATION DISORDERS (56)
315-31 Expressive Language Disorder (56)
315-32 Mixed Receptive-Expressive Language Disorder (55)
315-39 Phonological Disorder (57)
307.0 Stuttering (58)
307.9 Communication Disorder NOS (59)

PERVASIVE DEVELOPMENTAL DISORDERS (59)
299.00 Autistic Disorder (59)
299.80 Rett's Disorder (61)
299.10 Childhood Disintegrative Disorder (62)
299.80 Asperger's Disorder (63)
299.80 Pervasive Developmental Disorder NOS (64)

ATTENTION-DEFICIT AND DISRUPTIVE BEHAVIOR DISORDERS (65)
314.xx Attention-Deficit/Hyperactivity Disorder (65)
  .01 Combined Type
  .00 Predominantly Inattentive Type
  .01 Predominantly Hyperactive-Impulsive Type

314.9 Attention-Deficit/Hyperactivity Disorder NOS (67)
312.xx Conduct Disorder (68)
  .81 Childhood-Onset Type
  .82 Adolescent-Onset Type
  .89 Unspecified Onset
313.81 Oppositional Defiant Disorder (70)
312.9 Disruptive Behavior Disorder NOS (71)

FEEDING AND EATING DISORDERS OF INFANCY OR EARLY CHILDHOOD (71)
307-52 Pica (71)
307.53 Rumination Disorder (72)
307.59 Feeding Disorder of infancy or Early Childhood (72)

TIC DISORDERS (73)
307.23 Tourette's Disorder (73)
307.22 Chronic Motor or Vocal Tic Disorder (73)
307.21 Transient Tic Disorder (74)
    Specify if: Single Episode/Recurrent
307.20 Tic Disorder NOS (75)

ELIMINATION DISORDERS (75)
___.__ Encopresis (75)
787.6 With Constipation and Overflow Incontinence
307.7 Without Constipation and Overflow Incontinence
307.6 Enuresis (Not Due to a General Medical Condition) (76)
    Specify type: Nocturnal Only/Diurnal Only/Nocturnal and Diurnal

OTHER DISORDERS OF INFANCY, CHILDHOOD, OR ADOLESCENCE (76)
309.21 Separation Anxiety Disorder (76)
    Specify if: Early Onset
313.23 Selective Mutism (78)
313.89 Reactive Attachment Disorder of Infancy or Early Childhood (78)
    Specify type: Inhibited Type/Disinhibited Type
307.3 Stereotypic Movement Disorder (80)
    Specify if: With Self-Injurious Behavior

(Reprinted with permission from *Diagnosic and Statistical Manual of Mental Disorders*, 2000.)

313.9 Disorder of Infancy, Childhood, or Adolescence NOS (81)

Delirium, Dementia, and Amnestic and Other Cognitive Disorders (83)

DELIRIUM (83)

293.0 Delirium Due to . . . [Indicate the General Medical Condition] (83)

___._ Substance Intoxication Delirium (refer to Substance-Related Disorders for substance-specific codes) (84)

___._ Substance Withdrawal Delirium (refer to Substance-Related Disorders for substance-specific codes) (85)

___._ Delirium Due to Multiple Etiologies (code each of the specific etiologies) (86)

780.09 Delirium NOS (87)

DEMENTIA (88)

294.xx Dementia of the Alzheimer's Type, With Early Onset (also code 331. 0 Alzheimer's disease on Axis III) (88)

.10 Without Behavioral Disturbance

.11 With Behavioral Disturbance

294.xx Dementia of the Alzheimer's Type, With Late Onset (also code 331. 0 Alzheimer's disease on Axis III) (88)

.10 Without Behavioral Disturbance

.11 With Behavioral Disturbance

290.xx Vascular Dementia (90)

.40 Uncomplicated

.41 With Delirium

.42 With Delusions

.43 With Depressed Mood

Specify if: With Behavioral Disturbance

Code presence or absence of a behavioral disturbance in the fifth digit for Dementia Due to a General Medical Condition:

0 = Without Behavioral Disturbance

1 = With Behavioral Disturbance

294.1x Dementia Due to HIV Disease (also code 042 HIV on Axis III) (91)

294.1x Dementia Due to Head Trauma (also code 854. 00 head injury on Axis III) (91)

294.1x Dementia Due to Parkinson's Disease (also code 332. 0 Parkinson's disease on Axis III) (91)

294.1x Dementia Due to Huntington's Disease (also code 333.4 Huntington's disease on Axis III) (91)

294.1x Dementia Due to Pick's Disease (also code 331.1 Pick's disease on Axis III) (91)

294.1x Dementia Due to Creutzfeldt-Jakob Disease (also code 046.1 Creutzfeldt-Jakob disease on Axis III) (91)

294.1x Dementia Due to . . . [Indicate the General Medical Condition not listed above] (also code the general medical condition on Axis III) (91)

___._ Substance-Induced Persisting Dementia (refer to Substance-Related Disorders for substance-specific codes) (93)

___._ Dementia Due to Multiple Etiologies (code each of the specific etiologies) (94)

294.8 Dementia NOS (95)

AMNESTIC DISORDERS (95)

294.0 Amnestic Disorder Due to . . . [Indicate the General Medical Condition] (95)

Specify if: Transient/Chronic

___._ Substance-Induced Persisting Amnestic Disorder (refer to Substance-Related Disorders for substance-specific codes) (96)

294.8 Amnestic Disorder NOS (97)

OTHER COGNITIVE DISORDERS (98)

294.9 Cognitive Disorder NOS (98)

Mental Disorders Due to a General Medical Condition Not Elsewhere Classified (99)

293.89 Catatonic Disorder Due to . . . [Indicate the General Medical Condition] (101)

310.1 Personality Change Due to . . . [*Indicate the General Medical Condition*] (101) *Specify type:* Labile Type/Disinhibited Type/ Aggressive Type/Apathetic Type/ Paranoid Type/Other Type/ Combined Type/Unspecified Type

293.9 Mental Disorder NOS Due to . . . [*Indicate the General Medical Condition*] (103)

Substance-Related Disorders (105)

The following specifiers apply to Substance Dependence as noted:

ᵃ With Physiological Dependence/Without Physiological Dependence

ᵇ Early Full Remission/Early Partial Remission/Sustained Full Remission/Sustained Partial Remission

ᶜ In a Controlled Environment

ᵈ On Agonist Therapy

The following specifiers apply to Substance-Induced Disorders as noted:

ᴵWith Onset During Intoxication
ᵂWith Onset During Withdrawal

ALCOHOL-RELATED DISORDERS (119)

Alcohol Use Disorders (119)
303.90 Alcohol Dependence[a,b,c] (110)
305.00 Alcohol Abuse (114)

Alcohol-induced Disorders (119)

303.00 Alcohol Intoxication (120)
291.81 Alcohol Withdrawal (121)
    Specify if: With Perceptual Disturbances
291.0 Alcohol Intoxication Delirium (84)
291.0 Alcohol Withdrawal Delirium (85)
291.2 Alcohol-Induced Persisting Dementia (93)
291.1 Alcohol-Induced Persisting Amnestic Disorder (96)
291.x Alcohol-Induced Psychotic Disorder (163)
    .5 With Delusions[L,W]
    .3 With Hallucinations[L,W]
291.89 Alcohol-Induced Mood Disorder[L,W] (192)

291.89 Alcohol-Induced Anxiety Disorder[L,W] (224)
291.89 Alcohol-Induced Sexual Dysfunction[I] (253)
291.89 Alcohol-Induced Sleep Disorder[L,W] (278)
291.9 Alcohol-Related Disorder NOS (120)

AMPHETAMINE (OR AMPHETAMINE-LIKE)–RELATED DISORDERS (122)

Amphetamine Use Disorders (122)

304.40 Amphetamine Dependence[a,b,c] (110)
305.70 Amphetamine Abuse (114)

Amphetamine-Induced Disorders (122)

292.89 Amphetamine Intoxication (124)
    Specify if: With Perceptual Disturbances
292.0 Amphetamine Withdrawal (125)
292.81 Amphetamine Intoxication Delirium (84)
292.xx Amphetamine-Induced Psychotic Disorder (163)
    .11 With Delusions[I]
    .12 With Hallucinations[I]
292.84 Amphetamine-Induced Mood Disorder[L,W] (192)
292.89 Amphetamine-Induced Anxiety Disorder[I] (224)
292.89 Amphetamine-Induced Sexual Dysfunction[I] (253)
292.89 Amphetamine-Induced Sleep Disorder[L,W] (278)
292.9 Amphetamine-Related Disorder NOS (123)

CAFFEINE-RELATED DISORDERS (126)

Caffeine-Induced Disorders (126).

305.90 Caffeine Intoxication (126)
292.89 Caffeine-Induced Anxiety Disorder[I] (224)
292.89 Caffeine-Induced Sleep Disorder[I] (278)
292.9 Caffeine-Related Disorder NOS (126)

CANNABIS-RELATED DISORDERS (127)

Cannabis Use Disorders (127)

304.30 Cannabis Dependence[a,b,c] (110)
305.20 Cannabis Abuse (114)

(Reprinted with permission from *Diagnosis and Statistical Manual of Mental Disorders*, 2000.)

Cannabis-induced Disorders (127)

292.89 Cannabis Intoxication (128)
Specify if: With Perceptual
Disturbances

292.81 Cannabis Intoxication
Delirium (84)

292.xx Cannabis-Induced Psychotic
Disorder (163)
.11 With Delusions[I]
.12 With Hallucinations[I]

292.89 Cannabis-Induced Anxiety
Disorder[I] (224)

292.9 Cannabis-Related Disorder
NOS (128)

COCAINE-RELATED DISORDERS (129)
Cocaine Use Disorders (129)

304.20 Cocaine Dependence[a,b,c] (110)
305.60 Cocaine Abuse (114)

Cocaine-Induced Disorders (129)

292.89 Cocaine Intoxication (131)
Specify if: With Perceptual
Disturbances

292.0 Cocaine Withdrawal (132)

292.81 Cocaine Intoxication Delirium
(84)

292.xx Cocaine-Induced Psychotic
Disorder (163)
.11 With Delusions[I]
.12 With Hallucinations[I]

292.84 Cocaine-Induced Mood
Disorder[I,W] (192)

292.89 Cocaine-Induced Anxiety
Disorder[I,W] (224)

292.89 Cocaine-Induced Sexual
Dysfunction[I] (253)

Cocaine-Induced Sleep Disorder[I,W]
(278)

292.9 Cocaine-Related Disorder
NOS (130)

HALLUCINOGEN-RELATED DISORDERS (132)
Hallucinogen Use Disorders (132)

304.50 Hallucinogen Dependence[b,c]
(110)

305.30 Hallucinogen Abuse (114)

Hallucinogen-Induced Disorders (133)

292.89 Hallucinogen Intoxication (134)

292.89 Hallucinogen Persisting
Perception Disorder
(Flashbacks) (135)

292.81 Hallucinogen Intoxication
Delirium (84)

292.xx Hallucinogen-Induced
Psychotic Disorder (163)
.11 With Delusions[I]
.12 With Hallucinations[I]

292.84 Hallucinogen-Induced Mood
Disorder[I] (192)

292.89 Hallucinogen-Induced Anxiety
Disorder[I] (224)

292.9 Hallucinogen-Related Disorder
NOS (133)

INHALANT-RELATED DISORDERS (135)
Inhalant Use Disorders (135)

304.60 Inhalant Dependence[b,c] (110)
305.90 Inhalant Abuse (114)

Inhalant-Induced Disorders (136)

292.89 Inhalant Intoxication (136)

292.81 Inhalant Intoxication Delirium
(84)

292.82 Inhalant-Induced Persisting
Dementia (93)

292.xx Inhalant-Induced Psychotic
Disorder (163)
.11 With Delusions[I]
.12 With Hallucinations[I]

292.84 Inhalant-Induced Mood
Disorder[I] (192)

292.89 Inhalant-Induced Anxiety
Disorder[I] (224)

292.9 Inhalant-Related Disorder
NOS (136)

NICOTINE-RELATED DISORDERS (137)
Nicotine Use Disorder (137)

305.1 Nicotine Dependence[a,b] (110)

Nicotine-Induced Disorder (138)

292.0 Nicotine Withdrawal (138)
292.9 Nicotine-Related Disorder
NOS (138)

OPIOID-RELATED DISORDERS (139)
Opioid Use Disorders (139)

304.00 Opioid Dependence[a,b,c,d] (110)
305.50 Opioid Abuse (114)

Opioid-Induced Disorders (139)

292.89 Opioid Intoxication (140)
Specify if: With Perceptual
Disturbances

(Reprinted with permission from *Diagnosic and Statistical Manual of Mental Disorders*, 2000.)

292.0   Opioid Withdrawal (141)
292.81 Opioid Intoxication Delirium
        (84)
292.xx Opioid-Induced Psychotic
        Disorder (163)
    .11   With Delusions[I]
    .12   With Hallucinations[I]
292.84 Opioid-Induced Mood
        Disorder[I] (192)
292.89 Opioid-Induced Sexual
        Dysfunction[I] (253)
292.89 Opioid-Induced Sleep
        Disorder[I,W] (278)
292.9   Opioid-Related Disorder NOS
        (140)

**PHENCYCLIDINE (OR PHENCYCLIDINE-LIKE)–
RELATED DISORDERS (142)**
Phencyclidine Use Disorders (142)
304.60 Phencyclidine Dependence[b,c]
        (110)
305.90 Phencyclidine Abuse (114)

Phencyclidine-Induced Disorders (142)
292.89 Phencyclidine Intoxication
        (143)
        Specify if: With Perceptual
        Disturbances
292.81 Phencyclidine Intoxication
        Delirium (84)
292.xx Phencyclidine-Induced
        Psychotic Disorder (163)
    .11   With Delusions[I]
    .12   Without Hallucinations[I]
292.84 Phencyclidine-Induced Mood
        Disorder[I] (192)
292.89 Phencyclidine-Induced Anxiety
        Disorder[I] (224)
292.9   Phencyclidine-Related
        Disorder NOS (143)

**SEDATIVE-, HYPNOTIC-, OR ANXIOLYTIC-RELATED DIS-
ORDERS (144)**
Sedative-, Hypnotic-, or Anxiolytic Use Disorders (145)
304.10 Sedative-, Hypnotic, or
        Anxiolytic Dependence[a,b,c]
        (110)
305.40 Sedative-, Hypnotic, or
        Anxiolytic Abuse (114)

**Sedative-, Hypnotic-, or Anxiolytic-Induced Disorders
(145)**
292.89 Sedative-, Hypnotic, or
        Anxiolytic Intoxification (146)

292.0   Sedative-, Hypnotic, or
        Anxiolytic Withdrawal (147)
        Specify if: With Perceptual
        Disturbances
292.81 Sedative-, Hypnotic, or
        Anxiolytic Intoxication
        Delirium (84)
292.81 Sedative-, Hypnotic, or Anxio-
        Anxiolytic Withdrawal
        Delirium (85)
292.82 Sedative-, Hypnotic-, or
        Anxiolytic-Induced Persisting
        Dementia (93)
292.83 Sedative-, Hypnotic-, or
        Anxiolytic-Induced Persisting
        Amnestic Disorder (96)
292.xx Sedative-, Hypnotic-, or
        Anxiolytic-Induced Psychotic
        Disorder (163)
    .11   With Delusions[L,W]
    .12   Without Hallucinations[L,W]
292.84 Sedative-, Hypnotic-, or
        Anxiolytic-Induced Mood
        Disorder[L,W] (192)
292.89 Sedative-, Hypnotic-, or
        Anxiolytic-Induced Anxiety
        Disorder[W] (224)
292.89 Sedative-, Hypnotic-, or
        Anxiolytic-Induced Sexual
        Dysfunction[I] (253)
292.89 Sedative-, Hypnotic-, or
        Anxiolytic-Induced Sleep
        Disorder[L,W] (278)
292.9   Sedative-, Hypnotic-, or
        Anxiolytic-Related Disorder
        NOS (146)

POLYSUBSTANCE-RELATED DISORDER (148)
304.80 Polysubstance
        Dependence[a,b,c,d] (148)

**OTHER (OR UNKNOWN) SUBSTANCE-RELATED
DISORDERS (149)**
Other (or Unknown) Substance Use Disorders (149)
304.90 Other (or Unknown) Sub-
        stance Dependence[a,b,c,d] (110)
305.90 Other (or Unknown)
        Substance Abuse (114)

**Other (or Unknown) Substance-Induced Disorders
(150)**
292.89 Other (or Unknown)
        Substance Intoxication (115)
        Specify if: With Perceptual
        Disturbances

(Reprinted with permission from *Diagnosic and Statistical Manual of Mental Disorders*, 2000.)

292.0 Other (or Unknown) Substance Withdrawal (116)
Specify if: With Perceptual Disturbances

292.81 Other (or Unknown) Substance-Induced Delirium (84)

292.82 Other (or Unknown) Substance-Induced Persisting Dementia (93)

292.83 Other (or Unknown) Substance-Induced Persisting Amnestic Disorder (96)

292.xx Other (or Unknown) Substance-Induced Psychotic Disorder (163)
.11 With Delusions[L,W]
.12 With Hallucinations[L,W]

292.84 Other (or Unknown) Substance–Induced Mood Disorder[L,W] (192)

292.89 Other (or Unknown) Substance–Induced Anxiety Disorder[L,W] (224)

292.89 Other (or Unknown) Substance–Induced Sexual Dysfunction[I] (253)

292.89 Other (or Unknown) Substance–Induced Sleep Disorder[L,W] (278)

292.9 Other (or Unknown) Substance–Related Disorder NOS (150)

Schizophrenia and Other Psychotic Disorders (153)

295.xx Schizophrenia (153)
The following Classification of Longitudinal Course applies to all subtypes of Schizophrenia:

Episodic With Interepisode Residual Symptoms (*specify if:* With Prominent Negative Symptoms)/ Episodic With No Interepisode Residual Symptoms

Continuous (*specify if:* With Prominent Negative Symptoms)

Single Episode In Partial Remission (*specify if:* With Prominent Negative Symptoms)/Single Episode In Full Remission

Other or Unspecified Pattern
.30 Paranoid Type (155)
.10 Disorganized Type (155)
.20 Catatonic Type (156)
.90 Undifferentiated Type (156)
.60 Residual Type (156)

295.40 Schizophreniform Disorder (158)
Specify if: Without Good Prognostic Features/With Good Prognostic Features

295.70 Schizoaffective Disorder (159)
Specify type: Bipolar Type/ Depressive Type

297.1 Delusional Disorder (159)
Specify type: Erotomanic Type/Grandiose Type/Jealous Type/Persecutory Type/Somatic Type/Mixed Type/Unspecified Type

298.8 Brief Psychotic Disorder (161)
Specify if: With Marked Stressor(s)/Without Marked Stressor(s)/With Postpartum Onset

297.3 Shared Psychotic Disorder (162)

293.xx Psychotic Disorder Due to . . . [*Indicate the General Medical Condition*] (162)
.81 With Delusions
.82 With Hallucinations

___._ Substance-Induced Psychotic Disorder (*refer to Substance-Related Disorders for substance-specific codes*) (163)
Specify if: With Onset During Intoxication/With Onset During Withdrawal

289.9 Psychotic Disorder NOS (165)

Mood Disorder (167)

Code current state of Major Depressive Disorder or Bipolar I Disorder in fifth digit.

1 = Mild
2 = Moderate
3 = Severe Without Psychotic Features
4 = Severe With Psychotic Features
Specify: Mood-Congruent Psychotic Features/Mood-Incongruent Psychotic Features
5 = In Partial Remission
6 = In Full Remission
0 = Unspecified

(Reprinted with permission from *Diagnosic and Statistical Manual of Mental Disorders*, 2000.)

The following specifiers apply (for current or most recent episode) to Mood Disorders as noted:

[a]Severity/Psychotic/Remission Specifiers/ [b]Chronic/ [c]With Catatonic Features/ [d]With Melancholic Features/ [e]With Atypical Features/ [f]With Postpartum Onset

The following specifiers apply to Mood Disorders as noted:

[g] With or Without Full Interepisode Recovery/ [h]With Seasonal Pattern/ [i]With Rapid Cycling

DEPRESSIVE DISORDERS (173)

296.xx Major Depressive Disorder (173)
   .2x Single Episode[a,b,c,d,e,f]
   .3x Recurrent[a,b,c,d,e,f,g,h]
300.4 Dysthymic Disorder (176)
   Specify if: Early Onset/Late Onset
   Specify: With Atypical Features
311 Depressive Disorder NOS (178)

BIPOLAR DISORDERS (179)

296.xx Bipolar I Disorder, (180)
   .0x Single Manic Episode[a,c,f] (173)
   Specify if: Mixed
   .40 Most Recent Episode Hypomanic[g,h,i]
   .4x Most Recent Episode Manic[a,c,f,g,h,i]
   .6x Most Recent Episode Mixed[a,c,f,g,h,i]
   .5x Most Recent Episode Depressed[a,b,c,d,e,f,g,h,i]
   .7 Most Recent Episode Unspecified[g,h,i]
296.89 Bipolar II Disorder[a,b,c,d,e,f,g,h,i] (187)
   Specify (current or most recent episode): Hypomanic/Depressed
301.13 Cyclothymic Disorder (189)
296.80 Bipolar Disorder NOS (190)
293.83 Mood Disorder Due to . . . [*Indicate the General Medical Condition*] (191)
   Specify type: With Depressive Features/With Major Depressive–

Like Episode/With Manic Features/With Mixed Features
___.___ Substance-Induced Mood Disorder (*refer to Substance-Related Disorders for substance-specific codes*) (192)
   Specify type: With Depressive Features/With Manic Features/With Mixed Features
   Specify if: With Onset During Intoxication/With Onset During Withdrawal
Mood Disorder NOS (195)

Anxiety Disorders (209)

300.01 Panic Disorder Without Agoraphobia (211)
300.21 Panic Disorder With Agoraphobia (212)
300.22 Agoraphobia Without History of Panic Disorder (213)
300.29 Specific Phobia (213)
   Specify type: Animal Type/Natural Environment Type/Blood-Injection-Injury Type/Situational Type/Other Type
300.23 Social Phobia (215)
   Specify if: Generalized
300.3 Obsessive-Compulsive Disorder (217)
   Specify if: With Poor Insight
309.81 Posttraumatic Stress Disorder (209)
   Specify if: Acute/Chronic
   Specify if: With Delayed Onset
308.3 Acute Stress Disorder (221)
300.02 Generalized Anxiety Disorder (222)
293.84 Anxiety Disorder Due to . . . [*Indicate the General Medical Condition*] (223)
   Specify if: With Generalized Anxiety/With Panic Attacks/With Obsessive-Compulsive Symptoms
___.___ Substance-Induced Anxiety Disorder (*refer to Substance-Related Disorders for substance-specific codes*) (224)
   Specify if: With Generalized Anxiety/With Panic Attacks/With Obsessive-Compulsive Symptoms/With Phobic Symptoms
   Specify if: With Onset During

(Reprinted with permission from *Diagnosic and Statistical Manual of Mental Disorders*, 2000.)

Intoxication/With Onset During
Withdrawal
300.00 Anxiety Disorder NOS (226)

Somatoform Disorders (229)

300.81 Somatization Disorder (229)
300.82 Undifferentiated Somatoform
Disorder (230)
300.11 Conversion Disorder (231)
Specify type: With Motor Symptom
or Deficit/With Sensory Symptom
or Deficit/With Seizures or
Convulsions/With Mixed
Presentation
307.xx Pain Disorder (232)
.80 Associated With Psychological
Factors
.89 Associated With Both
Psychological Factors and a
General Medical Condition
Specify if: Acute/Chronic
300.7 Hypochondriasis (234)
Specify if: With Poor Insight
300.7 Body Dysmorphic Disorder
(235)
300.82 Somatoform Disorder NOS
(236)

Factitious Disorders (237)

300.xx Factitious Disorder (237)
.16 With Predominantly
Psychological Signs and
Symptoms
.19 With Predominantly
Physical Signs and
Symptoms
.19 With Combined
Psychological and Physical
Signs and Symptoms
300.19 Factitious Disorder NOS
(228)

Dissociative Disorders (239)

300.12 Dissociative Amnesia (239)
300.13 Dissociative Fugue (240)
300.14 Dissociative Identity Disorder
(240)
300.6 Depersonalization Disorder
(241)
300-15 Dissociative Disorder NOS
(242)

Sexual and Gender Identity Disorders (245)

SEXUAL DYSFUNCTIONS (245)
*The following specifiers apply to all
primary Sexual Dysfunctions:*

Lifelong Type/Acquired Type
Generalized Type/Situational Type
Due to Psychological Factors/Due
to Combined Factors

Sexual Desire Disorders (245)
302.71 Hypoactive Sexual Desire
Disorder (245)
302.79 Sexual Aversion Disorder
(246)

Sexual Arousal Disorders (246)
302.72 Female Sexual Arousal
Disorder (246)
302.72 Male Erectile Disorder (247)

Orgasmic Disorders (247)
302.73 Female Orgasmic Disorder
(247)
302.74 Male Orgasmic Disorder (248)
302.75 Premature Ejaculation (249)

Sexual Pain Disorders (249)
302.76 Dyspareunia (Not Due to a
General Medical Condition)
(249)
306.51 Vaginismus (Not Due to a
General Medical Condition)
(250)

Sexual Dysfunction Due to a General Medical Condition (252)
625.8 Female Hypoactive Sexual
Desire Disorder Due to . . .
*[Indicate the General Medical
Condition]* (252)
608.89 Male Hypoactive Sexual Desire
Disorder Due to . . . *[Indicate the
General Medical Condition]* (252)
607.84 Male Erectile Disorder Due to
. . . *[Indicate the General Medical
Condition]* (252)
625.0 Female Dyspareunia Due to . . .
*[Indicate the General Medical
Condition]* (252)

(Reprinted with permission from *Diagnosic and Statistical Manual of Mental Disorders*, 2000.)

608.89 Male Dyspareunia Due to . . .
[*Indicate the General Medical Condition*] (252)

625.8 Other Female Sexual Dysfunction Due to . . .
[*Indicate the General Medical Condition*] (252)

608.89 Other Male Sexual Dysfunction Due to . . .
[*Indicate the General Medical Condition*] (252)

___.__ Substance-Induced Sexual Dysfunction (*refer to Substance-Related Disorders for substance-specific codes*) (253)
Specify if: With Impaired Desire/With Impaired Arousal/With Impaired Orgasm/With Sexual Pain
Specify if: With Onset During Intoxication

302.70 Sexual Dysfunction NOS (255)

PARAPHILIAS (255)

302.4 Exhibitionism (255)
302.81 Fetishism (256)
302.89 Frotteurism (256)
302.2 Pedophilia (256)
Specify if: Sexually Attracted to Males/Sexually Attracted to Females/Sexually Attracted to Both
Specify if: Limited to Incest
Specify type: Exclusive Type/Nonexclusive Type

302.83 Sexual Masochism (257)
302.84 Sexual Sadism (258)
302.3 Transvestic Fetishism (258)
Specify if: With Gender Dysphoria

302.82 Voyeurism (258)
302.9 Paraphilia NOS (259)

GENDER IDENTITY DISORDERS (259)

302.xx Gender Identity Disorder (259)
.6 in Children
.85 in Adolescents or Adults
Specify if: Sexually Attracted to Males/Sexually Attracted to Females/Sexually Attracted to Both/Sexually Attracted to Neither

302.6 Gender Identity Disorder NOS (261)
302.9 Sexual Disorder NOS (262)

Eating Disorders (263)

307.1 Anorexia Nervosa (263)
Specify type: Restricting Type: Binge-Eating/Purging Type

307.51 Bulimia Nervosa (264)
Specify type: Purging Type/Nonpurging Type

307.50 Eating Disorder NOS (265)

Sleep Disorders (267)

PRIMARY SLEEP DISORDERS (267)

Dyssomnias (267)

307.42 Primary Insomnia (267)
307.44 Primary Hypersomnia (268)
Specify if: Recurrent

347 Narcolepsy (269)
780.59 Breathing-Related Sleep Disorder (269)
307.45 Circadian Rhythm Sleep Disorder (270)
Specify type: Delayed Sleep Phase Type/Jet Lag Type/Shift Work Type/Unspecified Type

307.47 Dyssomnia NOS (271)

Parasomnias (272)

307.47 Nightmare Disorder (272)
307.46 Sleep Terror Disorder (273)
307.46 Sleepwalking Disorder (273)
307.47 Parasomnia NOS (274)

SLEEP DISORDERS RELATED TO ANOTHER MENTAL DISORDER (275)

307.42 Insomnia Related to . . .
[*Indicate the Axis I or Axis II Disorder*] (275)

307.44 Hypersomnia Related to . . .
[*Indicate the Axis I or Axis II Disorder*] (276)

OTHER SLEEP DISORDERS (277)

780.xx Sleep Disorder Due to . . .
[*Indicate the General Medical Condition*] (277)
.52 Insomnia Type
.54 Hypersomnia Type
.59 Parasomnia Type
.59 Mixed Type

___.__ Substance-Induced Sleep Disorder (*refer to Substance-Related Disorders for substance-specific codes*) (278)

(Reprinted with permission from *Diagnosic and Statistical Manual of Mental Disorders,* 2000.)

Specify type: Insomnia
Type/Hypersomnia
Type/Parasomnia Type/Mixed Type
Specify if: With Onset During
Intoxication/With Onset During
Withdrawal

Impulse-Control Disorders Not Elsewhere Classified (281)

312.34 Intermittent Explosive
Disorder (281)
312.32 Kleptomania (282)
312.33 Pyromania (282)
312.31 Pathological Gambling (283)
312.39 Trichotillomania (284)
312-30 Impulse-Control Disorder
NOS (284)

Adjustment Disorders (285)

309.xx Adjustment Disorder (285)
.0   With Depressed Mood
.24   With Anxiety
.28   With Mixed Anxiety and
Depressed Mood
.3   With Disturbance of Conduct
.4   With Mixed Disturbance of
Emotions and Conduct
.9   Unspecified
Specify if: Acute/Chronic

Personality Disorders (287)

Note: These are coded on Axis II.
301.0   Paranoid Personality Disorder
(288)
301.20 Schizoid Personality Disorder
(289)
301.22 Schizotypal Personality
Disorder (290)
301.7   Antisocial Personality Disorder
(291)
301.83 Borderline Personality
Disorder (292)
301-50 Histrionic Personality Disorder
(293)
301.81 Narcissistic Personality
Disorder (294)
301.82 Avoidant Personality Disorder
(295)
301.6   Dependent Personality
Disorder (295)

301.4   Obsessive-Compulsive
Personality Disorder (296)
301.9   Personality Disorder NOS
(297)

Other Conditions That May Be a Focus of Clinical Attention (299)

PSYCHOLOGICAL FACTORS AFFECTING MEDICAL CONDITION (300)

316   . . . *[Specified Psychological Factor]*
Affecting . . . *[Indicate the General
Medical Condition]* (300) *Choose
name based on nature of factors:*
Mental Disorder Affecting
Medical Condition

Psychological Symptoms
Affecting Medical Condition

Personality Traits or Coping
Style Affecting Medical
Condition

Maladaptive Health Behaviors
Affecting Medical Condition

Stress-Related Physiological
Response Affecting Medical
Condition

Other or Unspecified
Psychological Factors Affecting
Medical Condition

MEDICATION-INDUCED MOVEMENT DISORDERS (289)

332.1   Neuroleptic-Induced
Parkinsonism (302)
333.92 Neuroleptic Malignant
Syndrome (302)
333.7   Neuroleptic-Induced Acute
Dystonia (303)
333.99 Neuroleptic-Induced Acute
Akathisia (303)
333.82 Neuroleptic-Induced Tardive
Dyskinesia (303)
333.1   Medication-Induced Postural
Tremor (304)
333-90 Medication-Induced
Movement Disorder NOS
(304)

OTHER MEDICATION-INDUCED DISORDER (304)

995.2   Adverse Effects of Medication
NOS (304)

(Reprinted with permission from *Diagnosic and Statistical Manual of Mental Disorders, 2000.*)

RELATIONAL PROBLEMS (305)

V61.9 Relational Problem Related to a Mental Disorder or General Medical Condition (305)

V61.20 Parent-Child Relational Problem (306)

V61.10 Partner Relational Problem (306)

V61.8 Sibling Relational Problem (306)

V62.81 Relational Problem NOS (306)

PROBLEMS RELATED TO ABUSE OR NEGLECT (307)

V61.21 Physical Abuse of Child (307)
       (*code 995.54 if focus of attention is on victim*)

V61.21 Sexual Abuse of Child (307)
       (*code 995.53 if focus of attention is on victim*)

V61.21 Neglect of Child (308)
       (*code 995.52 if focus of attention is on victim*)

___.___ Physical Abuse of Adult (308)

V61.12 (if by partner)

V62.83 (if by person other than partner)
       (*code 995.81 if focus of attention is on victim*)

___.___ Sexual Abuse of Adult (308)

V61.12 (if by partner)

V62.83 (if by person other than partner)
       (*code 995.83 if focus of attention is on victim*)

ADDITIONAL CONDITIONS THAT MAY BE A FOCUS OF CLINICAL ATTENTION (309)

V15.81 Noncompliance With Treatment (309)

V65.2 Malingering (309)

V71.01 Adult Antisocial Behavior (310)

V71.02 Child or Adolescent Antisocial Behavior (310)

V62.89 Borderline Intellectual Functioning (311)
       Note: This is coded on Axis II.

780.9 Age-Related Cognitive Decline (311)

V62.82 Bereavement (311)

V62.3 Academic Problem (312)

V62.2 Occupational Problem (313)

313.82 Identity Problem (313)

V62.89 Religious or Spiritual Problem (313)

V62.4 Acculturation Problem (313)

V62.89 Phase of Life Problem (313)

Additional Codes (315)

300.9 Unspecified Mental Disorder (nonpsychotic) (315)

V71.09 No Diagnosis or Condition on Axis I (315)

799.9 Diagnosis or Condition Deferred on Axis I (316)

V71.09 No Diagnosis on Axis II (316)

799.9 Diagnosis Deferred on Axis II (316)

Multiaxial System

Axis I Clinical Disorders
        Other Conditions That May Be a Focus of Clinical Attention

Axis II Personality Disorders
         Mental Retardation

Axis III General Medical Conditions

Axis IV Psychosocial and Environmental Problems

Axis V Global Assessment of Functioning

(Reprinted with permission from *Diagnosic and Statistical Manual of Mental Disorders*, 2000.)

Appendix D

Minimum Data Set (MDS)— Version 2.0

The following Material Data Set (MDS) is reprinted with permission of Briggs Corporation, Des Moines, IA 50306. (800) 247-2343.

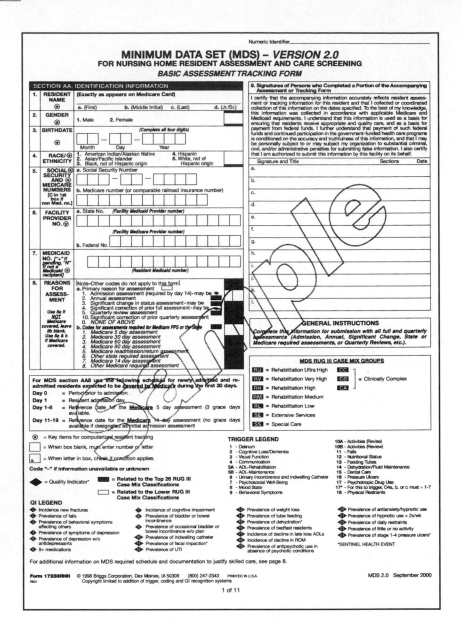

Resident _____   Numeric Identifier _____

MINIMUM DATA SET (MDS) – *VERSION 2.0*
FOR NURSING HOME RESIDENT ASSESSMENT AND CARE SCREENING
BACKGROUND (FACE SHEET) INFORMATION AT ADMISSION

SECTION AB. DEMOGRAPHIC INFORMATION

1. DATE OF ENTRY — Date the stay began. Note – Does not include readmission if record was closed at time of temporary discharge to hospital, etc. In such cases, use prior admission date.

Do NOT change this date on readmission

☐☐ — ☐☐ — ☐☐☐☐
Month   Day   Year

2. ADMITTED FROM (AT ENTRY)
1. Private home/apt. with no home health services
2. Private home/apt. with home health services
3. Board and care/assisted living/group home
4. Nursing home
5. Acute care hospital   *(Not SNF unit of acute care hospital)*
6. Psychiatric hospital, MR/DD facility
7. Rehabilitation hospital
8. Other

3. LIVED ALONE (PRIOR TO ENTRY)   0. No   1. Yes   2. In other facility

4. ZIP CODE OF PRIOR PRIMARY RESIDENCE   ☐☐☐☐☐

5. RESIDEN-TIAL HISTORY 5 YEARS PRIOR TO ENTRY   *(Check all settings resident lived in during 5 years prior to date of entry given in item AB1 above.)*
Prior stay at this nursing home	a.
Stay in other nursing home	b.
Other residential facility – board and care home, assisted living, group home	c.
MH/psychiatric setting	d.
MR/DD setting	e.
NONE OF ABOVE	f.

6. LIFETIME OCCUPA-TION(S) *(Put "/" between two occupations)*

7. EDUCATION *(Highest level completed)*
1. No schooling   5. Technical or trade school
2. 8th grade/less   6. Some college
3. 9-11 grades   7. Bachelor's degree
4. High School   8. Graduate degree

8. LANGUAGE *(Code for correct response)*
a. Primary Language
0. English   1. Spanish   2. French   3. Other
b. If other, specify

9. MENTAL HEALTH HISTORY — Does resident's RECORD indicate any history of mental retardation, mental illness, or developmental disability problem?   0/ No   1. Yes

10. CONDITIONS RELATED TO MR/DD STATUS — *Check all conditions that are related to MR/DD status that were manifested before age 22, and are likely to continue indefinitely.*
Not applicable – no MR/DD (Skip to AB11)	a.
MR/DD with organic condition	
Down's syndrome	b.
Autism	c.
Epilepsy	d.
Other organic condition related to MR/DD	e.
MR/DD with no organic condition	f.

11. DATE BACK-GROUND INFORMA-TION COMPLETED   *(This date must NOT be earlier than date of entry)*
☐☐ — ☐☐ — ☐☐☐☐
Month   Day   Year

SECTION AC. CUSTOMARY ROUTINE

1. CUSTOMARY ROUTINE *(Check all that apply. If all information UNKNOWN, check last box only.)*

(In year prior to this nursing home, or year last in community if now being admitted from another nursing home)

Review for possible care plan approaches

CYCLE OF DAILY EVENTS
Stays up late at night (e.g., after 9 pm)	a.
Naps regularly during day (at least 1 hour)	b.
Goes out 1+ days a week	c.
Stays busy with hobbies, reading, or fixed daily routine	d.
Spends most of time alone or watching TV	e.
Moves independently indoors (with appliances, if used)	f.
Use of tobacco products at least daily	g.
NONE OF ABOVE	h.

EATING PATTERNS
Distinct food preferences	i.
Eats between meals all or most days	j.
Use of alcoholic beverage(s) at least weekly	k.
NONE OF ABOVE	l.

ADL PATTERNS
In bedclothes much of day	m.
Wakens to toilet all or most nights	n.
Has irregular bowel movement pattern	o.
Showers for bathing	p.
Bathing in PM	q.
NONE OF ABOVE	r.

INVOLVEMENT PATTERNS
Daily contact with relatives/close friends	s.
Usually attends church, temple, synagogue (etc.)	t.
Finds strength in faith	u.
Daily animal companion/presence	v.
Involved in group activities	w.
NONE OF ABOVE	x.
UNKNOWN – Resident/family unable to provide information	y.

END

SECTION AD. FACE SHEET SIGNATURES

SIGNATURES OF PERSONS COMPLETING FACE SHEET:

a. Signature of RN Assessment Coordinator _____ Date ____

I certify that the accompanying information accurately reflects resident assessment or tracking information for this resident and that I collected or coordinated collection of this information on the dates specified. To the best of my knowledge, this information was collected in accordance with applicable Medicare and Medicaid requirements. I understand that this information is used as a basis for ensuring that residents receive appropriate and quality care, and as a basis for payment from federal funds. I further understand that payment of such federal funds and continued participation in the government-funded health care programs is conditioned on the accuracy and truthfulness of this information, and that I may be personally subject to or may subject my organization to substantial criminal, civil, and/or administrative penalties for submitting false information. I also certify that I am authorized to submit this information by this facility on its behalf.

Signature and Title	Sections	Date
b.		
c.		
d.		
e.		
f.		
g.		

☐ = When box blank, must enter number or letter

a. = When letter in box, check if condition applies

Code "-" if information unavailable or unknown

NOTE: Normally, the MDS Face Sheet is completed once, when an individual first enters the facility. However, the face sheet is also required if the person is readmitted to the facility after a discharge where return had not previously been expected. It is not completed following temporary discharges to hospitals or after therapeutic leaves/home visits.

Form 17233RHH   © 1998 Briggs Corporation, Des Moines, IA 50306   (800) 247-2343   PRINTED IN U.S.A.
Copyright limited to addition of trigger, coding and QI recognition systems

MDS 2.0   September 2000

2 of 11

Resident _____   Numeric Identifier _____

MINIMUM DATA SET (MDS) – VERSION 2.0
FOR NURSING HOME RESIDENT ASSESSMENT AND CARE SCREENING
FULL ASSESSMENT FORM
(Status in last 7 days, unless other time frame indicated)

SECTION A. IDENTIFICATION AND BACKGROUND INFORMATION

1. RESIDENT NAME (Exactly as appears on Medicare Card)

a. (First)   b. (Middle Initial)   c. (Last)   d. (Jr./Sr.)

2. ROOM NUMBER

3. ASSESSMENT REFERENCE DATE
a. Last day of MDS observation period

Month — Day — Year

b. Original (0) or corrected copy of form (enter number of correction)

4a. DATE OF REENTRY Date of reentry from most recent temporary discharge to a hospital in last 90 days (or since last assessment or admission if less than 90 days)

Month — Day — Year

5. MARITAL STATUS
1. Never married   3. Widowed   5. Divorced
2. Married   4. Separated

6. MEDICAL RECORD NO.

7. CURRENT PAYMENT SOURCES FOR N.H. STAY (Billing Office to indicate; check all that apply in last 30 days)
- Medicaid per diem a.
- Medicare per diem b.
- Medicare ancillary part A c.
- Medicare ancillary part B d.
- CHAMPUS per diem e.
- VA per diem f.
- Self or family pays for full per diem g.
- Medicaid resident liability or Medicare co-payment h.
- Private insurance per diem (including co-payment) i.
- Other per diem j.

8. REASONS FOR ASSESSMENT
[Note—If this is a discharge or reentry assessment, only a limited subset of MDS items need be completed]

See Section AA8 for explanation

a. Primary reason for assessment
1. Admission assessment (required by day 14)—may be
2. Annual assessment
3. Significant change in status assessment—may be
4. Significant correction of prior full assessment—may be
5. Quarterly review assessment
6. Discharged—return not anticipated
7. Discharged—return anticipated
8. Discharged prior to completing initial assessment
9. Reentry
10. Significant correction of prior quarterly assessment
0. NONE OF ABOVE
b. Codes for assessments required for Medicare PPS or the State
1. Medicare 5 day assessment
2. Medicare 30 day assessment
3. Medicare 60 day assessment
4. Medicare 90 day assessment
5. Medicare readmission/return assessment
6. Other state required assessment
7. Medicare 14 day assessment
8. Other Medicare required assessment

9. RESPONSIBILITY/ LEGAL GUARDIAN (Check all that apply)
- Legal guardian a.
- Other legal oversight b.
- Durable power of attorney/health care c.
- Durable power of attorney/ financial d.
- Family member responsible e.
- Patient responsible for self f.
- NONE OF ABOVE g.

10. ADVANCED DIRECTIVES (For those items with supporting documentation in the medical record, check all that apply)
- Living will a.
- Do not resuscitate b.
- Do not hospitalize c.
- Organ donation d.
- Autopsy request e.
- Feeding restrictions f.
- Medication restrictions g.
- Other treatment restrictions h.
- NONE OF ABOVE i.

SECTION B. COGNITIVE PATTERNS

1. COMATOSE (Persistent vegetative state/no discernible consciousness)
1 = CC   0. No   O4b   1. Yes (If yes, skip to Section G)

2. MEMORY (Recall of what was learned or known)
a1 = B / A   a. Short-term memory OK—seems/appears to recall after 5 minutes
0. Memory OK   1. Memory problem 2
a1 = C7   b. Long-term memory OK—seems/appears to recall long past
0. Memory OK   1. Memory problem 2

3. MEMORY/RECALL ABILITY (Check all that resident was normally able to recall during last 7 days)
- Current season a.
- Location of own room b.
- Staff names/faces c.
- That he/she is in a nursing home d.
- NONE OF ABOVE are recalled

4. COGNITIVE SKILLS FOR DAILY DECISION-MAKING (Made decisions regarding tasks of daily living) 1,2,3 = O
0. INDEPENDENT–decisions consistent/reasonable
1. MODIFIED INDEPENDENCE–some difficulty in new situations only 2
2. MODERATELY IMPAIRED–decisions poor; cues/ supervision required 2
2,3= B / A
3. SEVERELY IMPAIRED–never/rarely made decisions 2, 5B

5. INDICATORS OF DELIRIUM– PERIODIC DISORDERED THINKING/ AWARENESS (Code for behavior in the last 7 days.) [Note: Accurate assessment requires conversations with staff and family who have direct knowledge of resident's behavior over this time.]
0. Behavior not present
1. Behavior present, not of recent onset
2. Behavior present, over last 7 days appears different from resident's usual functioning (e.g., new onset or worsening)

a. EASILY DISTRACTED–(e.g., difficulty paying attention; gets sidetracked) 2 = 1, 17*
b. PERIODS OF ALTERED PERCEPTION OR AWARENESS OF SURROUNDINGS–(e.g., moves lips or talks to someone not present; believes he/she is somewhere else; confuses night and day) 2 = 1, 17*
c. EPISODES OF DISORGANIZED SPEECH–(e.g., speech is incoherent, nonsensical, irrelevant, or rambling from subject to subject; loses train of thought) 2 = 1, 17*
d. PERIODS OF RESTLESSNESS–(e.g., fidgeting or picking at skin, clothing, napkins, etc.; frequent position changes; repetitive physical movements or calling out) 2 = 1, 17*
e. PERIODS OF LETHARGY–(e.g., sluggishness; staring into space; difficult to arouse; little body movement) 2 = 1, 17*
f. MENTAL FUNCTION VARIES OVER THE COURSE OF THE DAY–(e.g., sometimes better, sometimes worse; behaviors sometimes present, sometimes not) 2 = 1, 17*

6. CHANGE IN COGNITIVE STATUS Resident's cognitive status, skills, or abilities have changed as compared to status of 90 days ago (or since assessment if less than 90 days)
0. No change   1. Improved   2. Deteriorated 1, 17*

SECTION C. COMMUNICATION/HEARING PATTERNS

1. HEARING (With hearing appliance, if used)
0. HEARS ADEQUATELY–normal talk, TV, phone
1. MINIMAL DIFFICULTY when not in quiet setting 4
2. HEARS IN SPECIAL SITUATIONS ONLY–speaker has to adjust tonal quality and speak distinctly 4
3. HIGHLY IMPAIRED/absence of useful hearing 4

2. COMMUNICATION DEVICES/ TECHNIQUES (Check all that apply during last 7 days)
- Hearing aid, present and used a.
- Hearing aid, present and not used regularly b.
- Other receptive comm. techniques used (e.g., lip reading) c.
- NONE OF ABOVE d.

3. MODES OF EXPRESSION (Check all used by resident to make needs known)
- Speech a.
- Writing messages to express or clarify needs b.
- American sign language or Braille c.
- Signs/gestures/sounds d.
- Communication board e.
- Other f.
- NONE OF ABOVE

4. MAKING SELF UNDERSTOOD (Expressing information content–however able)
0. UNDERSTOOD
1. USUALLY UNDERSTOOD–difficulty finding words or finishing thoughts 4
2. SOMETIMES UNDERSTOOD–ability is limited to making concrete requests 4
2,3= B / A
3. RARELY/NEVER UNDERSTOOD 4

5. SPEECH CLARITY (Code for speech in the last 7 days)
0. CLEAR SPEECH–distinct, intelligible words
1. UNCLEAR SPEECH–slurred, mumbled words
2. NO SPEECH–absence of spoken words

6. ABILITY TO UNDERSTAND OTHERS (Understanding verbal information content–however able)
0. UNDERSTANDS
1. USUALLY UNDERSTANDS–may miss some part/ intent of message 2, 4
2. SOMETIMES UNDERSTANDS–responds adequately to simple, direct communication 2, 4
3. RARELY/NEVER UNDERSTANDS 2, 4

7. CHANGE IN COMMUNICATION/ HEARING Resident's ability to express, understand, or hear information has changed as compared to status of 90 days ago (or since last assessment if less than 90 days)
0. No change   1. Improved   2. Deteriorated 17*

= Quality Indicator*

TRIGGER LEGEND
1 - Delirium
2 - Cognitive Loss/Dementia
4 - Communication
5B - ADL Maintenance
17* - Psychotropic Drugs
(For this to trigger, O4a, b, or c must = 1-7)

☐ = When box blank, must enter number or letter.   ■ = Related to the Top 26 RUG III Case Mix Classifications
a = When letter in box, check if condition applies   ☐ = Related to the Lower RUG III Case Mix Classifications
Code "–" if information unavailable or unknown

Form 17233RHH   © 1998 Briggs Corporation, Des Moines, IA 50306   (800) 247-2343   PRINTED IN U.S.A.
Copyright limited to addition of trigger, coding and QI recognition systems

MDS 2.0 September 2000

3 of 11

(Reprinted with permission of Briggs Corporation, Des Moines, IA 50306. (800) 247-2343)

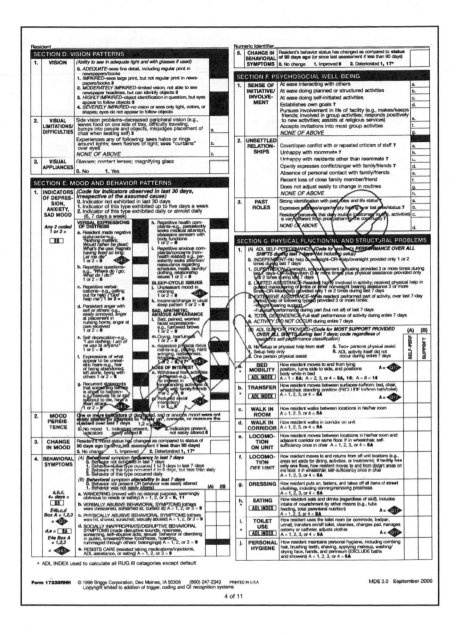

Form 17233RHH   © 1998 Briggs Corporation, Des Moines, IA 50306   (800) 247-2343   PRINTED IN U.S.A.
Copyright limited to addition of trigger, coding and QI recognition systems

MDS 2.0   September 2000

Resident _____ Numeric Identifier _____

| 2. | BATHING | How resident takes full-body bath/shower, sponge bath, and transfers in/out of tub/shower (EXCLUDE washing of back and hair). Code for most dependent in self-performance and support. A = 1, 2, 3 or 4 = **5A** (A) BATHING SELF-PERFORMANCE codes appear below. 0. Independent–No help provided 1. Supervision–Oversight help only 2. Physical help limited to transfer only 3. Physical help in part of bathing activity 4. Total dependence 8. Activity itself did not occur during entire 7 days (Bathing support codes are as defined in Item 1, code B above) | (A) (B) |

3.	TEST FOR BALANCE (See training manual)	(Code for ability during test in the last 7 days) 0. Maintained position as required in test 1. Unsteady, but able to rebalance self without physical support 2. Partial physical support during test; or stands (sits) but does not follow directions for test 3. Not able to attempt test without physical help	
		a. Balance while standing	
		b. Balance while sitting–position, trunk control 1, 2, or 3 = 17*	

4.	FUNCTIONAL LIMITATION IN RANGE OF MOTION (see training manual) ↑ Loss a-f = 0 but sum of a-f is <12 = **O16**	(Code for limitations during last 7 days that interfered with daily functions or placed resident at risk of injury) (A) RANGE OF MOTION (B) VOLUNTARY MOVEMENT 0. No limitation 0. No loss 1. Limitation on one side 1. Partial loss 2. Limitation on both sides 2. Full loss (A) (B)	
		a. Neck	
		b. Arm–Including shoulder or elbow	
		c. Hand–Including wrist or fingers	
		d. Leg–Including hip or knee	
		e. Foot–Including ankle or toes	
		f. Other limitation or loss	

5.	MODES OF LOCOMO-TION	(Check all that apply during last 7 days)	
		Cane/walker/crutch a.	Wheelchair primary mode of locomotion d.
		Wheeled self b.	
		Other person wheeled c.	NONE OF ABOVE e.

6.	MODES OF TRANSFER # = **O18** Transfer Included in ADL Index	(Check all that apply during last 7 days)	
		Bedfast all or most of time 16 a.	Lifted mechanically d.
		Bed rails used for bed mobility or transfer b.	Transfer aid (e.g., slide board, trapeze, cane, walker, brace) e.
		Lifted manually c.	NONE OF ABOVE f.

| 7. | TASK SEGMEN-TATION | Some or all of ADL activities were broken into subtasks during last 7 days so that resident could perform them 0. No 1. Yes | |

8.	ADL FUNCTIONAL REHABILITA-TION POTENTIAL	Resident believes he/she is capable of increased independence in at least some ADLs **5A**	a.
		Direct care staff believe resident is capable of increased independence in at least some ADLs **5A**	b.
		Resident able to perform tasks/activity but is very slow	c.
		Difference in ADL Self-Performance or ADL Support, comparing mornings to evenings	d.
		NONE OF ABOVE	e.

| 9. | CHANGE IN ADL FUNCTION | Resident's ADL self-performance status has changed as compared to status of 90 days ago (or since last assessment if less than 90 days) 0. No change 1. Improved 2. Deteriorated | |

SECTION H. CONTINENCE IN LAST 14 DAYS

1.	CONTINENCE SELF-CONTROL CATEGORIES (Code for resident's PERFORMANCE OVER ALL SHIFTS) 0. CONTINENT–Complete control (includes use of indwelling urinary catheter or ostomy device that does not leak urine or stool) 1. USUALLY CONTINENT–BLADDER, incontinent episodes once a week or less; BOWEL, less than weekly 2. OCCASIONALLY INCONTINENT–BLADDER, 2 or more times a week but not daily; BOWEL, once a week 3. FREQUENTLY INCONTINENT–BLADDER, tended to be incontinent daily, but some control present (e.g., on day shift); BOWEL, 2-3 times a week 4. INCONTINENT–Had inadequate control. BLADDER, multiple daily episodes; BOWEL, all (or almost all) of the time		
a.	BOWEL CONTI-NENCE	Control of bowel movement, with appliance or bowel continence programs, if employed 1, 2, 3 or 4 = **16** 3,4 = **O6** 2,3 = **O9**	
b.	BLADDER CONTI-NENCE	Control of urinary bladder function (if dribbles, volume insufficient to soak through underpants, with appliances (e.g., foley) or continence programs, if employed 2, 3 or 4 = **6** 3,4 = **O6** 2,3 = **O9**	
c.	BOWEL ELIMIN-ATION PATTERN	Bowel elimination pattern regular–at least one movement every three days a.	Diarrhea c.
			Fecal impaction 17* **O11** d.
		Constipation 17* b.	NONE OF ABOVE e.

3.	APPLIANCES AND PROGRAMS a,b, no? /2 = **O5**	Any scheduled toileting plan a.	Did not use toilet room/commode/urinal f.
		Bladder retraining program b.	Pads/briefs used 6 g.
		External (condom) catheter 6 c.	Enemas/irrigation h.
	*	Indwelling catheter 6 **O16** d.	Ostomy present i.
	*	Intermittent catheter 6 e.	NONE OF ABOVE

| 4. | CHANGE IN URINARY CONTI-NENCE | Resident's urinary continence has changed as compared to status of 90 days ago (or since last assessment if less than 90 days) 0. No change 1. Improved 2. Deteriorated | |

* H3 a & b included in Nursing Rehab calculation

SECTION I. DISEASE DIAGNOSES

Check only those diseases that have a relationship to current ADL status, cognitive status, mood and behavior status, medical treatments, nursing monitoring, or risk of death. (Do not list inactive diagnoses)

1.	DISEASES	(If none apply, CHECK the NONE OF ABOVE box)	
		ENDOCRINE/METABOLIC/NUTRITIONAL	Hemiplegia/Hemiparesis **CC** v.
Insulin → 14 days & 2 order changes = **CC**		Diabetes mellitus a.	Multiple sclerosis **SS** w.
		Hyperthyroidism b.	Paraplegia x.
		Hypothyroidism c.	Parkinson's disease y.
		HEART/CIRCULATION	Quadriplegia **SS** z.
		Arteriosclerotic heart disease (ASHD) d.	Seizure disorder aa.
		Cardiac dysrhythmias e.	Transient ischemic attack (TIA) bb.
		Congestive heart failure f.	Traumatic brain injury cc.
		Deep vein thrombosis g.	PSYCHIATRIC/MOOD
		Hypertension h.	Anxiety disorder dd.
		Hypotension 17* i.	Depression 1 17* CB, CA codes ee.
		Peripheral vascular disease 16 j.	Manic depression (bipolar disease) ff.
		Other cardiovascular disease k.	Schizophrenia gg.
		MUSCULOSKELETAL	PULMONARY
		Arthritis l.	Asthma hh.
		Hip fracture m.	Emphysema/COPD ii.
		Missing limb (e.g., amputation) n.	SENSORY
		Osteoporosis o.	Cataracts 3 jj.
		Pathological bone fracture p.	Diabetic retinopathy kk.
		NEUROLOGICAL	Glaucoma 3 ll.
		Alzheimer's disease q.	Macular degeneration mm.
		Aphasia r.	OTHER
		Cerebral palsy **SS** s.	Allergies nn.
		Cerebrovascular accident (stroke) t.	Anemia oo.
		Dementia other than Alzheimer's disease u.	Cancer pp.
			Renal failure qq.
			NONE OF ABOVE rr.

2.	INFECTIONS	(If none apply, CHECK the NONE OF ABOVE box)	
		Antibiotic resistant infection (e.g., Methicillin resistant staph) a.	Septicemia **CC** g.
		Clostridium difficile (c. diff.) b.	Sexually transmitted disease h.
		Conjunctivitis c.	Tuberculosis i.
		HIV infection d.	Urinary tract infection in last 30 days 17* j.
W/Fever → **SS**		Pneumonia **CC** e.	Viral hepatitis k.
		Respiratory infection f.	Wound infection l.
			NONE OF ABOVE m.

3.	OTHER CURRENT OR MORE DETAILED DIAGNOSES AND ICD-9 CODES	Dehydration 276.5 = 14 **O16**	Fever & dehydration = **SS**
		a.	
		b.	
		c.	
		d.	

SECTION J. HEALTH CONDITIONS

1.	PROBLEM CONDITIONS	(Check all problems present in last 7 days unless other time frame is indicated)	
		INDICATORS OF FLUID STATUS	Dizziness/Vertigo 11, 17* f.
W/Fever → **SS**		Weight gain or loss of 3 or more pounds within a 7 day period 14 a.	Edema g.
			Fever 14 w/dehyd. **SS** h.
		Inability to lie flat due to shortness of breath b.	Hallucinations 17* **RA** i.
			Internal bleeding 14 **CC** j.
W/Fever → **SS**		Dehydrated; output exceeds input 14 **CC O16** c.	Recurrent lung aspirations in last 90 days 17* k.
			Shortness of breath l.
		Insufficient fluid; did NOT consume all/almost all liquids provided during last 3 days 14 d.	Syncope (fainting) 17* m.
			Unsteady gait 17* n.
		OTHER	Vomiting w/wt. loss & fever **SS** o.
		Delusions **RA** e.	NONE OF ABOVE **SS** p.

MDS 2.0 September 2000

(Reprinted with permission of Briggs Corporation, Des Moines, IA 50306. (800) 247-2343)

Resident _____ Numeric Identifier _____

2.	PAIN SYMPTOMS	*(Code the highest level of pain present in the last 7 days)*

a. FREQUENCY with which resident complains or shows evidence of pain

0. No pain *(skip to J4)*
1. Pain less than daily
2. Pain daily

b. INTENSITY of pain
1. Mild pain
2. Moderate pain
3. Times when pain is horrible or excruciating

3.	PAIN SITE	*(If pain present, check all sites that apply in last 7 days)*	
		Back pain	a.
		Bone pain	b.
		Chest pain while doing usual activities	c.
		Headache	d.
		Hip pain	e.
		Incisional pain	f.
		Joint pain (other than hip)	g.
		Soft tissue pain (e.g., lesion, muscle)	h.
		Stomach pain	i.
		Other	j.

4.	ACCIDENTS	*(Check all that apply)*	
a = ○2		Fell in past 30 days 11, 17*	a.
c,d = ○1		Fell in past 31-180 days 11, 17*	b.
		Hip fracture in last 180 days 17*	c.
		Other fracture in last 180 days	d.
		NONE OF ABOVE	e.

5.	STABILITY OF CONDITIONS		
		Conditions/diseases make resident's cognitive, ADL, mood or behavior patterns unstable (fluctuating, precarious, or deteriorating)	a.
		Resident experiencing an acute episode or a flare-up of a recurrent or chronic problem	b.
		End-stage disease, 6 or fewer months to live	c.
		NONE OF ABOVE	d.

SECTION K. ORAL/NUTRITIONAL STATUS

1.	ORAL PROBLEMS		
		Chewing problem	a.
		Swallowing problem 17*	b.
		Mouth pain 15	c.
		NONE OF ABOVE	d.

2.	HEIGHT AND WEIGHT	*Record (a.) height in inches and (b.) weight in pounds. Base weight on most recent measure in last 30 days; measure weight consistently in accord with standard facility practice–e.g., in a.m. after voiding, before meal, with shoes off, and in nightclothes.*	
		a. HT (in.)	b. WT (lb.)

3.	WEIGHT CHANGE	**a. Weight loss**–5% or more in **last 30 days**; or 10% or more in **last 180 days** 0. No 1. Yes 12 SS ○3 ○5 ○13	a.
		b. Weight gain–5% or more in **last 30 days**; or 10% or more in **last 180 days** 0. No 1. Yes	b.

4.	NUTRITIONAL PROBLEMS	Complains about the taste of many foods 12	a.	Leaves 25% or more of food uneaten at most meals 12	c.
		Regular or repetitive complaints of hunger	b.	NONE OF ABOVE	d.

5.	NUTRITIONAL APPROACHES	*(Check all that apply in last 7 days)*			
Tube Fed & Fever or Aphasia = SS		Parenteral/IV 12, 14 SE	a.	Dietary supplement between meals	e.
		Feeding tube 13, 14 CC ○13	b.	Plate guard, stabilized built-up utensil, etc.	f.
		Mechanically altered diet 12	c.	On a planned weight change program 12	g.
		Syringe (oral feeding) 12	d.	NONE OF ABOVE	h.
		Therapeutic diet 12			

6.	PARENTERAL OR ENTERAL INTAKE	*(Skip to Section L if neither 5a nor 5b is checked)*

a. Code the proportion of **total calories** the resident received through parenteral or tube feedings in the **last 7 days**
If a,b≥2,3,4 = SS Off CC
0. None   1. 1% to 25%   2. 26% to 50%   3. 51% to 75%   4. 76% to 100%

b. Code the average **fluid intake** per day by IV or tube in **last 7 days**
0. None   1. 1 to 500 cc/day   2. 501 to 1000 cc/day   3. 1001 to 1500 cc/day   4. 1501 to 2000 cc/day   5. 2001 or more cc/day

SECTION L. ORAL/DENTAL STATUS

1.	ORAL STATUS AND DISEASE PREVENTION		
		Debris (soft, easily movable substances) present in mouth prior to going to bed at night 15	a.
		Has dentures or removable bridge	b.
		Some/all natural teeth lost–does not have or does not use dentures (or partial plates) 15	c.
		Broken, loose, or carious teeth 15	d.
		Inflamed gums (gingiva); swollen or bleeding gums; oral abscesses; ulcers or rashes 15	e.
		Daily cleaning of teeth/dentures or daily mouth care–by resident or staff Not ✓ = 15	f.
		NONE OF ABOVE	g.

TRIGGER LEGEND
10A – Activities (Revise)
10B – Activities (Review)
11 – Falls
12 – Nutritional Status
13 – Feeding Tubes
14 – Dehydration/Fluid Maintenance
15 – Dental Care
16 – Pressure Ulcers
17* – Psychotropic Drugs
(*For this to trigger, O4a, b, or c must = 1-7)

SECTION M. SKIN CONDITION

1.	ULCERS (Due to any cause)	*(Record the number of ulcers at each ulcer stage–regardless of cause. If none present at a stage, record "0" (zero). Code all that apply during last 7 days. Code 9 = 9 or more.) [Requires full body exam.]*	Number of Stages
2+ sites any stage or any stage 3 or 4 = SS		a. **Stage 1.** A persistent area of skin redness (without a break in the skin) that does not disappear when pressure is relieved.	
		b. **Stage 2.** A partial thickness loss of skin layers that presents clinically as an abrasion, blister, or shallow crater.	
		c. **Stage 3.** A full thickness of skin is lost, exposing the subcutaneous tissues–presents as a deep crater with or without undermining adjacent tissue.	
		d. **Stage 4.** A full thickness of skin and subcutaneous tissue is lost, exposing muscle or bone.	

2.	TYPE OF ULCER	*(For each type of ulcer, code for the highest stage in the last 7 days using scale in item M1–i.e., 0=none; stages 1, 2, 3, 4)*	
a = SS		a. Pressure ulcer–any lesion caused by pressure resulting in damage of underlying tissue 1 = 16; 2, 3, or 4 = 12, 16	
a > 0 = ○24		b. Stasis ulcer–open lesion caused by poor circulation in the lower extremities	

3.	HISTORY OF RESOLVED ULCERS	Resident had an ulcer that was resolved or cured in LAST 90 DAYS 0. No 1. Yes 16	

4.	OTHER SKIN PROBLEMS OR LESIONS PRESENT	*(Check all that apply during last 7 days)*	
		Abrasions, bruises	a.
		Burns (second or third degree) CC	b.
		Open lesions other than ulcers, rashes, cuts (e.g., cancer lesions) SS	c.
		Rashes–e.g., intertrigo, eczema, drug rash, heat rash, herpes zoster	d.
		Skin desensitized to pain or pressure 14	e.
		Skin tears or cuts (other than surgery)	f.
		Surgical wounds	g.
		NONE OF ABOVE	h.

5.	SKIN TREATMENTS	*(Check all that apply during last 7 days)*	
		Pressure relieving device(s) for chair	a.
		Pressure relieving device(s) for bed	b.
a thru h = SS		Turning/repositioning program	c.
		Nutrition or hydration intervention to manage skin problems	d.
		Ulcer care	e.
		Surgical wound care	f.
		Application of dressings (with or without topical medications) other than to feet	g.
		Application of ointments/medications (other than to feet)	h.
		Other preventative or protective skin care (other than to feet)	i.
		NONE OF ABOVE	j.

6.	FOOT PROBLEMS AND CARE	*(Check all that apply during last 7 days)*	
		Resident has one or more foot problems–e.g., corns, calluses, bunions, hammer toes, overlapping toes, pain, structural problems	a.
		Infection of the foot–e.g., cellulitis, purulent drainage CC	b.
		Open lesions on the foot CC	c.
		Nails/calluses trimmed during last 90 days	d.
		Received preventative or protective foot care (e.g., used special shoes, inserts, pads, toe separators)	e.
		Application of dressings (with or without topical medications) CC	f.
		NONE OF ABOVE	g.

SECTION N. ACTIVITY PURSUIT PATTERNS

1.	TIME AWAKE	*(Check appropriate time periods over last 7 days)* Resident awake all or most of time (i.e., naps no more than one hour per time period) in the:	d = CC ○45	
10B only if BOTH N1a = 0 and N2 = 0		Morning ○45	a.	Evening ○15	c.
		Afternoon ○45	b.	NONE OF ABOVE	d.

(IF RESIDENT IS COMATOSE, SKIP TO SECTION O)

2.	AVERAGE TIME INVOLVED IN ACTIVITIES	*(When awake and not receiving treatments or ADL care)* 0. Most–more than 2/3 of time 10B 1. Some–from 1/3 to 2/3 of time 2. Little–less than 1/3 of time 10A 3. None 10A ○23

3.	PREFERRED ACTIVITY SETTINGS	*(Check all settings in which activities are preferred)*	
		Own room	a.
		Day/activity room	b.
		Inside NH/off unit	c.
		Outside facility	d.
		NONE OF ABOVE	e.

4.	GENERAL ACTIVITY PREFERENCES (Adapted to resident's current abilities)	*(Check all PREFERENCES whether or not activity is currently available to resident)*	
		Cards/other games	a.
		Crafts/arts	b.
		Exercise/sports	c.
		Music	d.
		Reading/writing	e.
		Spiritual/religious activities	f.
		Trips/shopping	g.
		Walking/wheeling outdoors	h.
		Watching TV	i.
		Gardening or plants	j.
		Talking or conversing	k.
		Helping others	l.
		NONE OF ABOVE	m.

Form 17233RHH   © 1998 Briggs Corporation, Des Moines, IA 50306   (800) 247-2343   PRINTED IN U.S.A.   MDS 2.0 September 2000
Copyright limited to addition of trigger, coding and QI recognition systems

Resident _____   Numeric Identifier _____

5.	PREFERS CHANGE IN DAILY ROUTINE	Code for resident preferences in daily routines 0. No change 1. Slight change 2. Major change
		a. Type of activities in which resident is currently involved 1 or 2 = **10A**
		b. Extent of resident involvement in activities 1 or 2 = **10A**

SECTION O. MEDICATIONS

1.	NUMBER OF MEDICATIONS	(Record the number of different medications used in the last 7 days; enter "0" if none used) 9+ = ◆
2.	NEW MEDICA-TIONS	(Resident currently receiving medications that were initiated during the last 90 days) 0. No 1. Yes
3.	INJECTIONS	(Record the number of DAYS injections of any type received during the last 7 days; enter "0" if none used) **CA**
4.	DAYS RECEIVED THE FOLLOWING MEDICATION c = Affects CC, CB, CA	(Record the number of DAYS during last 7 days; enter "0" if not used. Note–enter "1" for long-acting meds used less than weekly) (NOTE: For 17 to actually be triggered, O4a, b, or c MUST = 1–7 AND at least one additional item marked 17* must be indicated. See sections B, C, E, G, H, I, J, and K.)

a. Antipsychotic ≥ 1 = ◆   1-7 = 17   d. Hypnotic ≥ 1 = ◆
b. Antianxiety ≥ 1 = ◆   1-7 = 11, 17   2+ = ◆
c. Antidepressant 0 = ◆   1-7 = 11, 17   e. Diuretic 1-7 = **14**

SECTION P. SPECIAL TREATMENTS AND PROCEDURES

1.	SPECIAL TREAT-MENTS, PROCE-DURES, AND PROGRAMS	a. SPECIAL CARE–Check treatments or programs received during the last 14 days

TREATMENTS
Chemotherapy **CB**   a.
Dialysis **C9**   b.
IV medication **SE**   c.
Intake/output   d.
Monitoring acute medical condition   e.
Ostomy care   f.
Oxygen therapy **CC**   g.
Radiation **SS**   h.
Suctioning **SE**   i.
Tracheostomy care **CC**   j.
Transfusions   k.

PROGRAMS
Ventilator or respirator **SE**   l.
Alcohol/drug treatment program   m.
Alzheimer's/dementia special care unit   n.
Hospice care   o.
Pediatric unit   p.
Respite care   q.
Training in skills required to return to the community (e.g., taking medications, house work, shopping, transportation, ADLs)   r.
NONE OF ABOVE   s.

b. THERAPIES–Record the number of days and total minutes each of the following therapies was administered (for at least 15 minutes a day) in the last 7 calendar days (Enter 0 if none or less than 15 min daily) [Note–count only post admission therapies]

(A) = # of days administered for 15 minutes or more   **DAYS** (A)
(B) = total # of minutes provided in last 7 days   **MIN** (B)

a. Speech-language pathology and audiology services
b. Occupational therapy
c. Physical therapy
d. Respiratory therapy **SS**
e. Psychological therapy (by any licensed mental health professional)

2.	INTERVEN-TION PROGRAMS FOR MOOD, BEHAVIOR, COGNITIVE LOSS	(Check all interventions or strategies used in last 7 days–no matter where received)

Special behavior symptom evaluation program   a.
Evaluation by a licensed mental health specialist in last 90 days   b.
Group therapy   c.
Resident-specific deliberate changes in the environment to address mood/behavior patterns–e.g., providing bureau in which to rummage   d.
Reorientation–e.g., cueing   e.
NONE OF ABOVE   f.

3.	NURSING REHABILI-TATION/ RESTOR-ATIVE CARE	Record the NUMBER OF DAYS each of the following rehabilitation or restorative techniques or practices was provided to the resident for more than or equal to 15 minutes per day in the last 7 days (Enter 0 if none or less than 15 min. daily)

Any 2, 6x wk = **Nursing Rehab.** ◆   **RL** = 2
Nsg. rehab & therapy 3 days/45 min.

a. Range of motion (passive)
b. Range of motion (active)
c. Splint or brace assistance
TRAINING AND SKILL PRACTICE IN:
d. Bed mobility
e. Transfer
f. Walking
g. Dressing or grooming
h. Eating or swallowing
i. Amputation/prosthesis care
j. Communication
k. Other

◆ may affect IB, IA, BB, BA, PE, PD, PC, PB, PA

◆ = Quality Indicator

4.	DEVICES AND RESTRAINTS If c,d,e = 2 = ◆	(Use the following codes for last 7 days:) 0. Not used 1. Used less than daily 2. Used daily

Bed rails
a.–Full bed rails on all open sides of bed
b.–Other types of side rails used (e.g., half rail, one side)
c. Trunk restraint 1 = **11, 18**; 2 = **11, 16, 18**
d.Limb restraint 1 or 2 = **18**
e. Chair prevents rising 1 or 2 = **18**

5.	HOSPITAL STAY(S)	Record number of times resident was admitted to hospital with an overnight stay in last 90 days (or since last assessment if less than 90 days). (Enter 0 if no hospital admissions)
6.	EMERGENCY ROOM (ER) VISIT(S)	Record number of times resident visited ER without an overnight stay in last 90 days (or since last assessment if less than 90 days). (Enter 0 if no ER visits)
7.	PHYSICIAN VISITS	In the LAST 14 DAYS (or since admission if less than 14 days in facility) how many days has the physician (or authorized assistant or practitioner) examined the resident? (Enter 0 if none) **CB** **CA**
8.	PHYSICIAN ORDERS	In the LAST 14 DAYS (or since admission if less than 14 days in facility) how many days has the physician (or authorized assistant or practitioner) changed the resident's orders? Do not include order renewals without change. (Enter 0 if none) **IB**
9.	ABNORMAL LAB VALUES	Has the resident had any abnormal lab values during the last 90 days (or since admission)? 0. No 1. Yes

SECTION Q. DISCHARGE POTENTIAL AND OVERALL STATUS

1.	DISCHARGE POTENTIAL	a. Resident expresses/indicates preference to return to the community 0. No 1. Yes

b. Resident has a support person who is positive toward discharge 0. No   1. Yes
c. Stay projected to be of a short duration–discharge projected within 90 days (do not include expected discharge due to death) 0. No   1. Within 31-90 days   2. Within 31-90 days   3. Discharge status uncertain

2.	OVERALL CHANGE IN CARE NEEDS	Resident's overall self sufficiency has changed significantly as compared to status of 90 days ago (or since last assessment if less than 90 days) 0. No change 1. Improved–receives fewer supports, needs less restrictive level of care 2. Deteriorated–receives more support

SECTION R. ASSESSMENT INFORMATION

1.	PARTICI-PATION IN ASSESSMENT	a. Resident: 0. No 1. Yes
		b. Family: 0. No 1. Yes 2. No family
		c. Significant other: 0. No 1. Yes 2. None

2. SIGNATURE OF PERSON COORDINATING THE ASSESSMENT:

a. Signature of RN Assessment Coordinator (sign on above line)   completion date for full and quarterly assessments

b. Date RN Assessment Coordinator signed as complete

Month ___ Day ___ Year ___
Must NOT be dated before A3a (Assessment reference date)

Form 17233RHH   © 1998 Briggs Corporation, Des Moines, IA 50306   (800) 247-2343   PRINTED IN U.S.A.   MDS 2.0 September 2000
Copyright limited to addition of trigger, coding and QI recognition systems
7 of 11

(Reprinted with permission of Briggs Corporation, Des Moines, IA 50306. (800) 247-2343)

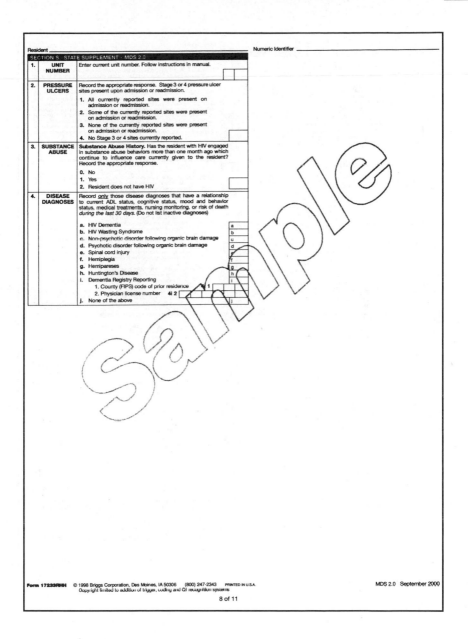

Resident _____ Numeric Identifier _____

SECTION T. THERAPY SUPPLEMENT FOR MEDICARE PPS		

1.	SPECIAL TREAT- MENTS AND PROCE- DURES	a. **RECREATION THERAPY**–*Enter number of days and total minutes of recreation therapy administered (for at least 15 minutes a day) in the last 7 days (Enter 0 if none)*

(A) = # of days administered for 15 minutes or more
(B) = total # of minutes provided in last 7 days

	DAYS (A)	MIN (B)

Skip unless this is a Medicare 5 day or Medicare readmission/return assessment.

b. **ORDERED THERAPIES**–*Has physician ordered any of following therapies to begin in FIRST 14 days of stay–physical therapy, occupational therapy, or speech pathology service?*
0. No   1. Yes

If not ordered, skip to Item 2

c. Through day 15, provide an estimate of the number of days when at least 1 therapy service can be expected to have been delivered.

d. Through day 15, provide an estimate of the number of therapy minutes (across the therapies) than can be expected to be delivered.

2.	WALKING WHEN MOST SELF SUFFICIENT	*Complete Item 2 if ADL self-performance score for TRANSFER (G.1.b.A) is 0, 1, 2, or 3 AND at least one of the following are present:*

- Resident received physical therapy involving gait training (P.1.b.c)
- Physical therapy was ordered for the resident involving gait training (T.1.b)
- Resident received nursing rehabilitation for walking (P.3.f)
- Physical therapy involving walking has been discontinued within the past 180 days
Skip to Item 3 if resident did not walk in last 7 days
FOR FOLLOWING FIVE ITEMS, BASE CODING ON THE EPISODE WHEN THE RESIDENT WALKED THE FARTHEST WITHOUT SITTING DOWN. INCLUDE WALKING DURING RE-HABILITATION SESSIONS.)

a. **Furthest distance walked** without sitting down during this episode.
0. 150+ feet   3. 10-25 feet
1. 51-149 feet   4. Less than 10 feet
2. 26-50 feet

b. **Time walked** without sitting down during this episode.
0. 1-2 minutes   3. 11-15 minutes
1. 3-4 minutes   4. 16-30 minutes
2. 5-10 minutes   5. 31+ minutes

c. **Self-Performance** in walking during this episode.
0. *INDEPENDENT*–No help or oversight
1. *SUPERVISION*–Oversight, encouragement or cueing provided
2. *LIMITED ASSISTANCE*–Resident highly involved in walking; received physical help in guided maneuvering of limbs or other nonweight bearing assistance
3. *EXTENSIVE ASSISTANCE*–Resident received weight bearing assistance while walking

d. **Walking support** provided associated with this episode (code regardless of resident's self-performance classification).
0. No setup or physical help from staff
1. Setup help only
2. One person physical assist
3. Two persons physical assist

e. **Parallel bars** used by resident in association with this episode.
0. No   1. Yes

3.	CASE MIX GROUP	Medicare [ ][ ][ ][ ][ ] State [ ][ ][ ][ ][ ]

The following criteria are used to classify residents in the RUG III classi-fication groups.

In Sections P of the MDS, record the number of days and minutes of PT, OT, ST received by the resident during the observation period that ends on the Assessment Reference Date (A3a).

How time the therapist spends evaluating the resident is counted, depends on whether it is an <u>INITIAL</u> evaluation or an evaluation performed after the course of therapy has begun. The time it takes to perform an initial evaluation and developing the treatment goals and plan of care for the resident CANNOT BE COUNTED AS MINUTES OF THERAPY received by the resident (P1a, b, c). However, reevaluations that are performed once a therapy regimen is under way may be counted as minutes of therapy received. Documentation time may not be counted in P1a, b, c.

RU = 720 minutes a week minimum, at least 2 disciplines, 1 discipline 5 days a week, 2nd 3 days a week

RV = 500 minutes a week minimum, at least 1 discipline 5 days a week

RH = 325 minutes a week minimum, at least 1 discipline 5 days a week. If this is a Medicare 5 day or a Medicare Readmission/Return Assessment, then the following apply:
- Ordered Therapies, T1b is checked
AND
- Received 65 or more more minutes, P1b (a,b,c)
AND
- In first 15 days from admission:
520 or more minutes expected, T1d
AND rehabilitation services expected on 8 or more days, T1c

RM = 150 minutes a week minimum, 5 days across 3 disciplines. If this is a Medicare 5 day or a Medicare Readmission/Return Assessment, then the following apply:
- Ordered therapies T1b is checked
AND
- In the first 15 days from admission:
240 or more minutes are expected, T1d
AND rehabilitation services expected on 8 or more days, T1c

RL = 3 days/45 min. a week minimum, Neg. rehab 6 days a week/2 restorative nursing activities. If this is a Medicare 5 day or a Medicare Readmission/Return Assessment, then the following apply:
- Ordered Therapies, T1b is checked
AND
- In the first 15 days from admission:
75 or more minutes are expected, T1d
AND rehabilitation services expected on 5 or more days, T1c
AND 2 or more nursing rehabilitation services received for at least 15 minutes each with each administered for 2 or more days, P3

RAPS MUST BE COMPLETED WITH THE 5 OR 14 DAY ASSESSMENT, WHICHEVER IS DESIGNATED AS INITIAL ADMISSION ASSESSMENT

Day 21-34 = Last day for assessment reference date for **Medicare** 30 day assessment (RAPs not required unless significant change in status occurred).

Day 50-64 = Last day for assessment reference date for **Medicare** 60 day assessment (RAPs not required unless significant change in status occurred).

Day 80-94 = Last day for assessment reference date for **Medicare** 90 day assessment (RAPs not required unless significant change in status occurred).

Day 100 = Last possible day of **Medicare** coverage.

RETURN TO THE STATE REQUIRED OR CLINICAL MDS ASSESSMENT SCHEDULE.

DOCUMENTATION REQUIRED TO JUSTIFY SKILLED CARE

[IB] [IA]	= Impaired Cognition (NOT AUTOMATIC MEDICARE SKILLED LEVEL OF CARE)
[BB] [BA]	= BEHAVIOR ONLY (NOT AUTOMATIC MEDICARE SKILLED LEVEL OF CARE)
[PE] [PD] [PC] [PB] [PA]	= Physical Function Reduced (NOT AUTOMATIC MEDICARE SKILLED LEVEL OF CARE)

MDS 2.0 September 2000

Resident _____ Numeric Identifier _____

SECTION U. MEDICATIONS

List all medications that the resident **received** during the last 7 days. Include scheduled medications that are used regularly, but less than weekly.

1. **Medication Name and Dose Ordered.** Record the name of the medication and dose ordered.

2. **Route of Administration (RA).** Code the Route of Administration using the following list:

1 = by mouth (PO)	5 = subcutaneous (SQ)	8 = inhalation
2 = sublingual (SL)	6 = rectal (R)	9 = enteral tube
3 = intramuscular (IM)	7 = topical	10 = other
4 = intravenous (IV)		

3. **Frequency (Freq.).** Code the number of times per day, week, or month the medication is administered using the following list:

PR = (PRN) as necessary	2D = (BID) two times daily	QO = every other day
1H = (QH) every hour	(includes every 12 hours)	4W = four times each week
2H = (Q2H) every two hours	3D = (TID) three times daily	5W = five times each week
3H = (Q3H) every three hours	4D = (QID) four times daily	6W = six times each week
4H = (Q4H) every four hours	5D = five times daily	1M = (Q month) once every month
6H = (Q6H) every six hours	1W = (Q week) once each week	2M = twice every month
8H = (Q8H) every eight hours	2W = two times every week	C = continuous
1D = (QD or HS) once daily	3W = three times every week	O = other

4. **Amount Administered (AA).** Record the number of tablets, capsules, suppositories or liquid (any route) **per dose** administered to the resident. Code 999 for topicals, eye drops, inhalants and oral medications that need to be dissolved in water.

5. **PRN-number of days (PRN-n).** If the frequency code for the medication is "PR", record the number of times during the last 7 days each PRN medication was given. Code STAT medications as PRNs given once.

6. **NDC Codes.** Enter the National Drug Code for each medication given. Be sure to enter the correct NDC code for the drug name, strength, and form. The NDC code must match the drug dispensed by the pharmacy.

9+= ◀▣

1. Medication Name and Dose Ordered	2. RA	3. Freq	4. AA	5. PRN-n	6. NDC Codes							

Required for Comprehensive Assessments
SECTION V. RESIDENT ASSESSMENT PROTOCOL SUMMARY Numeric Identifier_____

Resident's Name: | Medical Record No.:

1. Check if RAP is triggered.
2. For each triggered RAP, use the RAP guidelines to identify areas needing further assessment. Document relevant assessment information regarding the resident's status.
   - Describe:
     - Nature of the condition (may include presence or lack of objective data and subjective complaints).
     - Complications and risk factors that affect your decision to proceed to care planning.
     - Factors that must be considered in developing individualized care plan interventions.
     - Need for referrals/further evaluation by appropriate health professionals.
   - Documentation should support your decision-making regarding whether to proceed with a care plan for a triggered RAP and the type(s) of care plan interventions that are appropriate for a particular resident.
   - Documentation may appear anywhere in the clinical record (e.g., progress notes, consults, flowsheets, etc.).
3. Indicate under the Location of RAP Assessment Documentation column where information related to the RAP assessment can be found.
4. For each triggered RAP, indicate whether a new care plan, care plan revision, or continuation of current care plan is necessary to address the problem(s) identified in your assessment. The Care Planning Decision column must be completed within 7 days of completing the RAI (MDS and RAPs)

A. RAP Problem Area	(a) Check if Triggered	Location and Date of RAP Assessment Documentation	(b) Care Planning Decision–check if addressed in care plan
1. DELIRIUM			
2. COGNITIVE LOSS			
3. VISUAL FUNCTION			
4. COMMUNICATION			
5. ADL FUNCTIONAL/ REHABILITATION POTENTIAL			
6. URINARY INCONTINENCE AND INDWELLING CATHETER			
7. PSYCHOSOCIAL WELL-BEING			
8. MOOD STATE			
9. BEHAVIORAL SYMPTOMS			
10. ACTIVITIES			
11. FALLS			
12. NUTRITIONAL STATUS			
13. FEEDING TUBES			
14. DEHYDRATION/FLUID MAINTENANCE			
15. ORAL/DENTAL CARE			
16. PRESSURE ULCERS			
17. PSYCHOTROPIC DRUG USE			
18. PHYSICAL RESTRAINTS			

B. _____
1. Signature of RN Coordinator for RAP Assessment Process

2. [ ] [ ] – [ ] [ ] – [ ] [ ] [ ] [ ]
   Month   Day   Year

_____
3. Signature of Person Completing Care Planning Decision

4. [ ] [ ] – [ ] [ ] – [ ] [ ] [ ] [ ]
   Month   Day   Year

MDS 2.0 September 2000

Glossary

abnormal–behavior not practiced by the majority, considered weird or bizarre

abortion–the premature expulsion of a fetus from the womb which may be either spontaneous (miscarriage) or induced (removal of fetus from the womb per an operation)

abstraction–the ability to generalize and categorize things

acculturation–process that occurs when an individual or group from a given culture is required to adapt and adjust to another cultural group

active listening–being attentive, verifying by stating: "I heard you say"

acute–severe symptoms of a short duration

adaptation–the act of coping with or handling stressors

addiction–physical dependence on a drug to the extent that physical symptoms occur when the drug is withdrawn

Addiction Severity Index (ASI)–a tool to assess alcohol and drug use

adulteration–changing and weakening of a drug by mixing it with other substances

affect–range of mood or emotion (bright, blunted, flat)

affective–pertaining to feelings or emotions

aggression–destructive behavior that results from feelings of anger

agnosia–difficulty in recognizing familiar objects

agoraphobia–fear of going out into public places

AIDS–acquired immune deficiency

akathisia–extreme restlessness

alarm stage–the first stage in the body's adaptation to stress in which the body's forces are mobilized; *also called crisis stage*

Alcoholics Anonymous (AA)–organization run by recovering alcoholics whose personal experiences enable them to understand problems of people with alcoholism

481

alcoholism–physical dependence on the drug alcohol

alienation–separation from a former attachment

Alzheimer's disease–a form of progressive dementia that is characterized by the presence of tangles and plaques in the brain tissue

ambivalence–the existence of mutually conflicting emotions or thoughts about a person, object, or idea

amnesia–sudden and total memory loss; the loss may be for a short or extended time period

anal stage–second stage in the child's development in which bowel training is most important

anger–a strong feeling of displeasure

anhedonia–persistent loss of pleasure; inability to find enjoyment in daily activities

anorexia nervosa–extreme form of fasting that usually affects female adolescents

antisocial–engaging in behavior that violates conventional moral attitude

anxiety–reaction to stress ranging from a feeling of uneasiness to panic, usually brought about by a nonspecific cause

apathy–lack of feeling or emotion

aphasia–inability to recall words

assertive–able to meet one's needs while also considering the other person's needs

associative looseness–personalized interpretation of reality; usually disorganized and fragmented

attentiveness–effective communication by body posture and position

autism–preoccupation with fantasy over reality; withdrawal into one's own world

autonomy–development of a sense of self-determination and independence

awareness–noticing how the self behaves, thinks, and senses at any given time

bad trip–emotional experience that may result in panic reactions

barbiturates–sedatives or hypnotics

baseline–measurement of behavior under normal conditions; used to determine effectiveness of behavior modification techniques

bedlam–insane asylum; place with noise and confusion

behavioral flagging–recording charts or designating on computer entries when a client has a history of assaultive behavior

behaviorism–psychotherapy based on the concept that behavior is controlled by rewards and consequences in the environment

behavior modification–changing behavior by eliminating a reinforcer for undesirable behavior or increasing the reinforcer for desirable behavior

belief system–what an individual believes about events or circumstances

benzodiazepines–medication effective in treating various medical problems, often misused are Librium, Valium, and Xanax.

bias–personal distortion of judgment; prejudice

bicultural–two distinct cultures (values, norms, lifestyles)

blocking–making statements that stop communication

bonding–process of establishing an intimate attachment, primarily between mother and infant or father and infant

borderline–not quite average, standard, or normal

bulimia–an eating disorder characterized by the consumption of a large amount of food in a short period of time (binging) followed by self-induced vomiting (purging)

burnout–a reaction to accumulated stress that overwhelms the individual

caffeine intoxication–a disorder with some of the following symptoms: restlessness, nervousness, psychomotor agitation, rambling flow of thought/speech, and tachycardia

CAGE questionnaire–questionnaire to screen clients who have problems with alcohol

catastrophizing–personally viewing events as terrible

catharsis–a process of psychotherapy in which the individual is encouraged to talk and verbalize feelings

chemical dependency–substance abuse

child abuse–maltreatment of a child by the child's caretaker

clarification–to make clear; technique in communicating

cliché–trite expression or idea; stereotype

client-centered therapy–therapy based on the concept that every person wants to achieve self-actualization

cocaine–a refined, pure, white crystalline powder product of the coca plant

codependency–behavior whereby someone assumes responsibilty for someone else's behavior

cognitive–thinking processes such as judgment, reasoning, and understanding; factual knowledge

cohesion–the process of clinging together

coitus–sexual intercourse

cold turkey–withdrawal from heroin without the aid of medication

commitment–legal act; court order confining a person

communication–sending and receiving messages between two or more people

compensation–defense mechanism in which a person develops an alternate ability in order to overcome a real or imagined defect

competency–according to law, a person who is capable of making sound decisions and can manage his/her personal affairs and life circumstances

compulsion–irresistible urge to engage in a behavior

conditioning–continuously teaching a behavior until it becomes automatic

confidentiality–maintaining privacy of all client information; information shared only with client's consent

conflict–Freudian: a clash between opposing unconscious feelings; Behaviorism: a clash between two opposing conditioned behaviors

conflict resolution–method of resolving feelings of alienation and anger

confrontation–to come face to face with in a direct manner

confusion–responding inappropriately; being mixed up

conscience–the faculty of recognizing the difference between right and wrong with a sense of proper conduct

conservator–person appointed to handle the estate of someone judged to be incompetent

contraband–goods or items not permitted; can be confiscated

contract–a verbal or written agreement that is understood and the client voices a willingness to comply

conversion disorder–changing an emotional problem into physical symptoms

cope–ability to deal with problems and stress

crack–a form of cocaine termed freebase

crank–ßN-methylcathinone, a newer, potent psychomotor stimulant

Creutzfeld-Jakob's disease–a form of rapidly progressing dementia

crisis–the first stage in the body's adaptation to stress in which the body's forces are mobilized; overwhelming stress

cross-gender identification–desire to be a member of the opposite sex

cues–nonverbal behavior used to communicate feelings

culture–values, beliefs and norms learned and shared within a particular group

custodial care–caring for the client's routine daily needs without rehabilitation or therapy

data collection–collection of data and information

defense mechanism–method frequently used to lessen anxiety; defense mechanism

dehydration–loss of fluid from the intra- or intercellular spaces

delirium–acute change in cognition and consciousness (i.e., loss of memory, disorientation) that develops over a short period of time and is usually reversible

delerium tremens–extreme restlessness and possibly seizures from alcohol withdrawal

delusion–false ideas that cannot be changed by logical argument

denial–defense mechanism in which the person unconsciously rejects the truth

depression–condition of sadness or dejection usually not proportionate to circumstances

desensitization–the process of describing stressful events over and over until the individual is able to tolerate them

detoxification–the act of detoxifying

development disability–the lack of mental development

Diagnostic and Statistical Manual of Mental Disorders (DSM)–published by the American Psychiatric Association in an attempt to assist in the formation of reliable, accurate and objective diagnoses for mental disorders

direct message–clear message of what you want or do not want

displacement–Freudian: taking out hostility on someone other than the person for whom it is intended; Behaviorism: engaging in substitute behavior

dissociation–an unconscious escape from situations that cause anxiety; the individual is cut off from his or her own awareness

diversional activity–an activity planned to take an individual's mind off stressful situations

dream analysis–in therapy session, the therapist interprets the imagery that occurs during sleep

drives–a strong motivating tendency or instinct

drug abuser–a person who takes drugs for other than medical reasons

drug dependence–psychological or physical dependence on a drug

drug user–a person who takes drugs according to directions for medical reasons

Duty to Warn–duty to warn of a client's violent behavior

DWI–driving while intoxicated

dyspareunia–vaginal infection caused by diabetes, resulting in painful intercourse

echolalia–involuntary repetition of words spoken by others

echopraxia–involuntary imitation of the motions of others

ego–the part of the personality that deals with reality; the conscious self

Electra complex–development stage in which daughter grows closer to her father and is jealous of her mother; same as Oedipus complex in males

electroconvulsive therapy–method of treatment in which electrical impulses are used to produce seizures in the mentally ill client when the client does not respond to drugs or other therapy

electrolytes–chemicals necessary for the effective functioning of all cells, including the nerve cell

emote–to express feelings

empathy–understanding the feelings of others

encopresis–feces is passed in an unacceptable manner

endogenous depression–a depression caused by factors inside the affected person

enuresis–involuntary voiding (urine) by a child beyond an age that is socially acceptable

environment–circumstances, conditions, and objects that surround and influence an individual

euphoria–a sense of elation or well-being

exaggeration–purposefully making something larger, louder, or more important to increase self-awareness

exhibitionism–sexual disorder in which a person (usually male) obtains sexual pleasure by displaying his genitals in public

explicit norms–verbal, overt behaviors that are perceived to be appropriate or inappropriate to a particular culture

explore alternatives–consider alternatives and look at possible options

extinction–the stopping of a conditioned response

failure to thrive–infant fails to grow and develop when there is no physical cause

fantasy–creation of the imagination; daydream

fear–anxiety reaction toward a known stimulus

fetal alcohol syndrome (FAS)–damage to the central nervous system of the fetus caused by females who drink during pregnancy

fetishism–sexual excitement from touching or fondling certain objects or clothing

fetus–developing infant in utero from about the eighth week after conception to birth

flashback–reexperiencing the effects of an hallucinogenic drug days, weeks, or months after using it

flight of ideas–the rapid succession of ideas that do not necessarily have a connection

free association–method of counseling that allows the person to say whatever comes to mind

game—relationships in which an individual engages to make his or her script turn out as planned

gay—term usually refering to men whose sexual desire is directed toward men only

general adaptation syndrome (GAS)—the measurable changes produced in the body in response to stress

genuine—free from pretense; showing of sincere and honest feelings

gravely disabled—person who is unable to provide self with food, clothing, or shelter due to mental illness

grief—deep distress caused by a loss

group process—what is happening to the group (i.e., morale, feeling, tone, and atmosphere) and what is happening among the group members (i.e., influence, participation, cooperation, competition, and styles of leadership)

group work—listen to others and recognize the importance of developing openness

guardian—one legally responsible for the care and management of a person whom the law regards as incompetent to handle his/her own affairs

habituation—emotional need or strong desire

halfway house—residence for the client before he or she re-enters the community

hallucination—imaginary sense perception that may involve the five senses of hearing, seeing, feeling, smelling, or tasting

heredity base—acquirement of qualities from parents through the genes

heroin—a derivative of morphine

hierarchy—arrangement of needs, from lowest to highest

histrionic—excessive emotional expression and desire to be the center of attention

holistic—view of people as total beings, considering physical, social, and emotional aspects

homeostasis—condition of internal balance

homicide—act of purposefully taking another person's life

homosexuality—sexual preference for an individual of the same sex

hospice—program or center caring for the physical and emotional needs of terminally ill clients

hostility—feeling of anger and pent-up energy that erupts in aggression

human immunodeficiency virus (HIV)—virus transmitted though unprotected sexual contact and sharing intravenous needles

humanism—pertaining to and concern for human beings

hypnosis—a sleeplike condition in which an individual is receptive to suggestions

hypochondriasis—preoccupation with the fear of having a serious disease, thereby misinterpreting minor body symptoms

hypothermia—loss of body heat and a lowering of body temperature

hypoxia—loss of oxygen to the brain cells

hysteria—maladaptive behavior due to overwhelming anxiety characterized by dissociation and conversion reactions

id—part of the personality that controls physical needs and instincts

incest—sexual activity between children and blood relatives

inhalants—volatile hydrocarbons that are highly soluble in fats commonly found in model glue, gasoline, nail polish lacquers, cooking and hair sprays, paints, aerosols, and butane fuel.

illusion–mistaken perception of reality

implicit norm–unspoken, covert behaviors that are perceived to be appropriate or inappropriate to a particular culture

implosive therapy–attempts to arouse as much anxiety in the individual as possible

impotence–having a sexual desire but lacking physiologic response

impulse control–history of substance abuse, difficulty keeping a job, multiple AMA (against medical advice)

incongruent–situation in which individuals see themselves as different from what they are experiencing; lacking internal harmony

instincts–inborn drive toward a behavior

intellectualization–defense mechanism in which one dissociates himself or herself from a stressful problem by overuse of intellectual processes

intervention–action taken by a helping person

introspection–evaluation of why the self reacts as it does

involuntary admission–a hospital in-patient admission not done willingly

irreversible confusion–caused by brain damage and not reversible

kleptomania–compulsion to steal

Kuru–a form of dementia found in cannibal tribes that is caused by a slow-acting virus

lesbian–woman whose sexual desire is directed toward women

libido–sexual energy available to an individual

lysosome–small body within the cell that contains destructive enzymes

macho image–tough, brave, fearless, volatile, abandonment, unpredictable

MADD–Mothers Against Drunk Driving

mainlining–injecting a drug directly into a vein

maladaptive behavior–energy-wasting response to stress

malformation–disability or serious illness

manipulate–to play on the emotions of others in order to get one's own way

marijuana (Cannabis sativa)–a mixture of dried up leaves, stems, flowers, and seeds of the Indian hemp plant

meditation–mind reflection; contemplation

mental health–considered to be learned behavior

mental illness–exhibit abnormal behaviors consistently

mental mechanism–way of coping with stress

mental status–mental assessment through observation and questioning

mesmerize–to hypnotize, enthrall

methadone–an opiate substitute taken orally, used in the treatment of opiate addicts

milieu therapy–technique used to help the client through the use of the environment

mindfulness–to be awake, aware, and focused in the present

modeling–being an example to be imitated or compared

motivation–something that causes a person to act

narcissistic–lacking empathy for others and possessing a grandiose sense of self-importance

natural consequence–something produced by a cause or necessarily following from a set of conditions

negative conditioning–rewarding an undesirable behavior

negativism–strong opposition to advice, direction, or suggestion

neologism–made-up word that has no meaning except to the person who has made it up

neuroleptic–antipsychotic medication

neuroleptic malignant syndrome–serious, life-threatening syndrome of sudden onset with the following symptoms: increased temperature and blood pressure, diaphoresis, tachycardia, disorientation, and confusion

neuropathy–abnormality of the nervous system

nod–to doze asleep (momentarily)

normal–actions that fit the social rules

norms–learned behaviors that are perceived to be appropriate or inappropriate to a particular culture

nursing process–process of achieving client care through deliberate systematic and individualized procedures; it consists of five major subprocesses: assessment, outcome identification, planning, intervention, and evaluation

obsession–recurring thought or feeling that is overpowering

Oedipus complex–a stage in development during which the boy falls in love with his mother and becomes extremely jealous of his father; same as Electra complex in females

opium–the dried milklike juice from the pod of the unripe opium poppy

oral stage–first stage in development in which the infant receives all of its pleasure through the mouth

organic brain syndrome–condition in which there is behavior change caused by demonstrable brain damage

orientation–an awareness of time, place and person

palliative–to make less intense or severe

panic–disorganized behavior as a response to severe anxiety

paranoia–psychotic state characterized by delusions of persecution

passive–suppresses his or her own desires in favor of others

passive aggression–use of passive behavior, such as pouting, producing guilt feelings, or intentional ineffectiveness, to express hostility

pathogenic–disease producing

payoff–reward for behavior

pedophilia–sexual desire directed toward children

peer–belonging to the same group in society

perception–ability to view, discern, notice

perfectionism–need to behave correctly at all times; inability to accept mistakes made by the self

perpetrator–to commit against someone; to be guilty of an act

personality disorder–maladaptive behavior created by defects in the development of the personality

phallic stage–stage in which the child begins to develop sexual identity

phenomenon–fact or event

phobia–abnormal excessive fear of a specific situation or object

physiological–pertaining to the body's physical reactions

PI–public intoxication

plaques–starchlike deposits in the brain tissue of Alzheimer's clients

play therapy–therapy in which children are helped to express themselves through play

poetry therapy–therapy using poetry to help clients express themselves

positive conditioning–reinforcing a desirable behavior

positive regard–acceptance of the client as he or she is

postacute withdrawal (PAW)–withdrawal symptoms that begin seven days into abstinence and may peak at 6 months after abstinence begins

postpartum depression depression during pregnancy and lactation

premenstrual dysphoric disorder (PMDD)–intense emotional and behavioral changes during the premenstrual phase of the menstrual cycle

presentizing–bringing past experiences into the present to increase self-awareness

primary bonding–process of establishing an intimate interdependent attachment among mother, father, and infant

projection–defense mechanism whereby the individual places blame for shortcomings on someone else

pseudo dementia–condition that mimics the symptoms of dementia

psychedelic–capable of producing hallucinations

psychiatrist–doctor of medicine who specializes in the diagnosis and treatment of mental illness

psychoanalysis–psychotherapy developed by Freud that attributes maladaptive behavior to repressions in the subconscious mind; technique involves bringing these repressed feelings and experiences to the conscious level where they can be dealt with

psychodrama–method of treatment allowing clients to act out their problems

psychologist–person who specializes in testing, diagnosis, and treatment of individuals with mental health problems; the person is not a medical doctor

psychophysiological–physical manifestations of emotional problems

psychosis–severe mental disorder with or without organic damage marked by degeneration of normal intellectual and social functioning and by complete or partial withdrawal from reality

psychosocial environment an environment consisting of nurturing, support, and opportunities

psychosocial history–a client medical history and past behaviors

psychosurgery–surgery on the brain for the purpose of relieving overwhelming stress when an incapacitating mental disorder does not respond to other therapies

psychotherapy–treatment of mental and emotional disorders

quaalude–synthetic, nonbarbiturate also known as ludes or soapers

quickening–stage of pregnancy when the fetus can be felt to move

rape–sexual intercourse by force, without the consent of the partner; an act of aggression, a violent sexual crime

rapport–relationship of mutual trust

rational–able to reason and understand

rational emotive therapy–psychotherapy based on the theory that problems are not caused by events that happen but are a direct result of what the person believes about the events

rationalization–defense mechanism whereby the individual denies his or her real thoughts by excusing behavior with more socially acceptable reasons

reactive depression–depression that results from some outside event

reality orientation–type of therapy that brings people back to awareness of reality

reality therapy–therapy developed by William Glasser in which clients are expected to take responsibility for changing their behavior

reflection–repeating the client's thoughts and feelings as understood by the helping person

regression–reversion to an earlier mental or behavioral level

rehabilitation–restoring to health or to useful, acceptable behavior

reinforcement–reward that continues a behavior

rejection–turning away from

REM (rapid eye movement)–movement of the eye during periods of sleep

reminiscing–thinking about and expressing events of the past as a starting point; used to bring the elderly back to reality

replacement therapy–treatment that reduces the desire to drink by producing an unpleasurable effect

repression–unconscious defense mechanism that keeps unpleasant experiences from awareness

resistance–attempts to block the movement of unconscious thoughts to the conscious level

response–action as a result of a stimulus

restraint–a means, force, or agency that restrains

retrograde ejaculation–dry ejaculation; sperm backs up into the bladder

reversible confusion–confusion caused by medical or environmental conditions that is treatable

reward–reinforcement for a specific behavior

role–the part one plays in society

rush–initial dose of heroin that creates an intense feeling of well-being followed by warmth and peacefulness

scapegoating–an individual or group bearing blame for others

schizoid–detachment, lack of emotion toward persons and events

schizotypal–inability to form close relationships, eccentric; pattern of cognitive and perceptual distortions

script–the pattern of behavior an individual follows

seclusion–a treatment intervention where the client is placed alone, in a specifically designated, lockable room where he/she can be directly observed

self-actualization—reach one's maximum potential

self-awareness—noticing how the self feels, thinks, behaves, and senses at any given time

self-concept—the way in which a person feels, views, and thinks of himself or herself; self-disclosure—process of letting people get to know one

self-fulfilling prophecy—attaining the results that were expected or foretold about you (i. e, you'll be a failure)

senior citizen—term referring to persons sixty-five and older

separation anxiety—inappropriate and excessive anxiety concerning separation from home or those one has become close to

sexism—belief that one sex is inferior to and exists for the benefit of the other

sexuality—a facet of personality that is self-affirming, encompasses the individual's personal value system, philosophy of life and is an integral part of self-concept

shaken-baby syndrome—occurs when a caretaker violently shakes an infant or young baby causing severe head trauma

skin pop—term for taking drugs subcutaneously

social skills—ability to interact with other people

soma—the body

standards of care—a means of determining the quality of care received

status—position or rank within a social group

stillborn—infant born dead

stimulus—something that causes action; may be internal or external

stress—nonspecific response to any demand made on the body

stressor—demand that causes the stress reaction

stressors of pregnancy—anxiety and/or negative feelings during pregnancy

sublimation—defense mechanism in which unacceptable instincts are substituted for socially acceptable behavior

suicidal ideation—to form an idea of killing oneself

suicide—act of purposefully taking one's own life

superego—internalized parental value system that is partly conscious

suppression—defense mechanism in which stressful events and feelings are deliberately blocked from awareness

systematic relaxation—method developed by behavioral psychologists to relieve anxiety

talking down—verbal deescalation

tangential—speech marked by failure to reach a goal or stick to a particular subject (switches topics, fails to complete sentence)

tangles—a characteristic of Alzheimer's disease; the axons and dendrites of the nerve cell wrap themselves around the atrophied nerve cell

tardive dyskinesia—serious movement disorder characterized by repetitive movements (i.e., chewing, facial grimacing, mouth movements)

teratogenic—causing fetal malformation

theory base—systematic, organized knowledge base that helps one analyze, predict, or explain a phenomenon

therapeutic neutrality—a response that is neutral: devoid of needs, value, morality

tolerance–body's ability to endure the effects of a drug without showing effect; after tolerance has developed, an increased amount of the drug is needed to produce the desired effect

tranquilizer–drug used to reduce anxiety and tension

transactional analysis–psychotherapy based on the study of interpersonal communication

transference–attributing characteristics of significant others in the client's life to another person

transsexual–one whose sex has been changed externally by surgery and by hormone injections

transvestism–cross dressing or fantasizing about cross dressing

validation–process by which one confirms a message by questioning the content

values–personal beliefs used in making decisions

Viagra (sildenafil)–medication used to help sexual dysfunction

victim–person harmed by another

victimization–the act of victimizing

violence–use of physical force or power against another person, against oneself, or against a group or community that results in injury, death, or deprivation

voyeurism–sexual pleasure is obtained by observing other people undressing, naked, or engaged in sexual activity

vulnerable–open to attack or damage

waxy flexibility–waxlike rigid condition of the extremities that is characteristic of catatonic schizophrenia; extremities remain in any position they are placed, no matter how uncomfortable the position may be

withdrawal–group of symptoms that occurs as a result of stopping the intake of an addictive drug

withdrawn–form of behavior that characterizes a retreat from reality

word salad–words or phrases that have no logical connection or meaning

CHAPTER 1 HISTORY, TRENDS AND STANDARDS
BOOKS

Aiken, T. D., & Catalano, P. (1994). *Legal, ethical and political issues in nursing.* Philadelphia: FA Davis.

Varvolis, E. M. (Eds.). (1998). *Foundations of psychiatric mental health nursing* (3rd ed.). Philadelphia: WB Saunders.

ARTICLES

Clarke, S. (1995). Let the caring show. *Imprint* 42(3): 67.

Denmen, J. (1995). Caring in the nursing profession is being forgotten. *Journal of Nursing Care Quaity,* 9(4), 86 87.

Offer, P. A. (1994). Nurse and patients rights: Can both be protected? *Journal of Psychosocial Nursing and Mental Health Services* 32(12): 48.

Oldover, S. (1995). Legal and ethical issues: Ethics in academia. *Journal of Professional Nursing* 11(5): 261.

Olsen, D. P. (1995). Ethical cautions in the use of outcomes for resources allocation in the managed care environment of mental health. *Archives of Psychiatric Nursing* 9(4): 173–178.

Sullivan, E. J. (1995). Ensuring clinical experiences: Is managed care a threat? *Journal of Professional Nursing* 11(5): 262.

Wilt, D. L., Evans, G. W., et al. (1995). Teaching with entertainment films: An empathic focus. *Journal of Psychosocial Nursing and Mental Health Services* 33(60): 5–14.

CHAPTER 2 STRESS AND MENTAL HEALTH
BOOKS

Davis, M., et al. (1995). *The relaxation and stress reduction workbook* (4th ed.). New York: New Harbinger.

Lazarus, R., & Folkman, S. (1984). *Stress, appraisal and coping.* New York: Springer Publisher.

Liberman, R., & Yager, J. (Eds.). (1994). *Stress in psychiatric disorders.* New York: Springer Publisher.

ARTICLES

Emrich, K. (1989). Helping or hurting? Interacting in the psychiatric milieu. *Journal of Psychosocial Nursing and Mental Health Services 27*(12): 26.

Kemper, B. J. (1992). Therapeutic listening: Developing the concept. *Journal of Psychosocial Nursing and Mental Health Services 30*(7): 12.

Manderino, M. A., & Brown, M. C. (1992). A practical step-by-step approach to stress management for women. *Nurse Practitioner 127*(7): 18.

Morse, J. M. (1992). Exploring empathy: A conceptual fit for nursing practice. *Image 24*(4): 273.

Selye, H. History and present status of the stress concept. In A. Motat & R. S. Lazarus (Eds.) *Stress and coping* (3rd ed.). New York: Columbia University Press.

CHAPTER 3 UNDERSTANDING SELF AND OTHERS

BOOKS

Bolles, R. N. (1996). *What color is your parachute? A practical guide for job hunters and career changers.* Berkley, CA: Ten Speed Press.

Frisch, N., & Frisch, L. (1998). *Psychiatric mental health nursing.* Albany, NY: Delmar.

ARTICLE

Trubowitz, J. (1994). Historical overview personality theories and classification of mental illness. In E. M. Varcolis (Ed.). *Foundations of psychiatric mental health nursing* (2nd ed). Philadelphia: WB Saunders.

CHAPTER 4 EFFECTIVE COMMUNICATION

BOOKS

Balzer-Riley, J. N. (1996). *Communications in nursing* (3rd ed.). St. Louis: Mosby.

Hill, S. S., & Howlett, H. A. (1997). *Success in practical nursing: Personal and vocational issues* (3rd ed.). Philadelphia: WB Saunders.

McKay, M., Davis, M., & Fanning, P. (1995). *Messages, the communication skills book* (2nd ed.). Oakland, CA: New Harbinger.

CHAPTER 5 RELIEVING ANXIETY

ARTICLES

Borintz-Wintz, C. J. (1994). Problematic issues in cross-cultural psychotherapy: Emotional conflicts occurring during acculturation. *Journal of Multicultural Nursing 1*: 6–11.

Bulmer, C. A. (1994, June). Maximum insight with minimal dependence: Brief therapy in psychiatric nursing. *Professional Nursing 9*: 621–625.

Montgomery, C. L., et al. (1994, October). Caring, curing and brief therapy: A model for nurse-psychotherapy. *Archives of Psychiatric Nursing 8*: 291–297.

Rockland, L. H. (1993, November). A review of supportive psychotherapy, 1986–1992. *Hospital and Community Psychiatry 44*: 1053–1060.

Sabin, J. E. (1995, January). Psychotherapy and managed care. *Harvard Mental Health Letter 11*: 4–7.

Zegans, L. S., et al. (1994, March). Psychotherapy for the client with HIV disease. *Psychiatric Clinics of North America 17*: 149–162.

CHAPTER 6 PSYCHOTHERAPIES
BOOKS

Antai-Otong, D. (Ed.). (1995). *Psychiatric nursing: Biological and behavioral concepts.* Philadelphia: WB Saunders.

Ellis, A. (1994). *Reasons and emotions in psychotherapy.* Secaucus, NJ: Birch Lane Press.

Tasman, A., Kay, J., & Liberman, J. A. (1997). *Psychiatry* (Vol. 1). Philadelphia: WB Saunders.

ARTICLES

Beck, J. S. (1996, February). Cognitive therapy for personality disorders. *Psychiatric Times.*

Beutler, L. E., & Hardwood, M. T. (1995). Prescriptive psychotherapies. *Applied & Preventive Psychology 4*: 89–100.

Webster, D., Vaughn, K., Webb, M., & Player, A. (1995). Modeling the client's world in brief solution-focused therapy. *Issues in Mental Health Nursing 16*: 505–518.

CHAPTER 7 GROUP PROCESS
BOOKS

Linehan, M. (1993). *Skills training manual for treating borderline personality disorders.* New York: Guilford Press.

Yalom, I. D. (1995). *The theory and practice of group psychotherapy* (4th ed.). New York: Basic Books.

ARTICLES

Bennett, J. B., & Jaquish, A. (1995). The winner's group: A self-help group for homeless chemically dependent persons. *Journal of Psychosocial Nursing 33*(4): 14–19.

LeBarge, E., & Trianj, F. (1995). A support group for people in the early stages of dementia of the Alzheimer type. *Journal of Applied Gerontology 14*(3): 289–301,

Miller, C. R. (1995). Creative coping: A cognitive-behavioral group for borderline personality disorders. *Archives of Psychiatric Nursing 8*(4): 280–285.

Nickerson, P. R. (1995). Solution-focused group therapy. *Social Work 40*(1): 132–133.

Owen, S. V., & Fullerton, M. L. (1995). Would it make a difference? A discussion group in behaviorally oriented in-patient eating disorder programs. *Journal of Psychosocial Nursing 33*(11): 35–40.

Pollack, L. E. Treatment of in-patients with bipolar disorders: A role for self management groups. *Journal of Psychosocial Nursing 33*: 11–16.

Wenckus, E. M. (1994). Storytelling: Using an ancient art to work with groups. *Journal of Psychosocial Nursing 32*: 30–32.

CHAPTER 8 EMOTIONAL ASPECTS OF MATERNAL AND CHILD CARE

ARTICLES

Baum, A., & Misri, S. (1996, Sept.). Selective serontonin-reuptake inhibitors in pregnancy and lactation. *Harvard Review of Psychiatry* 4(3): 117–125.

Cogan, J. C. (1998, Fall). The consumers as expert: Women with serious mental illness and their relationship-based needs. *Psychiatric Rehabilitation Journal* 22(2): 142–154.

Jennings, K., Ross, S., Popper, S., & Elmer, M. (1999, July). Thoughts of harming infants in depressed and non-depressed mothers. *Journal of Affective Disorders* 54(1–2): 21–28.

Joseph, J., Joshi, S. V., Lewin, A. B., & Abrams, M. (1999, Oct.). Characteristics and perceived needs of mothers with serious mental illness. *Psychiatric Services* 50(10): 1357–1359.

McLennan, J. D., & Ganguli, R. (1999, Aug.). Family planning and parenthood needs of women with severe mental illness: Clinician perspective. *Community Mental Health Journal* 35(4): 369–380.

Mowbray, C., Schwartz, S., Bybee, D., et al. (2000, Mar./Apr.). Mothers with a mental illness: Stressors and resources for parenting and living. *Families in Society* 81(2): 118–129.

Nicholson, J., Sweeny, E., Geller, J. (1998, May). Mothers with mental illness I: The competing demands of mothering and living with mental illness. *Psychiatric Services* 49(5): 635–642.

Nicholson, J., Sweeny, E., Geller, J. (1998, May). Mothers with mental illness II: Family relationships and the context of parenting. *Psychiatric Services* 49(5): 643–649.

Padgett, D. K. (1997, Oct.). Women's mental health: Some directions for research. *American Journal of Orthopsychiatry* 67(4): 522–534.

Pinkosky, H. B. (1997, Sept.). Psychosis during pregnancy: Treatment considerations. *Annals of Clinical Psychiatry* 9(3): 175–179.

Pinkosky, H. B., Fitzgerald, M. J., & Reeves, R. R. (1997, May). Psychotropic treatment during pregnancy. *American Journal of Psychiatry* 154(5): 718–719.

Robert, E. (1996, Oct.). Treating depression in pregnancy. *New England Journal of Medicine* 335(14): 1056–1058.

Steiner, J., Hoff, R. A., & Mofett, C. (1998, May). Preventive health care for the mentally ill woman. *Psychiatric Services* 49(5): 696–698.

Stuart, S., Couser, G., Schider, K. (1998, July). Postpartum anxiety and depression: Onset and co-morbidity in a community sample. *Journal of Nervous & Mental Health* 186(7): 420–424.

Wirtz, C., & Boritz, J. (1999, Feb.). Difficult decisions: Women of childbearing age, mental illness and psychopharmologic therapy. *Journal of the American Nurses Association.* 5(1): 5–14.

CHAPTER 9 GERIATRIC MENTAL HEALTH

BOOKS

American Psychiatric Association. (1994). *Diagnostic and statistical manual of mental disorders* (4th ed.). Washington, DC: APA.

Andrews, M., & Boyle, J. (1995). *Transcultural concepts in nursing care* (2nd ed.). Philadelphia: Lippincott.

Asaad, C. (1996). *Psychosomatic disorders. Theoretical and clinical aspects.* New York: Brunner Mazel.

Bailey, D. S., & Bailey, D. R. (1997). *Therapeutic approaches in mental health psychiatric nursing* (4th ed.). Philadelphia: F. A. Davis.

Bourne, E. J. (1995). *The anxiety and phobia workbook* (2nd ed.). Oakland, CA: New Harbinger.

Brownell, K. C., & Fairburn, C. G. (Eds.). (1995). *Eating disorders and obesity. A comprehensive handbook.* New York: The Guilford Press.

Deglin, J. H., & Vallerand, A. H. (1997). *Davis' drug guide for nurses* (5th ed.). Philadephia: F. A. Davis.

Karch, A. M. (1996). *Lippincott's nursing drug guide.* Philadelphia: Lippincott Raven.

Kramer, P. D. (1993). *Listening to Prozac.* New York: Viking Press.

Guzzetta, C., & Dossey, B. (1995). *Spiritual assessment tools: Holistic nursing: A handbook for practice.* Gaitherburg, MD: Aspen.

Lacy, C., Armstrong, L., Lipsey, R., & Lance, L. (1995). *Drug information handbook* (2nd ed.). Hudson, OH: Lexi-Comp.

Lipson, J, Dribbe, S., & Minaril, P. (Eds.). (1996). *Culture and nursing care. A pocket guide.* San Francisco: UCSF Nursing Press.

Neeb, K. (1997). *Fundamentals of mental health nursing.* Philadelphia: F. A. Davis.

Reiss, B. S., & Evans, M. E. (1996). *Pharmacological aspects of nursing care* (5th ed.). Albany, NY: Delmar.

ARTICLES

Benhan, E. (1995). Coping strategies: A psychoeducational approach to post-traumatic symptomatology. *Journal of Psychosocial Nursing* 33(6): 30–35.

Blise, M. L. (1995). Everything I learned, I learned from patients: Radical positive reframing. *Journal of Psychiatric Nursing and Mental Health Services* 33(12): 18–25.

Buchanan, J. (1995). Social support and schizophrenia: A review of the literature. *Archives of Psychiatric Nursing* 9(2): 68–76.

Calabrese, J. R., & Woyshville, M. J. (1994). A medication algorithm for bipolar rapid cycling. *Journal of Clinical Psychiatry* 56(3): 11–18.

Clark, C. C. (1997). Post-traumatic Stress Disorder: How to support healing. *American Journal of Nursing* 97(8): 27–32.

Covington, H., & Crosby, C. (1997). Music therapy as a nursing intervention. *Journal of Psychosocial Nursing* 35(3): 34–37.

DeGroot, J. M., Rodin, G., & Olmstead, M. P. (1995). Alexithymia, depression and treatment outcomes in bulimia nervosa. *Comprehensive Psychiatry* 36(1): 53–60.

DeLeo, D., et al. (1999, June). Pharmacological and psychotherapeutic treatment of personality disorders in the elderly. *International Psychogeriatrics* 11(2): 191–206.

Gerchufsky, M. (1996, Feb.). Helping families cope with ADHD. *Advance for Nurse Practitioners.*

Gillberg, C., Rastam, M., & Gillberg, C. (1995). Anorexia Nervosa 6 years after onset. Part I. Personality disorders. *Comprehensive Psychiatry* 36(1): 61–69.

Gray-Vickrey, P. (2000, July). Combating abuse, part I: Protecting the older adult. *Nursing* 30(7): 34–38.

Hoover, S. D. (1995). Impaired personal boundaries: A nursing diagnosis. *Perspectives in Psychiatric Care* 31(3): 9–13.

Lester, R., & Petrie, T. A. (1995). Personality and physical correlates of bulimic symptomatology among Mexican-American female college students. *Journal of Counseling Psychology* 42(2): 199–203.

Long, K., & Long, R. (1995). Treating obsessive-compulsive disorder. *Nursing Practitioner* 6(3): 136–137.

Malinckrody, B., McCreary, B. A., & Roberton, A. K. (1995). Co-occurrence of eating disorders and incest: The role of attachment, family environment and social competencies. *Journal of Counseling Psychiatry* 42(2): 178–186.

McFarlane, A. C. (1994). Individual psychotherapy for post-traumatic stress disorder. *Psychiatric Clinics of North America* 17(2): 393–408.

Miller, S. G. (1994). Borderline personality disorder from the patient's perspective. *Hospital & Community Psychiatry* 22(7): 1215–1219.

Mizsur, G. L. (1995). Depression and paranoia: Is your patient at risk? *Nursing* 25(2): 66–67.

O'Connell, K. L. (1995). Schizo-affective disorder. A case study. *Journal of Psychosocial Nursing* 33(4). 5–8.

Roberts, S. J. (1994). Somatization in primary care: The common presentation of psychosocial problems through physical complaints. *Nurse Practitioner* 19(5): 47–56.

Ross, C. A., Anderson, G., Heber, S., & Norton, G. R. (1990). Dissociation and abuse among multiple personality patients, prostitutes and exotic dancers. *Hospital & Community Psychiatry* 41: 328.

Scott, A. L. (1995). Personal space boundaries: Clinical applications in psychiatric mental health nursing. *Perspectives in Psychiatric Care* 32(3): 14–19.

Siever, L. J., et al. (1994). Eye movement impairment and schizotypal psychopathology. *American Journal of Psychiatry* 151(8). 1209–1215.

Silver, M., et al. (1998, Dec.). Stress and coping with challenging behavioral disturbances in residential settings. *Journal of Psychiatric Nursing and Mental Health Services* 2(4): 128–131.

CHAPTER 10 ALCOHOLISM

BOOKS

American Medical Association. (1995) *Diagnosis and treatment guidelines on mental health effects of family violence.* Chicago: Author.

Nelson, M. (1996). *Domestic violence: A nursing concern* (3rd ed.). South Eaton, MA: Western Schools Press.

Thompson, J. A., & Mays, G. L. (1991). *American jails: Public policy issues.* Chicago: Nelson-Hall.

ARTICLES

Badger, J. N. (1995, March). Reaching out to the suicidal patient. *American Journal of Nursing* 95(3): 24–32.

Buchanon, D., Farran, D., & Clark, D. (1995). Suicidal thought and self-transcendence in older adults. *Journal of Psychiatric Nursing & Mental Health Services* 33(10): 31–34.

Burgess, A. W., Fehdur, W. P., & Harman, C. R. (1995). Delayed reporting of the rape victim. *Journal of Psychiatric Nursing & Mental Health Services* 33(9): 21–29.

Cooper, C. (1995). Patient suicide and assault: Their impact on psychiatric hospital staff. *Journal of Psychosocial Nursing* 33(6): 26–29.

Denham, S. (1995). Confronting the monster of family violence. *Nursing Forum* 30(3): 12–19.

Ehmann, T. S., Higgs, E., Sith, G. N., et al. (1995). Routine assessment of patient progress: A multi-format, change-sensitive nurses' method for assessing psychotic in-patients. *Comprehensive Psychiatry* 36(4):289–295.

Ellis, G. M. (1994). Acquaintance rape. *Perspectives in Psychiatric Care* 30(1): 11–16.

Harris, D., & Morrison, E. F. (1995). Managing violence without coercion. *Archives of Psychiatric Nursing* 9(4): 203–210.

Kaplan, M. L., Asnis, G. M., Lipschitz, D. S., & Chorney, P. (1995). Suicidal behavior and abuse in psychiatric outpatients. *Comprehensive Psychiatry* 36(3): 229–235.

King, M. K., Schmalin, K. B., Cowley, D. S., & Dunner, D. L. (1995). Suicide attempt history in depressed patients with and without a history of panic attacks. *Comprehensive Psychiatry* 36(1): 25–30.

Linehan, M. M., Tutek, D. A., Heard, H. L., & Armstrong, H. E. (1994). Interpersonal outcome of cognitive behavioral treatment for chronically suicidal borderline patients. *American Journal of Psychiatry* 151(12): 1771–1776.

Lynch, S. H., (1997). Older abuse: What to look for, how to intervene. *American Journal of Nursing* 97(1): 27–33.

Maier, G. J. (1996). Managing threatening behavior: The role of talk down and talk up. *Journal of Psychosocial Nursing* 34(6): 25–30.

Martin, K. H. (1995). Improving staff safety through an aggressive management program. *Archives of Psychiatric Nursing* 9(4): 211–215.

Morales, E., & Duphorne, P. L. (1995). Least restrictive measures: Alternative to four point restraints and seclusion. *Journal of Psychosocial Nursing* 33(10): 13–16.

Musto, S. M. (1995). Trauma junkie: Taking charge of my survival. *Journal of Psychosocial Nursing* 33(7): 11–13.

Rickelman, B. L., & Houfek, J. K. (1995). Toward an interactional model of suicidal behaviors: Cognitive rigidity, attributional style, stress, hopelessness and depression. *Archives of Psychiatric Nursing* (3): 158–168.

Short, L. M., Johnson, D., & Osattin, A. (1998). Recommended components of health care provider training programs on intimate partner violence. *American Journal of Preventive Medicine* 14: 283–288.

Simms, C. (1995, April). How to unmask the angry patient. *American Journal of Nursing* 95(4): 36–40.

Stevenson, S. (1991). Heading off violence with verbal de-escalation. *Journal of Psychosocial Nursing and Mental Health Services* 29(9): 6–15.

CHAPTER 11 DRUG DEPENDENCY

ARTICLES

Abraham, I. L., Holyroyd, S., Snustad, D. G., Manning, C.A., & Brasher, H. R. (1994). Multi-disciplinary assessment of patients with Alzheimer's disease. *Nursing Clinics of North America* 29(1): 113–128.

Adamek, M., & Kaplan, M. (1996). Firearm suicide among older men. *Psychiatric Services* 47(3): 304–306.

Agnostinelli, B., Demers, K., Garrigan, D., & Waszynski, C. (1994). Targeted interventions: Use of the mini-mental status exam. *Journal of Gerontology Nursing* 20(8): 15–23.

Brandt, B., & Ugarriza, D. (1996). Electro-convulsive therapy and the elderly client. *Journal of Gerontology Nursing* 22(2): 6–15.

Connor, K., Duberstein, P., & Conwell, Y. (1999). Age-related patterns of factors associated with completed suicide in men with alcohol dependence. *American Journal on Addictions* 8(4): 312–318.

Conwell, Y., Lyness, J. M., et al. (2000, Jan.). Completed suicide among older patients in primary care practices: A controlled study. *Journal of the American Geriatric Society* 48(1): 23–29.

Copenhaver, M. (1995). Better late than never: Of reminiscing and resolution. *Journal of Psychosocial Nursing* 33(7): 17–22.

Devons, C. (1996). Suicide in the elderly: How to identify and treat patients at risk. *Geriatrics* 51(3): 67–72.

Foreman, M. D., & Zane, D. (1996, April). Nursing strategies for acute confusion in the elders. *American Journal of Nursing*.

Grossberg, G. T., & Manapa, I. J. (1995). The older patient with psychotic symptoms. *Psychiatric Services* 46(1): 55–59.

Harwood, D., Hawton, K., et al. (2000, Aug.). Suicide in older people: Mode of death, demographic factors, and medical contact before death. *International Journal of Geriatric Psychiatry* 15(8): 736–743.

Hundley, J. (1991). Pet project: The use of pet facilitated therapy among the chronically mentally ill. *Journal of Psychiatric Nursing and Mental Health Services* 29(9): 16–21.

Johnson, B. K. (1996). Older adults and sexuality. A multidimensional perspective. *Journal of Gerontology Nursing* 22(2): 6–15.

Keltner, N. (1994). Tacrine: A pharmacological approach to Alzheimer's disease. *Journal of Psychosocial Nursing* 32(3): 37–39.

Kimball, M. J., & Williams-Burgess, C. (1995, April). Failure to thrive: The silent epidemic of the elderly. *Archives of Psychiatry* 9(2): 99–105.

Krach, P. (1995). Nursing implications: Functional status of older persons with schizophrenia. *Journal of Gerontology Nursing* 19(8): 21–27.

Levine, D. (1995). Your aging parents: Choosing a nursing home. *American Health* 1: 82.

Lynch. S. H. (1998). Elder abuse: What to look for, how to intervene. *American Journal of Nursing* 97(1): 27–32.

Malphurs, J., Eisdorfer, C., & Cohen, D. (2001). A comparison of antecedents of homicide-suicide and suicide in older married men. *American Journal of Geriatric Psychiatry* 9(1): 49–51.

Richter, J. M., Roberto, K. A., & Bottenberg, D. J. (1995). Communicating with persons with Alzheimer's disease: Experiences of family and formal caregivers. *Archives of Psychiatric Nursing* 9(5): 279–285.

Salvatore, T. (2000). Elder suicide: A preventable tragedy. *Caring* 19(3): 34–37.

Solomon, R. (1996). Coping with stress: A physician's guide to mental health in aging. *Geriatrics* 51(7): 46.

Sullivan-Marx, E. M. (1995). Psychological responses to physical restraint use in older patients. *Journal of Psychiatric Nursing and Mental Health Services*, 33(6): 20–25.

CHAPTER 12 MALADAPTIVE BEHAVIORS

ARTICLES

Antai-Otong, D. (1995, Aug.). Helping the alcoholic patient recover. *American Journal of Nursing*.

Foroud, T., & Lin, T. K. (1999). Genetics of alcoholism: A review of recent studies in human and animal models. *The American Journal of Addictions* 8: 261–278.

O'Neil, A. (1995, Sept.). Identifying alcohol dependence in women. *Advance for Nurse Practitioners*.

Salloum, I. M., Mezzich, J. E., Cornelius, J., Day, W. I., et al. (1995). Clinical profiles of co-morbid depressions and alcohol use disorders in an initial psychiatric evaluation. *Comprehensive Psychiatry* 36(4): 260–266.

CHAPTER 13 VIOLENCE AND DISTURBED BEHAVIORS
BOOK

Beattie, M. (1989). *Beyond co-dependency and getting better all the time.* New York: Harper/Hazelden-Harper & Row, the Hazelden Foundation.

ARTICLES

Blank-Reid, C. (1996, Feb.). How to have a stroke at an early age: The effects of crack, cocaine and other illicit drugs. *Journal of Neuroscience Nursing 28*(1): 19–27.

Deren, S., Beardsley, M., et al. (1999, Spring). Predictors of change in frequency of crack cocaine use in a street-recruited sample. *American Journal on Addictions 8*(2): 94–100.

Goldenberg, I. M., Mueller, T., Fierman, S. J., et al. (1995). Specificity of substance use in anxiety-disordered subjects. *Comprehensive Psychiatry 36*(5): 319–328.

Hoffman, J. A., Klein, H., et al. (2000, March). Frequency and intensity of crack use as predicators of women's involvement in HIV-related sexual risk behaviors. *Drug-Alcohol-Dependence 58*(3): 227–236.

Kokkevi, A., & Stefanis, C. (1995). Drug abuse and psychiatric comorbidity. *Comprehensive Psychiatry 36*(5): 329–337.

Kranzler, H. R., Kadden, R. M., Burelson, J. A., et al. (1995). Validity of psychiatric diagnosis in patients with substance use disorders: Is the interview more important than the interviewer? *Comprehensive Psychiatry 36*(4): 278–288.

Magura, S., & Rosenblum, A. (2000, Jan./Feb.). Modulating effects of alcohol use on cocaine use. *Addictive Behaviors 25*(1): 117–122.

Maseola, M. A., Vunakis, B., et al. (1998). Exposure of young infants to environmental tobacco smoke: Breast feeding among smoking mothers. *American Journal of Public Health 88*: 893–896.

Navarra, T. (1995, Jan.). Enabling behavior: The tender trap. *American Journal of Nursing.*

Riley, J. A. (1994). Dual-diagnosis. *Nursing Clinics of North America 29*(1): 29–33.

Shaw, V., Hser, Y., et al. (1999). Sequences of powder cocaine and crack use among arrestees in Los Angeles County. *American Journal of Drug & Alcohol Abuse 25*(1): 47–66.

Tortu, S., Goldstein, M., et al. (1998). Urban crack users: Gender differences in drug use, HIV risk and health status. *Women and Health 27*(1–2): 177–189.

Zust, B. L. (2000, April). Effects of cognitive therapy on depression in rural battered women. *Archives of Psychiatric Nursing 14*(2): 51–63.

CHAPTER 14 HUMAN SEXUALITY
BOOKS

Bass, E., & Davis, L. (1993). *Beginning to heal—A first book for survivors of child sexual abuse.* New York: Harper Perennial/Harper Collins.

Gilligan, C. (1982). *In a different voice: Psychological theory and women's development.* Cambridge, MA: Harvard University Press.

ARTICLES

Barstow, D. G. (1995). Self-injury and self mutilation. *Journal of Psychosocial Nursing 33*(2): 19–22.

Dockery, V. G., et al. (1999, April). Sexual dysfunction. *American Journal of Nursing 28-30*: 34–36.

Eurelings-Bontekoe, E. H., et al. (1998, Oct.).Personality disorders and personality dimensions among female patients with a history of sexual abuse. *Psychiatric Care 5*(9): 183–190.

Lewin, L. (1995). Interviewing the young child sexual abuse victim. *Journal of Psychosocial Nursing 33*(7): 5–10.

LeMone, P., & Weber, J. (1995). Validating of the defining characteristics of altered sexual patterns. *Nursing Diagnosis 6*: 64–69.

Pope, H. G., & Katz, D. L. (1994). Psychiatric and medical effects of anabolic-steroid use: A controlled study of 16 athletes. *Archives of General Psychiatry 51*: 375–382.

Thiel, A., Broocks, A., & Ohlmeier, M. (1995). Obsessive-compulsive disorder among patients with anorexia nervosa and bulimia. *American Journal of Psychiatry 152*: 72–75.

CHAPTER 15 GRIEVING AND PAIN

BOOKS

Achterberg, J., Dossey, B., & Kolkneier, L. (1994). *Rituals of healing: Using imagery for health and wellness*. New York: Bantam Books.

Backstrom, G. (1998). *When muscle pain won't go away: The relief handbook for fibromyalgia and chronic muscle pain*. Dallas: Taylor Publishing.

Catalano, E. M., & Hardin, K. N. (1996). *The chronic pain control workbook* (2nd ed.). New York: MJF Books.

Chopra, D. (1989). *Quantum healing*. New York: Bantam Books.

Eschelman, E., & McKay, M. (1995). *The relaxation and stress reduction workbook* (4h ed.). Oakland, CA: New Harbinger.

Gambill, A. (1996). *Do and don't suggestions for bereaved and their caregivers*. Colorado Springs, CO: Bereavement Publishers.

Hover-Kramer, D. (Ed.). (1996). *Healing touch: A resource for health care professionals*. Albany, NY: Delmar.

Joint Commission on Accreditation of Healthcare Organizations (2000). *Pain assessment and management: An organizational approach*. Oakbrook Terrace, IL: JCAHO.

Melzak, R., & Wall, P. (1988). *The challenge of pain*. London: Penquin Books.

McCaffery, M., & Pasero, C. (1999). *Pain: Clinical manual* (2nd ed.). St. Louis, MO: Mosby.

Nichol, R. (1995). *Irritable bowel syndrome: A national approach*. Berkeley, CA: Ulysses Press.

Philips, H. C., & Rachman, S. (1996). *The psychological management of chronic pain: A treatment manual*. New York: Springer.

Rapoport, A. M., & Sheftell, F. D. (1995). *Headache relief for women: How you can manage and prevent pain*. Boston: Little, Brown.

Schwartz, M. S. (1995). *Biofeedback: A practitioner's guide* (2nd ed.). New York: Guilford.

Shames, K. (1996). *Creative imagery in nursing*. Albany, NY: Delmar.

Somer, E. (1996). *Food & mood: The complete guide to eating well and feeling your best.* New York: Henry Holt.

Starlanyl, D., & Copeland, M. E. (1996). *Fibromyalgia and chronic myofascial pain syndrome: A survivor manual.* Oakland, CA: New Harbinger.

Thich, N. H. (1987). *The miracle of mindfulness.* Boston: Beacon.

Walsh, M., & Carson, V. B. (1996). Mind-body-spirit therapies. In V. B. Carson & E. N. Arnold (Eds.). *Mental health nursing: The nurse-patient journey.* Philadelphia: WB Saunders.

Weil, A. (1997). *Eight weeks to optimum health.* New York: Alfred A. Knopf.

Worden, J. W. (1991). *Grief counseling and grief therapy* (2nd ed.). New York: Springer.

Worwood, V. (1996). *The fragrant kind: Aromatherapy for personality, mind, mood, and emotion.* Norato, CA: New World Library.

ARTICLES

Barba, B. E. (1995). The positive influence of animals. Animal assisted therapy in acute care. *Clinical Nurse Specialist 9:* 199–202.

French, M. S. (1996, Nov.). The mind-body-spirit connection: An introduction to alternative therapies, *Advance for Nurse Practitioners.*

Hilliard, D. (1995). Massage for the seriously mentally ill. *Journal of Psychiatric Nursing & Mental Health Services 33:* 20–30.

Holmberg, L. (1994, Aug. 22). Diet and breast cancer risk. *Archives of Internal Medicine 154.*

Mackey, R. B. (1995, April). CE credit: Discover the healing power of therpeutic touch. *American Journal of Nursing.*

Mornhinweg, G. C., & Voignier, R. R. (1995). Music for sleep disturbances in the elderly. *Journal of Holistic Nursing 13:* 248–254.

O'Connor, N. K. (1995, April 12). Physician-assisted death. *Journal of the American Medical Association 273:* 1088–1089.

Olsen, M., & Sneed, N. (1995). Anxiety and therapeutic touch. *Issues in Mental Health Nursing 16:* 97–108.

Sandmaier, M. (2000, May/June). The breakthrough. *Family Therapy Networker 24* (3): 27–37.

Sirloin, R. C., et al. (1995). When is cancer pain mild, moderate or severe? Grading pain severity by its interference with function. *Pain 61(2):* 277–284.

Sloman, R. (1995). Relaxation and the relief of cancer pain. *Nursing Clinics of North America 30:* 697–709.

Wooten, P. (1996). Humor: An antidote to stress. *Holistic Nursing Practice 10(2):* 49–56.

CHAPTER 16 FACILITATING MENTAL HEALTH AND REENTRY INTO THE COMMUNITY
BOOKS

Kupers, T. (1999). *Prison madness: The mental health crisis behind bars and what we must do about it.* New York: Jossey-Bass.

Rossi, P. H. (1989). *Down and out in America—The origins of homelessness.* Chicago: University of Chicago Press.

ARTICLES

Bunn, H. (1995). Preparing nurses for the challenge of the new focus on a community mental health nursing. *Journal of Continuing Education in Nursing* 26(2): 55–59.

Burns, B. J., & Santos, A. B. (1995). Assertive community treatment: An update of randomized trials. *Psychiatric Services* 45: 669–674.

Byrne, C., Brown, B., Voorberg, N., & Schofield, R. (1994). Wellness education for individuals with chronic mental illness living in the community. *Issues in Mental Health Nursing* 15(3): 239–252.

Chamberlain, J. (1995). Rehabilitating ourselves: The psychiatric survivor movement. *Mental Health* 24(1): 39–46.

Drake, R. E., & Burns, B. J. (1995). Special section on assertive community treatment: An introduction. *Psychiatric Services* 46(7): 667–668.

Erbs-Palmer, V. K. (1995). Incorporating psychiatric rehabilitation principles into mental health nursing. *Psychosocial Nursing* 8(3): 36–44.

Furlong-Norman, K., Erbs-Palmer, V. K., & Jonikas, J. (1997). Exploring the field: Strengthening psychiatric rehabilitation nursing practice with new information and ideas. *Journal of Psychiatric Nursing and Mental Health Services* 35: 35–39.

Godin, P. (1996). The development of community psychiatric nursing: A professional project. *The Journal of Advanced Nursing* 23: 925–934.

Kales, J. P., Barone, M. A., & Bixler, E. O. (1995). Mental illness and substance abuse among sheltered homeless persons in lower-density population areas. *Psychiatric Services* 46: 592–595.

Morris, M. (1996). Patient's perceptions of psychiatric home care. *Archives of Psychiatric Nursing* 10: 176–183.

Murray, R., Baier, M., North, C., et al. (1995). Components of an effective transitional residential program for homeless mentally ill clients. *Archives of Psychiatric Nursing* 9: 152–157.

Parker, B. A. (1993). Living with mental illness: The family as caregivers. *Journal of Psychiatric Nursing & Mental Health Services* 31: 10–21.

Reding, G. R., & Raphelson, M. (1995). Around the clock psychiatric crisis intervention: Another effective alternative to psychiatric hospitalization. *Community Mental Health Journal* 31(2): 179–187.

Tuck, I., duMont, P., Evans, G., & Shupe, P. (1997). The experience of caring for an adult child with schizophrenia. *Archives of Psychiatric Nursing* 11(3) 118–125.

Tuck, I. (1997). The cultural context of mental health nursing. *Issues in Mental Health Nursing* 18: 269–281.

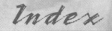

This book is useful for historical
reasons only. It does not contain
current medical information.